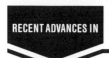

Cardiology

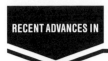

RECENT ADVANCES IN

Cardiology

Edited by

Derek J. Rowlands BSc MBChB FRCP MD FACC FESC

Consultant Cardiologist,
Manchester Area Health Authority;
Lecturer in Cardiology,
University of Manchester,
Manchester, UK

NUMBER ELEVEN

Presented by

of Cyanamid (Division of Lederle Laboratories)
As a service to Medicine

CHURCHILL LIVINGSTONE
EDINBURGH LONDON MADRID MELBOURNE NEW YORK AND TOKYO 1992

CHURCHILL LIVINGSTONE
Medical Division of Longman Group UK Limited

Distributed in the United States of America by Churchill
Livingstone Inc., 650 Avenue of the Americas, New York,
N.Y. 10011, and by associated companies, branches and
representatives throughout the world.

First published 1992

ISBN 0-443-04944-0
ISSN 0 265 1742

British Library Cataloguing in Publication Data
A catalogue record for this book is available from the British
Library

Library of Congress Cataloging in Publication Data
is available

Printed in Great Britain by The Bath Press, Avon

Preface

It is now five years since the previous issue of *Recent Advances in Cardiology*. A great deal has happened to clinical cardiology and to the practice of medicine during this period. This issue of *Recent Advances* differs substantially in form and style from the preceding 10 issues. It has moved a little away from reporting developments *primarily on the research front* to reporting developments *primarily in clinical areas*. It is no less research and development orientated but it is more practically based. It is hoped, therefore, that it will prove to be a valuable contribution for the practising physician. It addresses the common, the worrying, the controversial, the difficult and the evolving areas of cardiology. If it is aimed at any one group it is at the physician who may be called upon to handle cardiology patients and cardiology problems on a day-to-day basis.

Two of the areas of most rapid development during this period have been in relation to thrombolysis and to angioplasty. The previous issue appeared in 1987, the same year that the GISSI-1 trial was published and the year before ISIS-2. Intravenous coronary thrombolysis has (in the absence of contraindications) become standard practice in the management of acute myocardial infarction for those patients presenting early enough to obtain benefit. Professor de Bono has eloquently presented the current position and has given detailed practical advice on the use of these agents. The chapter on angioplasty is highly relevant to the physician who has to manage ischaemic heart disease. It is no longer sufficient to leave such matters to the Cardiologist. The physician needs to be able to advise his patients and to know when to refer the patient on. He needs to know the risks and the benefits of the procedure. In 1990 1000 angioplastics per million of the population were done in the USA, compared with 400–500 per million in Europe and 148 per million in the UK. In the USA the rate appears to have plateaued. In Europe and the UK it is still increasing.

Dr Durrington, with customary assurance and clarity, presents a very balanced view of the significance of lipid disturbances and of the approach to their management both in the patient and in their community. The question of hyperlipidaemia is one which is difficult to avoid.

Drs McMurray and Dargie present a comprehensive view of heart failure, its epidemiology, aetiology, pathophysiology and management. It seems to me to be a masterly review. According to the National Heart, Lung and Blood Institute, over two million Americans suffer from heart failure and it is estimated that 400 000 new cases of heart failure develop annually, requiring in excess of 900 000 hospital admissions. The probability is that in the UK the equivalent numbers would be about one-fifth of those in the USA—still very large numbers indeed compared with the size of the population.

The problem of the electrocardiographic recognition of tachycardias remains as important and as difficult as ever. Dr Creamer and I tackle that problem in what, it is hoped, is a practical and useful manner. It is still (regrettably) very common for broad QRS complex tachycardias to be misdiagnosed. When this mistake occurs it is almost always one way round—a ventricular tachycardia is misdiagnosed as 'supraventricular tachycardia with aberration'. Very rarely is the reverse mistake made. The error is serious and frequently results in the patient's being given intravenous verapamil (a drug with negative inotropic action) which has no chance of correcting the underlying true ventricular arrhythmia. The usual result is that the patient remains in ventricular tachycardia but now has (further) depression of left ventricular function. My own view is that the main reasons that this mistake is made are (1) because the doctor would *prefer* a diagnosis of supraventricular tachycardia with aberration to one of ventricular tachycardia, (2) because he mistakenly believes that all patients with ventricular tachycardia look moribund or (3) because of a combination of the above two.

Further pitfalls in relation to cardiac arrhythmias are highlighted by Dr Murgatroyd and Professor Camm who present an excellent review of a crucial topic, that of the pro-arrhythmic effects of anti-arrhythmic drugs. It is probably true to say that until the CAST study (first published in 1989) the majority of physicians were largely unaware of the potential of *all* anti-arrhythmic drugs to exert a pro-arrhythmic effect. There was general awareness that digitalis could act in this way and limited awareness that quinidine could. The CAST study revealed potential for worsening a patient's prognosis by giving an anti-arrhythmic drug for what seemed like perfectly satisfactory reasons. We are all now aware of the risk but confusion and uncertainty remain. We need further guidance of how to use (and perhaps more importantly when not to use) anti-arrhythmic agents.

One specific, large and evolving area of great clinical significance in relation to cardiac arrhythmias concerns the Wolff–Parkinson–White syndrome. I know of no one better qualified to address this topic than my good friend Doug Zipes. Open any modern American textbook or review of cardiology and look in the section relating to cardiac arrhythmias. There you will find his name. He is the most authoritative writer on this topic at the present time and he handles the chapter with his usual crystal clarity. An author can only write clearly if he can think clearly. The chapter speaks for itself.

Another area of arrhythmia management in which substantial progress has been made within the last five years concerns the field of permanent cardiac pacemakers. Although the simple ventricular demand (VVI) pacemaker is still the most commonly used pacing modality in the USA and Europe, its days as the leader in this respect are surely numbered. Clinicians are becoming increasingly convinced of the benefits of physiological pacing modalities. Dr Malcolm Clarke has a vast clinical experience and expertise in this field and he was a natural choice as author for the chapter on selection of pacemaker mode for the management of symptomatic bradycardia. His logical approach to the problem is highly illuminating and his classification of pacing modes as 'optimal', 'alternative' or 'inappropriate' for various clinical situations is exactly what is required.

Leaving the field of arrhythmias (now well covered) there are still many and various important topics outstanding. One of these is hypertrophic cardiomyopathy. This is no longer a rare diagnosis and no longer considered a piece of cardiological esoterica (though the condition is still often missed). It is an important cause of sudden death and the condition may present at any age. The chapter by Drs Stewart and McKenna comes from a world recognized centre for the study of this condition. The diagnosis, prognosis and management are presented authoritatively.

The surgical chapters are included at the end of the book. No value judgement is implied in this arrangement. It is for me a considerable privilege to work on a day-to-day basis with surgical colleagues of the calibre of Mr Grotte and Mr Keenan. In this book they approach their topics with the anticipated conviction and authority which is firmly based in extensive experience and success. Mr Keenan addresses the very important topic of aortic dissection (always a potential snare in relation to acute 'coronary' admissions) and the increasingly important topic of mitral valve repair (as opposed to replacement). Mr Grotte and I tackle the very large topic of the management of patients following prosthetic valve replacement. These patients cannot permanently be followed up by the cardiology or cardiothoracic surgery unit and most of them are inevitably cared for on a long-term basis by their local consultant physician. This chapter provides practical guidelines on when (and how quickly) such patients should be referred back to the Cardiothoracic Centre.

As Editor, I have been extremely fortunate in respects of my co-authors. I personally have been delighted with each contribution. Without exception they have shown discipline and organization in addressing their given topics.

I am grateful to my two secretaries, Jane Davies who typed and text-edited and text-edited and text-edited the chapters on angioplasty and the electrocardiographic diagnosis of tachycardia and Lesley Curtis who dealt with the extensive communications involving letters, faxes and telephone calls *ad nauseam* and looked after the overall organization. Each has a formidable on-going workload. If either of them felt any resentment or irritation as a result of the extra work, they were successful in hiding it from me. I doubt if I succeeded in hiding my own short temper from them.

The Publishers and I very much hope that you, the reader, enjoy the new style and the content of this issue. The next issue will follow this one in two years' time. Planning is now underway. What topics would you like to see addressed? And by whom? Who makes things clear to you when others cannot? Which chapters of this issue have you enjoyed and which have you not? Feedback would be very helpful. Any comments you send me will receive very careful consideration.

Department of Cardiology   Derek J. Rowlands
Manchester Royal Infirmary   1992
Oxford Road
Manchester M13 9WL

Contributors

A. John Camm MD FRCP
Professor of Clinical Cardiology and Chairman of Medicine, St George's
Hospital Medical School, London, UK

Malcolm Clarke FRCP FACC
Consultant Cardiologist, North Staffs Hospital, Stoke-on-Trent,
Staffordshire, UK

John E. Creamer BSc MBChB MRCP
Senior Registrar in Cardiology, Manchester Royal Infirmary, Manchester,
UK

H. J. Dargie FRCP FESC
Consultant Cardiologist, Western Infirmary, Glasgow, UK

David de Bono MA MD FRCP
Professor of Cardiology, British Heart Foundation, London, UK

Paul N. Durrington BSc MD FRCP
Senior Lecturer in Medicine, University of Manchester; Honorary
Consultant Physician, Manchester Royal Infirmary, Manchester, UK

Geir J. Grötte MBBS FRCS
Consultant Cardiothoracic Surgeon and Clinical Manager, Cardiothoracic
Surgery, Department of Cardiothoracic Surgery, Manchester Royal
Infirmary, Manchester, UK

Daniel J. M. Keenan BSc MB FRCS
Consultant Cardiac Surgeon, Manchester Royal Infirmary, Manchester,
UK

Lawrence S. Klein MD
Assistant Professor of Medicine, Indiana University School of Medicine;
Research Associate, Krannert Institute of Cardiology, Indianapolis,
Indiana, USA

William J. McKenna BA MD MRCP
Reader in Clinical Cardiology and Honorary Consultant Cardiologist, St
George's Hospital Medical School, London, UK

John McMurray BSc MB MRCP MD
Honorary Clinical Lecturer, University of Glasgow; British Heart
Foundation Research Fellow and Honorary Senior Registrar in
Cardiology, Western Infirmary, Glasgow, UK

William M. Miles MD
Associate Professor of Medicine, Indiana University School of Medicine;
Research Associate, Krannert Institute of Cardiology, Indianapolis,
Indiana, USA

Francis D. Murgatroyd MA MRCP
Research Fellow, Department of Cardiological Sciences, St George's
Hospital Medical School, London, UK

Derek J. Rowlands BSc MBChB FRCP MD FACC FESC
Consultant Cardiologist, Manchester Area Health Authority; Lecturer in
Cardiology, University of Manchester, Manchester, UK

Hue-Teh Shih
University of Texas Medical School at Houston, Houston, Texas, USA

James T. Stewart MB MRCP
Senior Registrar in Cardiology, St Thomas' Hospital, London, UK

Douglas P. Zipes MD
Professor of Medicine, Indiana University School of Medicine,
Indianapolis, Indiana, USA

Contents

Percutaneous transluminal coronary angioplasty

D. J. Rowlands

HISTORICAL PERSPECTIVE

The first coronary balloon angioplasty was performed by Dr Andreas Gruentzig in 1977. The development of percutaneous transluminal coronary angioplasty (PTCA), however, was dependent upon several major developments which took place over the preceding half century.

Development of cardiac catheterization

In 1929 Werner Forssman (in Germany) inserted a (urinary) catheter into his own left basilic vein and advanced it into the right atrium,[1] without the benefit of radiological visualization. He demonstrated his success with the aid of a chest X-ray. Local colleagues were sceptical and the achievement was largely ignored. Twelve years later the technique was rediscovered and developed by Cournand*[2] et al and by Richards et al.[3] In 1959 Mason Sones pioneered the technique of cine coronary angiography using a brachial artery cut-down technique.[4] This was a formidable achievement when one considers that open heart surgery, external defibrillation and external cardiopulmonary resuscitative techniques had not been developed.† In 1967 Judkins[5] described his femoral approach to coronary angiography – a technique which is now standard in most cardiac catheterization laboratories. With the advent of the Judkins technique, the procedure of coronary angiography became more widely practised. As a result, our knowledge of coronary disease increased enormously and successful coronary artery surgery (developed by Favaloro[6] and by Green[7] in 1968) became feasible.

---

* The author was privileged to meet André Cournand in 1985 at the fourth Eindhoven meeting at Leiden (Netherlands). At that time Dr Cournand was in his nineties and displayed a formidable intellect whether speaking in French (his native tongue) or in English. Retrograde extrapolation to the time when he won a Nobel Prize suggests a phenomenal intelligence.
† The author was fortunate to meet Mason Sones in Cleveland. Even on a brief acquaintance his incisive approach to problems was apparent. He also displayed a command of Anglo-Saxon expletives rare amongst citizens of the USA.

Development of transluminal angioplasty

In 1964 Dotter and Judkins[8] developed the technique of transluminal angioplasty in relation to large peripheral vessels. This was not well received and other investigators had difficulty in reproducing the results without significant complications. In Europe, however, Zeitler[9] in the early 1970s continued to develop the technique. In the mid-1970s Gruentzig developed and modified the available balloon catheter system and performed coronary angioplasty on human cadavers and in dogs.[10] In May 1977 the first coronary angioplasty on a living human was undertaken by Gruentzig, Myler, Hanna and Turina[11] in an operating room in San Francisco during the course of a multiple coronary artery bypass procedure. In September 1977, in Zurich, Gruentzig performed the first PTCA and reported it in a letter to the editor of the *Lancet*.[12] The era of PTCA had begun. In 1978 the first live demonstration course was given in Zurich – the forerunner of many similar courses now available around the world. The development of the technique has been explosive. In 1990 some 450 000 coronary angioplasties were performed world wide,[13] only 12 years after the first procedure was done. There is no sign of any slow-down in the growth of the procedure.

BASIC CONCEPTS AND PATHOLOGY

The concept of relieving an arterial narrowing by inflating a balloon positioned across the residual, constricted orifice in the vessel is not an easy one to comprehend. What happens to the atheromatous material? Is it embolized? These questions were foremost in the minds of Gruentzig et al when the first intraoperative human angioplasty was performed. During open heart surgery and before attachment of the coronary artery bypass graft a short balloon dilatation catheter was passed retrogradely through the coronary artery so as to place the dilatation balloon across the proximal stenosis. After inflation, deflation and subsequent removal of the balloon a cannula was inserted and the coronary artery flushed. The effluent was collected and was shown not to contain debri. Subsequent angiography showed reduction in the degree of stenosis.[11] A great deal of work has since been undertaken on the morphological and histological changes in the arteries following PTCA but despite this and despite the undoubted therapeutic success of the procedure, the precise mechanism by which coronary angioplasty improves vessel patency remains uncertain.[14] The probability is that several different mechanisms are involved.

Acute pathological changes following PTCA

Morphological and histological studies following PTCA are necessarily limited, being dependent upon the death of the patient and appropriate autopsy study. The possibility clearly exists that such studies may not provide information truly representative of the findings in survivors. In 1981 Block et al[15] reported on two patients with splitting of the atheromatous plaque. In one of the cases the split extended into the media, giving rise to a dissecting haematoma. Several other studies[16-19] have revealed tears, cracks, fractures or breaks in the intima, frequently with extension into the adjacent media. One case of rupture of the coronary artery during PTCA was reported by Saffitz et al.[20] In this case the disease-free wall of the artery ruptured at a point in the artery where there was a heavily calcified eccentric plaque.

Mechanism of increased luminal diameter in PTCA

The mechanism by which PTCA produces an increase in the effective cross-sectional area of a narrowed section of artery is likely to be multifactorial. Plaque compression, plaque remodelling, intimal splitting with plaque disruption and local aneurysm formation may all play a part. In each case more than one factor is likely to be important and individual factors are likely to have varying significance in different cases.

Plaque compression

Gruentzig[12] suggested that physical compression of the plaque might significantly contribute to the increased luminal diameter following successful PTCA. In this he was following the initial suggestion of Dotter et al.[8] Since liquids (and the arterial wall is effectively a liquid) and solids are virtually incompressible this was never a very plausible explanation.

Stretching of that part of the arterial circumference which is free from atheroma

This has also been suggested as the mechanism in relation to eccentric lesions. This mechanism can only apply to eccentric lesions. It is by no means always easy to recognize asymmetry of a stenosis by coronary angiography but Waller[21] has reviewed several pathological studies which show a high frequency (more than 70% in several series) of eccentric lesions in human coronary atheroma. Balloon dilatation of such an asymmetrical lesion may stretch the healthy (plaque-free) wall of the vessel without disrupting the plaque or the remaining portion of the arterial wall. Such a stretching of a plaque-free segment of the arterial diameter might easily result in a significant *initial* increase in the effective diameter without changing the disease process. It is not difficult to imagine that this over-stretched, healthy segment could regain its tone in a period of weeks and this might be one possible mechanism for early restenosis after a dilatation considered on angiographic evidence to be initially successful.[22,23] The high

high frequency (previously referred to) of asymmetrical lesions suggests that this mechanism for the observed increase in luminal diameter may not be uncommon.

Plaque fracture

Animal model experiments have clearly shown that plaque fracture is the common consequence of balloon dilatation. Pathological studies of the effect of balloon dilatation in human cadavers have shown cracking and dehiscence of the intima with permanent dilatation of the media.[24, 25] Furthermore, postmortem studies of human femoral and coronary arteries from patients who have undergone angioplasty have shown findings similar to those in the animal and cadaver experiments.[26] Block et al[27] suggested that splitting of the plaque occurs at its weakest point (often at its thinnest point) and that the split extends up to the internal elastic lamina, creating a 'wedge' widening of the artery at this point. Such a fracture of the intimal plaque may actually be necessary for a successful procedure.[27] In most cases of successful coronary angioplasty, close inspection of the post-dilatation cine-angiogram reveals a non-smooth outline to the vessel lumen. These irregular, shaggy borders reflect the intimal disruption. Plaque fracture is thought to increase the effective vessel patency by creating additional channels for blood flow.

Medial tears

Waller et al[28] reported the development of plaque fracture, intimal flaps and localized medial dissections as being a major mechanism of balloon angioplasty in man and commented that both immediate and sustained increase in the luminal diameter might *require* deep interval fractures with tears or dissections into the underlying media. In the absence of such dissections, he argued, restenosis may commonly occur.[21]

INDICATIONS AND PATIENT SELECTION

Clinical

The primary indication for PTCA is myocardial ischaemia due to localized coronary stenosis (or stenoses) deemed suitable (angiographically) for dilatation. The primary symptomatic indication is severe angina resistant to medical therapy. The threshold for intervention in such cases is lower than that for coronary artery bypass grafting (CABG); for example, elderly patients may more readily be accepted for PTCA than for CABG (although the possible need for urgent CABG following failed PTCA always has to be considered). One area in which the indications for PTCA are likely to increase is in patients experiencing a reccurence in angina sometime after successful CABG. Angioplasty may well be preferable to repeat surgery (but it has to be recalled that surgical back-up, in the event of early closure of the vessel, is not a readily available option in such situations). PTCA can also be used in unstable angina, acute myocardial infarction and post-infarction angina.

Angiographic

In all these clinical contexts, a decision on the advisability or otherwise of PTCA rests on the angiographic assessment. The angiographic criteria continue to evolve as techniques and equipment improve. Decisions should not be taken without high-quality, multiple-view angiographic data and the operator must base the decision in the context of his own (or at least his institution's) experience, capability and results rather than those obtained at some other centre. It is, for example, quite inappropriate to base a decision on the best internationally published results rather than the locally obtainable ones. Operators should resist the temptation to dilate a lesion because it is there – one is not climbing Everest! The joint American College of Cardiology/American Heart Association Task Force on PTCA classified stenoses angiographically into types A, B and C with differing risks and success rates (Table 1.1).[29] The type A lesion is the kind of lesion which constituted the original indication for angioplasty. Whilst, as

Table 1.1   Angiographic status of lesions and PTCA success rate

Type A lesions (high success rate (> 85%); low risk)	
Discrete (< 10 mm length)	Little or no calcification
Concentric	Less than totally occlusive
Readily accessible	Not ostial in location
Non-angulated segment < 45°	No major branch involvement
Smooth contour	Absence of thrombus

Type B lesions (moderate success rate (60–85%); moderate risk)	
Tubular (10–20 mm length)	Moderate to heavy calcification
Eccentric	Total occlusions <3 months old
Moderate tortuosity of proximal segment	Ostial in location
Moderately angulated segment > 45°, < 90°	Bifurcation lesions requiring double guidewires
Irregular contour	Some thrombus present

Type C lesions (low success rate (< 60%); high risk)	
Diffuse (> 2 cm length)	Total occlusion > 3 months old
Excessive tortuosity of proximal segment	Inability to protect major side branches
Extremely angulated segments > 90°	Degenerated vein grafts with friable lesions

Modified from Ryan TJ et al. Guidelines for percutaneous transluminal coronary angioplasty: American College of Cardiology/American Heart Association Task Force report. J Am Coll Cardiol 1988; 12: 538.

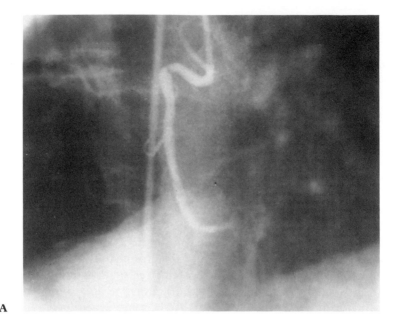

A

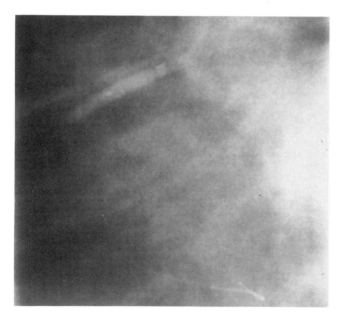

B

Fig. 1.1   PTCA to right coronary artery. **A** Pre-angioplasty appearance. The lesion is discrete, readily accessible, smooth, non-ostial in location and does not involve a side branch. There is no calcification and no evidence of thrombus. It would therefore be a 'type A' lesion if it were not for the fact that it involves a sharply angulated segment. **B** Inflated balloon and guide wire in situ. Note how the balloon has straightened out the affected segment of artery. **C** The immediate post-angioplasty film. Satisfactory dilatation. Residual stenosis 40%.

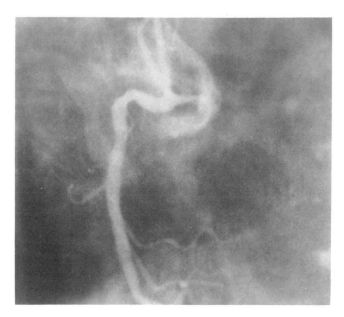

c

indicated in the table, more complex lesions can now be dilated, the success rate is less and the complication rate higher than with type A lesions (Fig. 1.1).

Single- and multivessel disease

In the early days of PTCA the procedure was virtually confined to patients with single-vessel disease. Multivessel angioplasty is no longer a rare procedure but single-vessel disease remains the favourite indication for PTCA for several reasons. There is usually a good correlation between the angiographic findings both before and after the intervention and the procedure itself is usually brief. Any complications are limited to a single area of myocardium and there are frequently contralateral (i.e. from the opposing coronary artery) or ipsilateral (from the same coronary artery) collaterals which substantially enhance safety. These factors also obtain in the case of single-vessel, multilesion disease although the acute complication rate, the complexity of the procedure and the chance of at least one restenosis are all increased. Multivessel disease does not necessarily require multivessel dilatation. In this respect the philosophy of the procedure differs radically from that of CABG. Repeat CABG is a very major undertaking involving a mortality rate about three times that of the initial procedure.[30] In contrast, repeat PTCA has a higher success rate and a lower mortality and infarction rate than the initial PTCA.[31, 32] Therefore, whereas it is accepted surgical policy to graft all arteries with stenoses of 50% or more (once a decision that CABG has justifiably been taken)[33] there is no such commitment in the philosophy of PTCA. Indeed, there is evidence from follow-up studies to suggest that when lesions of 60% (or less) diameter narrowing are dilated, restenosis is often more severe than the initial lesion and that the disease process may be accelerated.[34]

Complete revascularization

At this point it is convenient to discuss the concept of 'complete revascularization'. This concept arose in the surgical literature in the early 1980s.[35,36] It was demonstrated that patients with 'complete revascularization' were more likely to be asymptomatic at follow-up than those with incomplete revascularization. The assessment of adequacy of revascularization is, however, complex. When is a lesion sufficiently unimportant that not attempting to relieve does not constitute incomplete revascularization? Does a lesion in an artery supplying predominantly infarcted myocardium need to be dilated? Furthermore, do patients in whom complete revascularization is possible have less severe coronary disease and less severe ventricular damage and is their better prognosis therefore more related to their better baseline characteristics rather than to the revascularization intervention? Some authors feel that revascularization must be potentially as complete with PTCA as with CABG before PTCA can be comtemplated in multivessel disease.[37] Some follow-up studies have shown a reduced incidence of death, myocardial infarction and angina with complete as opposed to incomplete revascularization.[38] The need for complete revascularization in PTCA is, however, controversial. There is a restenosis rate and a complication rate in relation to each lesion dilated and it may be preferable to leave alone any less than critical lesion in patients with multivessel disease. The concept of the 'culprit lesion' or the 'target lesion' has arisen and this would be typified by, say, a 99% stenosis in the mid-portion of a dominant right coronary artery in the presence of a 60% stenosis in the anterior descending artery, a 50% stenosis in the diagonal and a 50% stenosis in a marginal branch in a patient who had inferior ST segment or T wave changes. It would seem unwise in such a patient to dilate anything other than the right coronary lesion, whereas if he were to go forward for surgery all four branches would presumably be grafted. It follows from these observations that, whilst there is still an obligation on the operator during PTCA to produce adequate revascularization, this is less constraining than during CABG. Arteries with 50–60% diameter stenosis (or with more critical narrowings) all tend to be grafted during CABG largely because of the high probability that the stenosis will increase combined with the known difficulty and increased risk of a second surgical procedure. If angioplasty is the preferred intervention in patients with multivessel disease it probably remains true to say that all *significant* lesions should be dilated, but 'significant' probably implies a diameter stenosis of 70% or more as against 50% or more for CABG. Furthermore, multivessel angioplasty can be 'staged', i.e. not all significant lesions need be attempted at the same session. The enthusiasm for multivessel angioplasty varies widely from one institution to another. Meier and colleagues from Geneva have provided an excellent set of guidelines for selecting patients for multivessel angioplasty.[35] Adherence to these principles and a conservative approach to multivessel angioplasty would seem to be prudent from most centres but there are undoubtedly those operators with very extensive experience who can achieve excellent results with a much more aggressive approach to the problem of multivessel disease.

TECHNIQUES

A detailed description of the procedure and technique of balloon angioplasty would be inappropriate here but a consideration of the general principles concerning technique and equipment is essential to an understanding of the place of angioplasty in patient management.

Patient preparation

This phase begins with a full and frank discussion with the patient concerning the pros and cons of angioplasty and of alternative strategies, including coronary artery bypass grafting and purely medical management. Unless circumstances preclude it, it is essential that the patient should understand that the procedure involves a mortality risk (which may be about 0.2% in a straightforward case or may be significantly higher in a complicated one), that the likelihood of a successful dilatation of the lesion will not exceed 90% (and may be significantly less in a complex case or when the operator is less experienced), that there is a 5% chance that emergency coronary artery bypass grafting would be required and that, even if all goes well with the initial procedure, there is a 25–30% chance of significant restenosis of the lesion(s) within six months. Usually the procedure is undertaken with full standby facilities for emergency coronary artery surgery. This implies the immediate availability of a cardiac surgeon and anaesthetist and a full complement of cardiac surgical personnel and equipment. In some special situations standby cardiac surgery may not be offered. A relatively common example of this is when the patient had previously had coronary artery bypass grafting and has remaining functional grafts. In such a situation it would not be possible safely to expose the heart and get onto cardiopulmonary bypass in time to preserve any myocardium, the viability of which is jeopardized by an acute coronary obstruction (the usual indication for emergency CABG). Other examples include situations where the patient's general condition will preclude open heart surgery at an acceptable risk, but would not preclude angioplasty (e.g. a patient with renal failure or systemic disease). In all cases where CABG standby is not a viable option this fact must be clearly explained to the patient together with the reasons. If acute vessel closure occurs during the procedure and if the vessel cannot be reopened the patient is likely to have a myocardial infarction unless the collateral supply is adequate. The infarction would have to be managed conventionally and an assessment of the mortality and morbidity risk of such an infarction must form part of the initial judgment of whether or not to undertake angioplasty in that particular case. Whether it is or is not feasible to offer standby CABG, it should be a clear principle of the process of recommending or rejecting angioplasty that the procedure should not be offered if it is perceived that the patient would not survive should acute occlusion occur in relation to the lesion (or any of the lesions) dilated.

From a practical point of view patients submitted for angioplasty should (unless there are contraindications) be receiving beta-blocking drugs (to help myocardial preservation), calcium channel blockers of the nifedipine variety to help prevent spasm (calcium channel blockers of the verapamil or diltiazem variety have powerful atrioventricular nodal blocking properties as well as relatively mild vasodilator action) and low-dose aspirin as a platelet antagonist. It is usual to give premedication prior to the procedure (e.g. lorazepam 1–2 mg orally). Atropine should be given at the start of the procedure if the heart rate is below 70 beats/min. Intravenous access has to be readily available throughout the procedure and the availability of plasma volume expanders and of blood (the latter in case surgery is needed) should be ensured. The patient should be fasting and fully prepared for open-heart surgery.

Most commonly the procedure is undertaken via the femoral artery but it can also be done via the brachial system. Formerly, it was very common to insert a temporary pacing system via the femoral vein, but since it is unusual to require pacing and since the insertion of a temporary pacemaker is, itself, not a completely risk-free procedure, most units no longer do this. Some insert a short sheath into the femoral vein to provide pacing access quickly if required. It is possible to pace down the guidewire when the tip is located in a coronary artery.

Equipment

The range and variety of equipment available for angioplasty is vast and is constantly evolving. Basically, however, there is a guiding catheter, a balloon dilatation catheter and a steerable guidewire. The *guiding catheter* is used to conduct the dilatation balloon and guidewire into the appropriate coronary orifice and also to monitor the (coronary) arterial pressure and to permit injection of contrast material selectively into the coronary artery to provide adequate visualization. The *guidewire* may be shaped by the oper-ator prior to the procedure and is steerable. It may be freely movable within the balloon and physically separate from it (an 'over-the-wire' system) or it may be fixed to the balloon tip (though possibly independently rotatable) – a fixed wire system. The over-the-wire systems give greater control and security during the procedure but are more complex to set up. They are also more bulky and, as a result of this, visualization (achieved via intracoronary contrast injection via the guiding catheter and over the balloon catheter) is less satisfactory. There are also monorail systems in which the balloon catheter passes over a pre-positioned guidewire. These differ from the conventional over-the-wire systems in that the guidewire lumen only extends for a short length of the distal part of the balloon catheter so that this catheter can be passed over a standard-length guidewire after the wire has been positioned. The system allows for rapid exchange of balloons. The *balloon catheters* vary enormously in the details of their construction. They range in inflated diameters from 1.5 mm to 4.5 mm and the size is chosen to match that of the native artery in the region of the stenosis. Oversizing a balloon gives a better dilatation but a greater risk of extensive dissection. Some balloons have a degree of compliance which permits slight adjustment of the effective size of the inflated balloon during the procedure. Important characteristics of the balloon system include the deflated profile, trackability (the ability to manoeuvre along a tortuous vessel), conformability (the ability to adopt the shape of the native vessel at the location of the lesion) and pushability (the ability to transmit push imparted by the operator to the distal, balloon-bearing end of the catheter).

SUCCESS RATES

The significance of any assessment of the success rate of PTCA depends on the definition of success employed. In clinical practice the main objective is the abolition or attenuation of angina but success in relation to PTCA is usually defined in angiographic terms. Initially, success was defined as an increase in the luminal diameter of 20% or more.[39] However, as Sowton and colleagues point out, it no longer seems reasonable to include as successes patients in whom a 90% diameter narrowing is reduced to a 70% stenosis.[40] More recently angiographic success has been defined as a residual stenosis of less than 50% diameter.[41]

Success rates have increased during the last decade from about 70% to about 90% in the case of *single-vessel disease*[42] and the success rate for repeat PTCA can be as high as 97%.[43]

In *multivessel disease* the Emory University Hospital experience showed a 91% success rate for at least one lesion being reduced to less than a 50% diameter stenosis and in 85% of patients all attempted lesions were successfully dilated.[44]

The success rate for dilating *total occlusions* depends on the age of the occlusion. For occlusions of less than one month duration the success rate is 69% and for occlusions of more than six months duration it is 11%.[45]

PTCA is increasingly used in *internal mammary artery grafts* – for

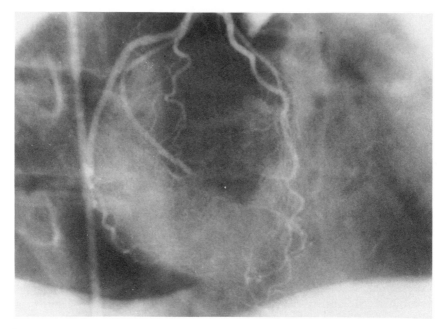

A

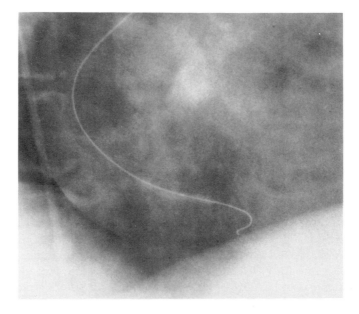

B

Fig. 1.2   PTCA to a completely occluded circumflex. **A** Pre-angioplasty appearance. Total occlusion of the circumflex. The distal circumflex is faintly outlined via collateral flow. **B** The guidewire and balloon in situ across the area of former occlusion. **C** The immediate post-angioplasty film. Satisfactory result. Residual stenosis about 30%.

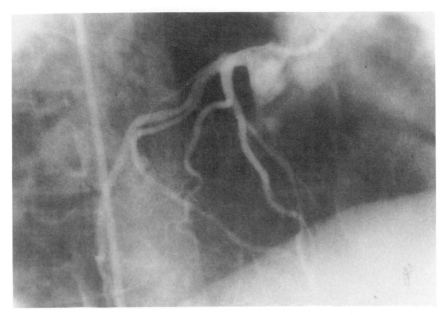

C

stenoses involving the body of the graft, for anastamotic lesions and for lesions of the native vessel distal to the graft. The success rate is 95% for all three locations.[48]

Lesions in *vein grafts* can be dilated by PTCA but the success rate depends upon the location of the stenosis, the age of the graft and the presence or absence of thrombus in the graft. Ostial stenoses generally do not respond well (as is the case for ostial stenosis of the native right coronary artery) but attempted dilatation of ostial stenoses within three years of surgery is generally safe.[47] In relation to discrete stenoses in the mid-portion of saphenous grafts less than three years after CABG the success rate is in the region of 90%. In older grafts the success with mid-graft lesions is less and such grafts are often diffusely abnormal. Many of them contain thrombotic material and attempted dilatation may risk distal coronary arterial embolism or acute occlusion.[48] Lesions at the distal anastamoses often occur within two months of CABG. Such lesions are generally easy to cross and dilate and the results of PTCA are good.[47] Lesions at the distal anastamosis developing some years after surgery give slightly less satisfactory results, more like those of angioplasty to native coronary arteries.[48]

ACUTE COMPLICATIONS

Minor complications

These include: (1) those related to vascular access via the femoral or

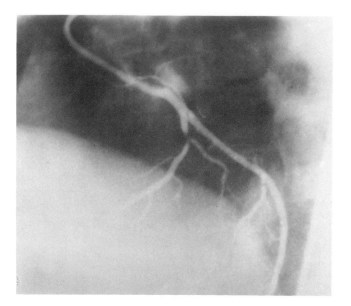

A

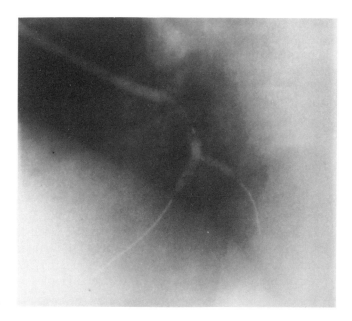

B

Fig. 1.3   The 'kissing balloon' technique. **A** Pre-angioplasty film. There is a critical stenosis in the anterior descending artery involving the diagonal branch. **B** Two balloons in situ and inflated. **C** The immediate post-angioplasty film. Satisfactory result in both arteries. Residual stenosis less than 20%.

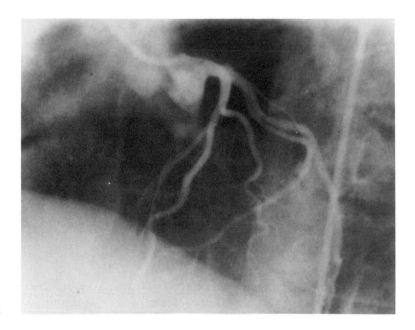

C

brachial arteries; (2) arrhythmias; and (3) complications of anticoagulation.

Femoral artery complications

Haematoma, pseudo-aneurysm or femoral arteriovenous fistula requiring surgical repair occur in 0.6% of patients and transfusion is necessary in fewer than 0.5% in Bredlau's series.[49]

Arrhythmias and conduction defects

In the same series (Bredlau's) ventricular arrhythmias requiring cardio-version were found in 1.5%. Atrial fibrillation and vasovagal reactions may also occur. The latter responds well to atropine and to head-down tilt but occasionally the use of plasma volume expanders may be required. New conduction defects were seen in 0.9% of Bredlau's series. Right bundle branch block is the commonest such abnormality, with first-degree heart rate block as the second commonest. Complete heart block is rare and it is no longer routine practice to place a pacing wire prophylactically into the right ventricle. Cardiac tamponade occurred in 0.1% of patients with a prophylactic pacemaker[4] (due to perforation of the right ventricle) and a pacing electrode is now only inserted when there is perceived to be a high risk of atrioventricular block.

Side branch occlusion

Important amongst the other minor complications of PTCA is occlusion of a side branch of the artery being dilated. Side branch occlusion occurred in 1.7% of patients in Bredlau's series. Meier studied the risk of side branch occlusion in a series in which 54% of the patients appeared angiographically to have side branches at risk. In 17% the side branch arose within the lesion and in 37% the side branch arose from an area discrete from the lesion but within the area of vessel compressed by the balloon. In the first group the incidence of side branch occlusion was 14% and in the second group 1%.[50] Side branch occlusion relatively rarely produces important complications but this obviously to a large extent depends on the size of the side branch. Modern techniques using 'kissing balloons' or protective guidewires have reduced the risks even further (Fig. 1.3).

Coronary emboli

Clinically recognizable coronary emboli are unusual after PTCA except when the dilatation is performed in the presence of obvious thrombus in the native vessel or in a diseased vein graft.

Guidewire emboli

Embolization of a fractured terminal part of the guidewire is rare. It may be caused by equipment failure or by fracture during an attempt to remove the guidewire from a total or critical stenosis. It may sometimes prove possible to remove the retained fragments with a bioptone. Sometimes it may be judged better to leave the fragment in situ, in which case the patient should be heparinized for several days and treated permanently with anti-coagulants.

Hypotension

Hypotension occurs not uncommonly after PTCA. This is hardly surprising in view of the usually rather generous use of intravenous nitrate and the possibility of myocardial damage during the balloon inflation. The former is the more important cause. Furthermore, most patients are receiving calcium channel blockers prior to the procedure (as antispasmodic agents) and sublingual nifedipine is frequently given immediately prior to the dilatation. Hypotension can also occur as a result of cardiac tamponade, groin bleeding, vasovagal reactions or from incidental problems such as gastrointestinal bleeding. Acute hypotension requires immediate attention by reducing the rate of administration of nitrates or calcium channel blockers, rectifying bradycardia and, if necessary, infusing plasma volume expanders. Sustained hypotension is to be avoided as it is likely to decrease coronary blood flow and increase the risk of thrombotic closure of the dilated vessel.

Cardiac tamponade

This is rare and when described has usually been related to the placing of a temporary pacing wire. In view of this, and because of the usually totally adequate response of bradycardia to atropine, pacing electrodes are not now routinely inserted prior to PTCA.

Major complications

The most important major acute complication of PTCA is acute vessel (coronary) closure with consequent prolonged myocardial ischaemia. The most important causes are: (1) dissection; (2) thrombus; (3) spasm; and any combination of these is possible.

Coronary artery spasm

It is our custom to pre-treat (for several days) all patients with nifedipine (unless contraindicated), to give 5 mg of sublingual nifedipine and 600 µg of nitroglycerin into the coronary artery immediately before the balloon catheter is passed into the coronary artery, and to use continuous intravenous nitrates during the procedure unless hypotension develops. It is sometimes, but not always, possible to recognize (angiographically) the occurrence of spasm. When in doubt further intravenous nitroglycerin is given unless the presence of hypotension precludes this.

Coronary artery dissection

This is a very frequent consequence of PTCA and is probably an important (possibly even an essential) part of a successful procedure. It has been argued that in the absence of such dissections restenosis is more common.[21,51] Coronary artery intimal dissection is recognized by: (1) the presence of angiographically evident intimal damage producing an intraluminal filling defect; or (2) extraluminal extravasation of contrast material; or (3) linear luminal density or luminal staining.[51] Coronary intimal dissection has been reported in up to 30–70% of arteries after PTCA. Current angiographic resolution does not permit the recognition of minor, superficial tears,[42] suggesting that they may be commoner still. Bredlau noted a 6.5-fold increase in the risk of developing a major complication (emergency CABG, myocardial infarction or death) when there was angiographic evidence of dissection at the time of PTCA.[49] In the series reported by Leimgruber,[51] 10% of patients with intimal dissection developed major complications, usually due to acute vessel occlusion. On the other hand, in the remaining 90% of cases with a non-occlusive intimal dissection and an uneventful PTCA the presence of intimal disruption was shown to be an indicator of long-term favourable outcome.

Acute vessel closure

This complication (Fig. 1.4) (due to dissection, thrombus or a combination of the two) is the most serious risk of PTCA. Ellis et al reviewed 4772 procedures performed at Emory University Hospital between 1982 and

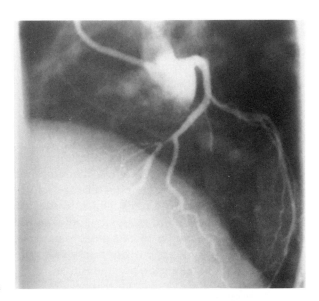

A

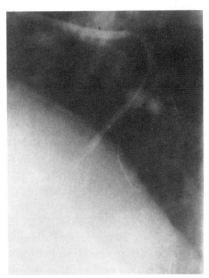

B

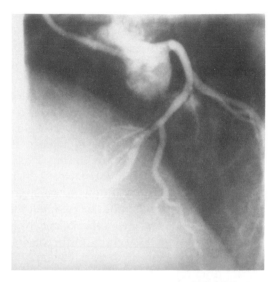

C

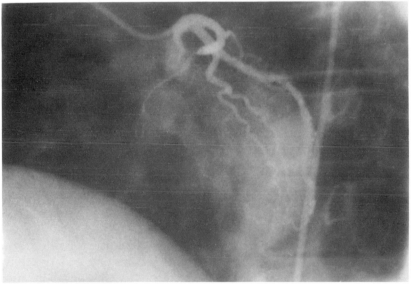

D

Fig. 1.4 Acute occlusion following PTCA. **A** Pre-angioplasty film. There is a smooth 95%
stenosis involving the anterior descending artery just distal to the origin of a large diagonal
branch. The diagonal artery does not appear to be involved in the disease process and this
looks like a straightforward type A lesion (Table 1.1). **B** The inflated balloon in the anterior
descending artery with a 'protecting' guidewire in the diagonal branch. **C** The immediate
post-angioplasty film. There has been a successful dilatation but this is an extensive
dissection in the anterior descending artery. This was not apparent until after the guidewire
was withdrawn from the anterior descending artery. The patient was painfree and
haemodynamically stable and had a satisfactory electrocardiogram. **D** Five hours after **C**. The
patient was experiencing severe cardiac pain and had ST segment elevation in the precordial
leads. Attempts at reopening the artery were unsuccessful and the patient went forward for
emergency coronary artery bypass grafting.

1986 and reported an acute closure rate of 4.4%.[52] Of these, 53% occurred before the patient left the cardiac catheterization laboratory. The important predictors of acute closure were intimal tear or dissection, percentage vessel stenosis (post-PTCA), branch or bend-point stenosis, other stenosis or stenoses in the vessel to be dilated and the presence of thrombus. The two most powerful predictors of complications were the length of the dissection and the residual stenosis after PTCA. When intracoronary thrombus is recognized prior to angioplasty the risk of acute vessel closure is increased and it is prudent to consider several days of heparin therapy prior to dilatation.[42] When dissection is recognized during PTCA the response depends on the overall situation. If a satisfactory dilatation has been achieved, if the patient is pain free and if flow in the appropriate vessel is satisfactory, adequate heparinization should be ensured, intracoronary and intravenous nitrates should be given, as appropriate, to minimize spasm and the patient should be observed carefully in the coronary care unit. If inappropriate chest pain develops or if there is haemodynamic or electro-cardiographic deterioration this patient should be returned to the catheter-ization laboratory for further angiography and appropriate intervention. If the patient has inappropriate chest pain, inappropriate hypotension (i.e. not that due to nitrates) or unsatisfactory ECG changes in the catheterization laboratory (either immediately after the PTCA or when they return to the laboratory from the coronary care unit) then repeat angiography should be undertaken to assess the adequacy of perfusion of the dilated vessel(s) and the undilated vessels. When there is acute vessel closure in the presence of an intimal tear it is highly likely that an intimal 'flap' is occluding the lumen. In such circumstances there are three possible approaches. The first is to attempt further dilatation; the second is to proceed to emergency coronary artery bypass grafting; and the third is to accept the ensuing infarction. This third approach should only be considered after attempted redilatation and then only if it is perceived that the risk/benefit ratio of acute CABG is greater than that of permitting infarction (e.g. where the vessel involved is small and therefore the mass of myocardium at risk is small or where the risk of surgery is high (e.g. in a patient with previous CABG). It is claimed that repeat dilatation (perhaps best undertaken with low inflation pressure, slightly oversized balloons and prolonged inflations) can reduce the need for emergency CABG by 44–85% of cases of acute coronary occlusion following PTCA.[53,54] It is said that 4–5 minutes in-flation in these circumstances can succeed in 'tacking up' a tear but such reports are anecdotal. If closure of the artery after PTCA occurs repeatedly a balloon perfusion catheter[55] may be used for further inflations. This catheter has side holes both proximal to and also distal to the balloon to allow auto-perfusion of the distal artery during prolonged balloon in-flations. This balloon can be left inflated for up to 20 minutes to try to secure adhesion of an intimal flap to the vessel wall. If closure still recurs despite prolonged balloon inflation (for up to 20 minutes with the Stack perfusion balloon or for up to 4 or 5 minutes with a conventional balloon), a 'bailout catheter' should be placed across the lesion.[56] This 'auto-perfusion catheter' has side holes arranged in a spiral fashion over the distal 10 cm. The segment with the side holes is placed (over an exchange wire) across the area of occlusion. It preserves myocardium while the patient is being prepared for emergency surgery and may even allow the surgeon enough time to construct an internal mammary artery graft instead of the (much quicker) saphenous vein graft. If a bailout catheter cannot be placed across the stenosis the placement of a guidewire alone may ensure sufficient flow to protect the myocardium whilst surgical revascularization is performed.[57]

The most important principle in dealing with acute occlusion following PTCA is that emergency surgery (if decided upon) should not be unduly delayed by vain or abortive efforts at re-establishing an effective lumen with further angioplasty attempts.

Need for on-site surgical standby

There is an ongoing debate at present about the level of surgical cover required for coronary angioplasty. Some hold that immediate cardiac surgery should be available at an operating theatre in the same building or at least on the same site as the catheterization laboratory where the PTCA takes place. Others feel that the availability of surgical facilities at a remote site is sufficient.[58] Clearly no one will choose off-site in preference to on-site surgical standby and the American College of Cardiology/American Heart Association Task Force report states that an experienced cardiovascular surgical team should be available within the institution for emergency surgery for all procedures.[59] The same view is held by the Society of Cardiothoracic Surgeons of Great Britain and Ireland and the International Society and Federation of Cardiology.[60] There is no doubt that on-site surgery is safer and highly desirable. The only question at issue is whether off-site surgery is acceptable. In some situations it may be argued that the distribution of facilities is such that the benefits of angioplasty might be denied to patients because of the lack of on-site surgical facilities. Those who undertake angioplasty without on-site surgical standby would seem to have an obligation to explain the situation fully and frankly to their patients prior to the procedure. It might also be considered reasonable for them to ask themselves if they would be prepared to submit to the procedure in the same circumstances. This argument is, of course, an emotional one but its relevance is difficult to refute.

If acute vessel closure occurs during or in the 24 hours immediately following PTCA, repeat angiographic assessment should immediately be undertaken. If reopening of the vessel is not successful within a very brief period of time patients should be transferred for emergency CABG unless this approach is felt to be contraindicated (see above).

Incidence of major complications

The inpatient morbidity and mortality in 3500 patients undergoing elective angioplasty at Emory University Hospital between 1980 and 1984 have been detailed by Bredlau et al.[49] Minor complications occurred in 6.9% and major complications (death, myocardial infarction, emergency CABG) in 4.1%. The rate of emergency CABG was 2.7% and that of myocardial infarction was 2.6%. The death rate was 0.1% (four cases out of 3500). In a large study combining the Emory University Hospital and the San Francisco Heart Institute experiences, the cardiac mortality rate after elective PTCA was 0.16%.[61] The pre-procedural predictors of a major complication are multivessel disease, eccentric lesions, calcified lesions, long lesions, extent of myocardium supplied by the target vessel and female gender.

The most important principle in the management of acute occlusion following PTCA is minimization of the delay time for revascularization. If revascularization cannot be achieved rapidly (within 30 minutes or so) of acute occlusion the patient should be sent for emergency CABG, preferably with perfusion balloon, bailout catheter or guidewire across the lesion. Cowley et al[62] in 1984 reported the death and Q wave myocardial infarction rate in the initial NHLBI PTCA Registry of 202 patients who underwent emergency CABG after failed angioplasty to be 6.6% and 25.7%, respectively. More recent studies show a smaller death rate but no change in the rate of Q wave infarction. Thus Talley et al[63] in 1989 reported a surgical mortality rate of 2.5% (compared with 0.9% for elective surgery not associated with failed PTCA) and a Q wave infarction rate of 27% (compared with 4% for elective surgery not associated with failed PTCA).

RESTENOSIS: THE CHRONIC PROBLEM

Restenosis following initially successful PTCA is the major long-term problem with the technique (just as acute occlusion is the major acute problem). The two difficulties which bedevil the assessment of restenosis are: (1) lack of uniformity of definition of what constitutes restenosis; and (2) lack of extensive detailed angiographic follow-up after successful PTCA. Since restudy rates in all the major surveys have been incomplete it is likely that the instance of restenosis has been overestimated (trouble-free patients being less likely to come to restudy). The angiographic criteria for restenosis have included: (1) a 50% or more diameter stenosis at the time of restudy; (2) an increase of 30% or more diameter stenosis compared with the immediate PTCA result; and (3) a loss of 50% or more of the initial gain.[42] Leimgruber et al[64] found no significant difference in the restenosis rate using any of these three definitions. In most studies restenosis rates have been between 17% and 40%.[65-68] It seems that restenosis begins early. In one serial angiographic study a 14.6% restenosis (50% or more loss of diameter gain) occurred within 24 hours.[69] The studies available seem to suggest that restenosis is an early phenomenon which peaks within six months.[65,68-70] If restenosis is absent in the first six months late restenosis is unlikely.[42]

All attempts at preventing or radically reducing the rate of restenosis have so far failed. The following regimes and devices have been tried (without success) in an attempt to reduce the rate of restenosis: (1) aspirin plus dipyridamole; (2) oral anticoagulants; (3) nifedipine; (4) diltiazem; (5) methyl prednisolone; (6) fish oil; (7) colestipol; (8) lovastatin; (9) platelet-derived growth factor (PDGF); (10) prostacyclin analogues; (11) serotonin (5-hydroxytryptamine) inhibitors; (12) low-molecular-weight heparin.[42] Direct coronary artherectomy has not improved on balloon angioplasty in relation to restenosis.[71] The restenosis rates after using heat-producing lasers are disappointingly high.[72,73] Intra-arterial stents may prove more helpful. If there is no thrombosis in the acute phase of their use then restenosis seems to be rare.[74,75] The technique of the angioplasty itself seems to have significance in relation to subsequent restenosis. In general it is felt that the use of relatively larger balloons (i.e. relative to the vessel size) might reduce restenosis (a retrospective assessment which postulated this is the explanation for the reduced rate of restenosis in women and in right coronary arteries).[76] It has to be remembered, however, that oversizing balloons increases the risk of acute complications (dissection and acute closure).

The *mechanism* of restenosis appears most commonly to be excessive local proliferation of smooth muscle cells, i.e. fibromuscular intimal hyper-plasia.[77]

The problem of restenosis is the major challenge facing the procedure of angioplasty. A 30% recurrence of the initial problem within six months of the procedure is a severe indictment of that procedure.

THE CURRENT PERSPECTIVE

As seems inevitably to be the case with regard to any new technique applied in medicine, angioplasty has been received enthusiastically and put into widespread and committed use long before controlled trials have demon-strated effectiveness in comparison with other techniques or with non-intervention. It always seems that the initial enthusiastic period is always followed by a more sober period of assessment before it can clearly be seen in the full perspective of all available methods of managing a given clinical problem – again including non-intervention. Coronary angioplasty is now clearly in this second phase. It is still a new technique offering an approach to management which might be the only one available in some circum-stances (e.g. in a patient with severe, disabling angina despite maximum medical therapy and in whom coronary artery surgery is contraindicated) or which might be one of several possible options (e.g. a patient with disabling angina who has not yet received maximal medical therapy and for whom cardiac surgery is not contraindicated). It is clear that angioplasty is here to stay and that the indications for it are likely to increase.[77] Multivessel coronary angioplasty is also likely to increase[77] and it is likely that an increasing number of patients in whom surgery is known to be contra-indicated will, if their symptoms warrant it, be investigated by coronary angiography with a view to contemplating the possibility of angioplasty for symptomatic relief. Several important comparative trials are now under way, including the Coronary Artery Bypass Revascularization Investi-gation (CABRI), the Randomized Interventional Trial of Angina (RITA), the Bypass Angioplasty Revascularization Investigation (BARI), the Emory Angioplasty Surgery Trial (EAST) and the German Angioplasty Bypass Intervention trial (GABI).[77] It is important to remember that, at present, there is no completed prospective study comparing PTCA with CABG and that the ongoing studies are not going to be completed and available for some years. The retrospective study by Akins et al[78] reviewed the case records of 1000 consecutive patients undergoing CABG and 389 patients currently undergoing PTCA. The CABG patients were older, were more symptomatic and had more prior infarctions, more left main-stem and multivessel disease and poorer left ventricular function. The in-hospital mortality rates for PTCA and CABG were 0.5% and 0.4%, respectively, and the acute infarction rates were 5.1% and 1.7%. The actuarial five-year survival rates were 96.3% for PTCA and 92.3% for CABG. Since this is a totally uncontrolled study it is not possible to draw reliable conclusions from it. The study is interesting and it clearly high-lights the need for results from controlled trials.

One powerful argument usually advanced in favour of angioplasty is its lower cost (compared with that of surgery). However, the differences are not as great as they might at first appear. Three to five per cent of PTCA patients require urgent CABG, 30% of patients develop restenosis after PTCA and need a repeat procedure (doubling the cost for one-third of the group) and 3–5% of the group will require CABG urgently. Thus Kelly reported that PTCA costs were 43% less than CABG costs (per patient) over one year in patients with single-vessel disease. In another study, conducted over five years, the PTCA costs were only 17% lower than when CABG was chosen as the initial strategy.[80]

AREAS OF CURRENT INVESTIGATION AND FUTURE PERSPECTIVES

Although the use of angioplasty continues to expand, the growth (at least in the USA) is slowing. The increase from 1988 to 1989 was 9%, a much smaller increase than in earlier years.[81] New techniques are evolving, including the use of lasers, atherectomy devices and stents. Laser ablation has had limited exposure. Although the rate of initial problems has been acceptable the restenosis rate for heat-producing lasers has been high.[72]

The restenosis rates with the Excimer laser are currently unknown.[81] Various mechanical procedures for removal of atheroma are under evaluation, including fluid jet systems, drills and shavers.[81] As yet, there is insufficient experience of these procedures for a balanced evaluation of their value and limitations.

Coronary artery stents were first used in 1986. Stents are used for three indications: (1) acute coronary occlusion after PTCA; (2) restenosis after PTCA; (3) stenoses within aorto-coronary bypass grafts. Sigwart[82] cited three contraindications to emergency stenting: (1) vessel diameter less than 3 mm; (2) contraindications to long-term anticoagulant therapy; (3) haemodynamic collapse. In relation to acute occlusion during PTCA, stent implantation is only considered if several attempts at repeat PTCA have failed and the patient continues to have chest pain or ECG changes or both. It has to be remembered, however, that experience with stents is not widespread and that units without this experience should probably send patients early for emergency CABG rather than delay with multiple attempts at repeat PTCA acutely. In experienced hands the results with stents are encouraging.[81] If the acute phase of stenting passes without thrombosis the restenosis seems to be rare.[75,81,82]

Predicting the future is a notoriously dangerous hobby. It seems inevitable, however, that angioplasty is here to stay and that it will evolve and develop. Atherectomy, angioscopy and stenting seem likely to develop and consolidate but conventional balloon angioplasty (which has a proven track record) is likely to expand numerically in England and Europe in the next ten years, until it reaches the American situation in which there are currently as many PTCA procedures as CABG procedures undertaken per annum.

REFERENCES

1 Forssman W. Die Sonderrung des rechten Hertzens. Klin Wochensohre 1929; 8: 2085
2 Cournand AF, Ranges HS. Catheterisation of the right auricle in man. Proc Soc Exp Biol Med 1942; 45: 462
3 Richards DW. Cardiac output in the catheterisation laboratory in various clinical conditions. Fed Proc 1945; 4: 45
4 Sones FM Jr, Shirey EK, Proudfit WL, Westcott RN. Cine coronary angiography. Circulation 1959; 20: 773
5 Judkins MP. Selective coronary arteriography: a percutaneous transfemoral technique. Radiology 1967; 89: 815
6 Favaloro RG. Saphenous vein autograft replacement of severe segmental coronary artery occlusion: operative technique. Ann Thorac Surg 1968; 5: 334
7 Green GE, Stertzer SH, Reppert EH. Coronary artery by-pass grafts. Ann Thorac Surg 1968; 5: 443
8 Dotter CT, Judkins MP. Transluminal treatment of arteriosclerotic obstruction: description of a new technique and preliminary report of its application. Circulation 1964; 30: 654
9 Zeitler E, Schoop W, Zahnow W. The treatment of occlusive arterial disease by transluminal catheter angioplasty. Radiology 1971; 99: 19
10 Gruentzig AR, Turina MF, Scheider JA. Experimental percutaneous dilatation of coronary artery stenosis. Circulation 1976; 54: 81

11 Gruentzig AR, Myler RK, Hanna EH, Turina MI. Coronary transluminal angioplasty. Circulation 1977; 55–56: III-84 (abstr)
12 Gruentzig AR. Transluminal dilatation of coronary artery stenosis. Lancet 1978; i: 263 (letter)
13 Myler RK. Cardiovascular intervention: an editorial. Cardiol Clin 1989; 7: 41
14 Waller BF. Pathology of transluminal balloon angioplasty used in the treatment of coronary heart disease. Cardiol Clin 1989; 7: 4
15 Block PC, Myler RK, Stertzer S, Fallon JT. Morphology after transluminal angioplasty in human beings. N Engl J Med 1981; 305: 382
16 Mizuno K, Jurita A, Imazeki N. Pathological findings after percutaneous transluminal coronary angioplasty. Br Heart J 1984; 52: 588
17 Soward AL, Essed CE, Serruys PW. Coronary arterial findings after accidental death immediately after successful percutaneous transluminal coronary angioplasty. Am J Cardiol 1985; 56: 974
18 Waller BF. Early and late morphological changes in human coronary angioplasty. Clin Cardiol 1983; 6: 363
19 Waller BF, Dillon JC, Cowley MH. Plaque haematoma and coronary dissection with percutaneous transluminal coronary angioplasty (PTCA) of severely stenotic lesions: morphological coronary observations in five men within 30 days of PTCA. Circulation 1983; 68 (Suppl III): III-144
20 Saffitz JE, Rose TE, Oaks JB, Roberts WC. Coronary arterial rupture during coronary angioplasty. Am J Cardiol 1983; 51: 902
21 Waller BF. Pathology of coronary balloon angioplasty and related topics. In: Topol EJ, ed. Textbook of interventional cardiology. Philadelphia: Saunders, 1990 : pp 395–451
22 Waller BF. Coronary luminal shape and the arc of disease-free wall: morphological observations and clinical relevance. J Am Coll Cardiol 1985; 6: 1100–1101
23 Waller BF. The eccentric coronary atheromatous plaque: morphological observations and clinical relevance. Clin Cardiol 1988; 12: 14–20
24 Casteneda-Zuniga WR, Formanek A, Tadavarthy M et al. The mechanism of balloon angioplasty. Radiology 1980; 135: 565–571
25 Baughmann K, Pasternak R, Fallon J et al. Transluminal coronary angioplasty of post mortem human hearts. Am J Cardiol 1981; 48: 1044–1047
26 Mizuno K, Kurita A, Imazeki N. Pathological findings after acute percutaneous transluminal coronary angioplasty. Br Heart J 1984; 52: 588–590
27 Block PC, Myler RK, Stertzer S et al. Morphology after transluminal angioplasty in human beings. N Engl J Med 1981; 305: 382–386
28 Waller BF, Dillon JC, Cowley MH. Plaque haematoma and coronary dissection with percutaneous transluminal angioplasty (PTCA) of severely stenotic lesions: morphological coronary observations in 5 men within 30 days of PTCA. Circulation 1983; 68: (Suppl III): III-144 (abstr)
29 Ryan TJ et al. Guidelines for percutaneous transluminal coronary angioplasty: American College of Cardiology/American Heart Association Task Force report. J Am Coll Cardiol 1988; 12: 538
30 Little WB, Loop FD, Cosgrove DM et al. Fifteen hundred coronary re-operations. J Thorac Cardiovasc Surg 1987; 93: 847–859
31 Myler RK, Topol EJ, Shaw RE et al. Multivessel coronary angioplasty: classification, results and patterns of restenosis in 494 consecutive patients. Cathet Cardiovasc Diagn 1987; 13: 1–15
32 Myler RK, Stertzer SH, Cumberland DC et al. Coronary angioplasty: indications, contraindications and limitations: historical perspectives and technological determinants. J Intervent Cardiol 1989; 3: 179–185
33 Cooley DA, Duncan JM. Coronary bypass surgery: the total experience at the Texas Heart Institute. In: Hurst J, ed. Clinical essays on the heart, Vol 2. New York: McGraw-Hill, 1984, pp 207–217
34 Ischinger T, Gruentzig AR, Hollman J et al. Should coronary arteries with less than 60% diameter stenosis be treated by angioplasty? Circulation 1983; 68: 148–154
35 Cukingnan RA, Carey JS, Wittig JH, Brown BG. Influence of complete revascularisation on relief of angina. J Thorac Cardiovasc Surg 1980; 79: 188
36 Jones EL, Craver JM, Guyton RA, Bone DK, Hatcher CR Jr, Riechwald N. Importance

of complete revascularisation in performance of the coronary bypass operation. Am J Cardiol 1983; 51: 7

37 Meyer B. Indications: angiographic indications. In: Coronary angioplasty. Orlando, FL: Grune and Stratton, 1987: pp 49–76

38 Vandormael MG, Chaitman BR, Ischinger T et al. Immediate and short term benefit of multi-vessel coronary angioplasty: influence of degree of revascularisation. J Am Coll Cardiol 1985; 6: 983

39 Levy RI, Mock MB, William VI et al. Percutaneous transluminal coronary angioplasty: a status report. N Engl J Med 1981; 305: 399–400

40 Sowton E, Timmis AD, Crick JCP et al. Early results after percutaneous transluminal coronary angioplasty in 400 patients. Br Heart J 1986; 56: 115–120

41 Savage MP, Goldberg S, Hirshfield JW et al. Clinical and angiographic determinants of primary coronary angioplasty success. J Am Coll Cardiol 1991; 17: 22–28

42 Ghazzal ZMB, King SB. Coronary angioplasty: a review. Prog Cardiol 1990; 3(2): 45–63

43 Qigley PJ et al. Repeat percutaneous transluminal coronary angioplasty and predictions of recurrent restenosis. Am J Cardiol 1989; 63: 409

44 Roubin GS et al. Percutaneous transluminal coronary angioplasty in patients with multi-vessel coronary artery disease. I. Spectrum of anatomy and initial outcome. In preparation (cited in ref 42)

45 Melchior JP et al. Percutaneous transluminal coronary angioplasty for chronic total coronary artery occlusion. Am J Cardiol 1987; 59: 535

46 Shimshak TM et al. Application of percutaneous transluminal coronary angioplasty to the internal mammary artery graft. J Am Coll Cardiol 1988; 12: 1205

47 Douglas JS. Angioplasty of saphenous vein and internal mammary artery bypass grafts. In: Topol EJ, ed. Textbook of interventional cardiology. Philadelphia: Saunders, 1990: pp 327–343

48 Douglas J, Robinson K, Schlumpf M. Percutaneous transluminal angioplasty in aorto coronary venous graft stenoses: immediate results and complications. Circulation 1986; 74 (Suppl II): II-281

49 Bredlau CE, Roubin GS, Leimgruber PP et al. In-hospital morbidity and mortality in patients undergoing elective coronary angioplasty. Circulation 1985; 72: 1044–1052

50 Meier B. Kissing balloon angioplasty. Am J Cardiol 1984; 54: 918–920

51 Leimgruber PP et al. Influence of intimal dissection on restenosis after successful coronary angioplasty. Circulation 1985; 72: 530–535

52 Ellis SG et al. Angiographic and clinical predictors of acute closure after native vessel coronary angioplasty. Circulation 1988; 77: 372

53 Hollman J, Gruentzig AR, Douglas JS Jr, King SB, Ischinger T, Meier B. Acute occlusion after percutaneous transluminal coronary angioplasty: a new approach. Circulation 1983; 68: 725–732

54 Palazzo AM, Gustafson GM, Santilli E, Kemp MC. Unusually long inflation times during percutaneous transluminal coronary angioplasty. Cathet Cardiovasc Diagn 1988; 14: 154–158

55 Stack RS, Quigley PJ, Collins G, Phillips MR. Perfusion balloon catheter. Am J Cardiol 1988; 61: 77G–80G

56 Hinohara T, Simpson JB, Phillips MR, Stack RS. Transluminal intracoronary reperfusion catheter: a device to maintain coronary perfusion between failed coronary angioplasty and emergency coronary bypass surgery. J Am Coll Cardiol 1988; II: 977–982

57 Tommaso CL, Singleton RT. Management of coronary occlusion during angioplasty: stabilisation using a guide wire. Cathet Cardiovasc Diagn 1987; 13: 391–393

58 Richardson SG, Morton P, Murtagh JG, O'Keefe DB, Murphy P, Scott ME. Management of acute coronary occlusion during percutaneous transluminal coronary angioplasty: experience of complications in a hospital without on site facilities for cardiac surgery. Br Med J 1990; 300: 355–358

59 Ryan TJ, Faxon DP, Funner RM et al. Guidelines for percutaneous transluminal coronary angioplasty: a report of the American College of Cardiology/American Heart Association Task Force on assessment of diagnostic and therapeutic cardiovascular procedures (Subcommittee on Percutaneous Transluminal Coronary Angioplasty). Circulation 1988; 2: 486–502

60 Report of the Joint International Society and Federation of Cardiology/World Health

Organization Task Force in coronary angioplasty. Eur Heart J 1989; 9: 1034–1045
61 Ellis SG et al. In-hospital cardiac mortality after acute closure after coronary angioplasty: analysis of risk factors from 8207 procedures. J Am Coll Cardiol 1988; 11: 211
62 Cowley MJ et al. Emergency coronary bypass surgery after coronary angioplasty: the National Heart, Lung and Blood Institute's Percutaneous Transluminal Coronary Angioplasty Registry experience. Am J Cardiol 1984; 5(3): 226
63 Talley JD et al. Coronary artery bypass surgery after failed elective percutaneous transluminal coronary angioplasty. Circulation 1989; 79 (Suppl I): 126
64 Leimgruber PP et al. Restenosis after successful coronary angioplasty in patients with a single vessel disease. Circulation 1986; 73: 710
65 Holmes DR Jr et al. Restenosis after percutaneous transluminal coronary angioplasty: a report from the Percutaneous Transluminal Coronary Angioplasty Registry of the National Heart, Lung and Blood Institute. Am J Cardiol 1984; 53: 77C–81C
66 Guiteras Val P et al. Restenosis after successful percutaneous transluminal coronary angioplasty: the Montreal Heart Institute experience. Am J Cardiol 1987; 60: 50B
67 Eliis SG et al. Importance of stenosis morphology in the estimation of restenosis risk after elective percutaneous transluminal coronary angioplasty. Am J Cardiol 1989; 63: 30
68 Gershlick AH, de Bono DP. Restenosis after angioplasty. Br Heart J 1990; 64: 351–353
69 Nobuyoshi M et al. Restenosis after successful percutaneous transluminal coronary angioplasty: serial angiographic follow-up of 229 patients. J Am Coll Cardiol 1988; 12: 616
70 Serruys PW, Luitjen HE, Beatt KJ et al. Incidence of restenosis after successful coronary angioplasty: a time related phenomenon. Circulation 1988; 77: 361–371
71 Simpson JB et al. Restenosis following successful dissectional coronary atherectomy. Circulation 1989; 80 (Suppl II): 582 (abstr)
72 Spears JR. Percutaneous transluminal coronary angioplasty restenosis: potential presentation with laser balloon angioplasty. Am J Cardiol 1987; 60: 61B–64B
73 Lee BI, Becker GJ, Waller BF et al. Thermal compression and molding with use of radiofrequency energy: implications for radiofrequency balloon angioplasty. J Am Coll Cardiol 1989; 13: 1167–1175
74 Sigwart U, Puel J, Mirkovitch V, Joffre F, Kappenberger L. Intravascular stents to present occlusion and restenosis after transluminal angioplasty. N Engl J Med 1987; 316: 201–206
75 Sigwart U, Kaufman U, Goy JJ et al. Prevention of coronary restenosis by stenting. Eur Heart J 1988; 9 (Suppl C): 31–37
76 Hollman J, Ischinger T. The problem of restenosis. In: Ischinger T, ed. Practice of coronary angioplasty. Berlin: Springer-Verlag, 1985, pp 211–222
77 Gerslick AH, de Bono DP. Restenosis after angioplasty. Br Heart J 1990; 64: 351–353
78 Akins CW, Block PC, Palacios IF et al. Comparison of coronary artery bypass grafting and percutaneous transluminal coronary angioplasty as initial treatment strategies. Ann Thorac Surg 1989; 47: 507–516
79 Kelly M, Taylor G, Moses H et al. Comparative cost of myocardial revascularisation: percutaneous transluminal angioplasty and coronary artery bypass surgery. J Am Coll Cardiol 1985; 5: 16–20
80 Wittels EH, Hay JW, Gotto AM. Medical cost of coronary artery disease in the United States. Am J Cardiol 1990; 65: 432–440
81 Sigwart U. Percutaneous transluminal coronary angioplasty. What next? Br Heart J 1990; 63: 321–322
82 Sigwart U, Puel J, Mirkovitch V, Joffre F, Kappenberg L. Intravascular stents to prevent occlusion and restenosis after transluminal angioplasty. N Engl J Med 1987; 316: 701–705

FURTHER READING

Chokshi SK, Myers S, Abi-Mansour P. Percutaneous transluminal coronary angioplasty: ten years experience. Prog Cardiovasc Dis 1987; XXX: 147–210
Ghuzzal ZMB, King SB. Coronary angioplasty: a review. Prog Cardiol 1990; 3(2): 45–63

2

Coronary thrombolysis

D. de Bono

At the end of the nineteenth century James Clerk Maxwell, the distinguished Edinburgh physicist, was asked what he thought the next important advances in physics would be. With becoming modesty, he replied that he thought everything important that could be known was now known, and any future advances would simply be a matter of filling in detail. An observer at the American College of Cardiology meeting in Atlanta in March 1991, having just listened to the presentation of the preliminary results of the ISIS-3 trial, could be forgiven for feeling much the same about coronary thrombolysis. Six years ago, the GISSI-1 trial[1] definitively established the role of thrombolytic therapy in the routine management of acute myocardial infarction. Subsequent controlled trials have repeatedly confirmed that thrombolytic therapy reduces mortality,[1-4] that the benefit is sustained, and that it does not depend on subsequent intervention by angioplasty or coronary bypass grafting.[5,6] Aspirin has been shown to enhance the benefit of streptokinase therapy, and is now a universal component of thrombolytic regimens.[2] Enormous enthusiasm and expense have gone into trials aimed at demonstrating the superiority of one thrombolytic agent over another, but no consistent overall survival benefit has yet been shown,[7-9] although these large trials have provided valuable insights into the natural history of coronary thrombosis. It seems unlikely that trials on this scale will again be contemplated in the near future, or perhaps ever – so the likelihood of radically new thrombolytic agents being introduced is presently remote.

But Maxwell was wrong, as every schoolboy knows, and 'answers' keep generating new questions. New dosage regimens may enhance the safety, efficacy and ease of use of existing agents. Humble ancillary treatments such as heparin have attracted increasing attention as it has been realised that they may, like aspirin, markedly affect outcome. Better understanding of the chemistry of blood coagulation and platelet aggregation has produced a whole new generation of antithrombotic agents, many of which have potential uses in conjunction with thrombolysis. Problems such as the nature and prevention of 'reperfusion injury' have been identified but not solved. Patients who develop cerebral haemorrhage after thrombolysis, or who receive thrombolytic therapy but do not recanalize an occluded vessel, continue to have a very poor prognosis. Thrombolytic therapy in practice still seems fated to carry an unacceptable delay in many clinical situations.

This review is divided into two parts: the first summarizes the 'state of the art' of clinical thrombolytic therapy; the second discusses experimental studies and developments which may have a bearing on the way we carry out thrombolysis in the future.

PART 1

CURRENT PRACTICE IN CLINICAL THROMBOLYSIS

Choice of patients for thrombolysis

Some of the early controlled trials of thrombolysis adopted 'restrictive' entry criteria, largely aimed at maximizing the difference between treatment and control groups by concentrating on patients perceived to be at the highest risk. Conversely, trials such as ISIS-2[2] and ASSET[3] adopted much looser entry criteria. The cost–benefit equation for each individual patient has to take account of three factors: the risk that the patient will die from the coronary thrombosis; the likelihood that thrombolytic therapy will reduce this risk; and the risk of side effects (Table 2.1). The quantity of data accumulated from several trials allows a sophisticated numerical approach to be made to decision taking,[10] but in practice most decisions will continue to be made clinically and to be based on a small number of factors.

Patient age

The risk of dying from an infarct increases steeply over the age of 65. Although the risks of thrombolytic side effects, in particular bleeding, also

Table 2.1   Factors affecting the cost–benefit equation for thrombolysis in acute myocardial infarction (MI)

	Risk of death	Efficacy of thrombolysis	Risk of side effects
Age > 65	+ + +	=	+
Previous MI	+	=	=
Early treatment	=	+ +	=
Late treatment	=	−	=
Anterior MI	+	=	=
Inferior MI	−	=	=
ST elevation	+	+ +	=
ST depression	+	−	=
Low body weight	=	? +	+
Previous anticoagulation	=	=	+
History of peptic ulcer etc.	=	=	+

+ (+ +), increased risk; = , average risk; − , reduced risk.

increase these are outweighed by the potential benefits, and unless 'survival would be an unreasonable burden' or there are clear contraindications, elderly patients with coronary thrombosis should always be considered for thrombolysis.

Time from onset of symptoms

For practical purposes, all clinical trials have shown that the earlier thrombolytic therapy is initiated after the onset of symptoms, the better the outcome. Although animal studies indicate no appreciable myocardial salvage on reperfusion after longer than 3 hours of total ischaemia, this is not applicable to the human situation, where intermittent occlusion, previous establishment of a collateral circulation, and myocardial conditioning may all apply. It is virtually always worth giving thrombolytic therapy if this can be done within 6 hours of the onset of major symptoms, and thrombolytic therapy should also be *considered* in anyone with clinical or electrocardiographic evidence of persisting ischaemia irrespective of the time of onset of symptoms. Patients with 'big bang' infarcts due to the proximal occlusion of a large coronary artery tend to present early with striking clinical symptoms and unequivocal electrocardiographic changes, and are a rewarding group for thrombolytic therapy. On the other hand older patients tend to present later after the onset of symptoms: in the AIMS trial[4] this led to a higher mortality, and proportionately greater mortality reduction with thrombolytic therapy, in a group treated between 3 and 6 hours after symptom onset than in patients presenting within 3 hours.

Electrocardiographic changes

The significance of electrocardiographic changes in predicting mortality and in predicting benefit from thrombolysis does not run quite in parallel. Patients with clear-cut ST segment elevation tend to show most benefit from thrombolysis; mortality risk in patients who reach hospital is higher with anterior than inferior infarcts, but the proportionate reduction in mortality with thrombolysis is similar.[11] Patients with ST segment depression as the dominant ECG manifestation tend to have a poor prognosis, and the proportionate benefit of thrombolysis is rather small. There is no really satisfactory explanation, but one of the better theories is that this group includes patients with multivessel coronary disease and perhaps pre-existing impairment of left ventricular function. Patients with bundle branch block have a high mortality, but thrombolytic therapy is worthwhile; in contrast, patients with other ECG changes such as isolated T wave inversion or Q waves without acute ST changes have a low mortality. To some extent the latter finding is an artefact of selection; when the different electrocardiographic groups are corrected for the proportion of patients with verified myocardial infarction there is little difference in mortality or in the proportionate benefit of thrombolysis.

Factors increasing the risk of side effects

All trials have confirmed that the major unwanted side effect of thrombolytic therapy is bleeding, and that the type of bleeding associated with the greatest mortality risk is intracranial haemorrhage. In a retrospective survey de Jaeghere and colleagues used multivariate analysis to identify pre-treatment factors which were associated with an increased risk of bleeding.[12] These were age greater than 65 years, weight less than 70 kg, previous anticoagulant therapy, and uncontrolled hypertension. Many would add to these a previous history of cerebrovascular accident, although the data on this point are less certain because most trials have excluded such patients. The possible relationship between haemorrhage risk and the choice of thrombolytic regimen, and the treatment of suspected intra-cerebral bleeding, are considered separately below.

Choice of thrombolytic agent

The three thrombolytic agents for which product licences or their equivalent are available in the United Kingdom and most other countries are streptokinase, alteplase (single-chain recombinant human tissue type plasminogen activator) and anistreplase (anisoylated plasminogen–streptokinase activator complex, APSAC). The chemistry and pharmacology of these agents have been described in detail elsewhere[13,14] and are summarized in Table 2.2. The ideal thrombolytic agent would combine efficacy, safety, and ease of use.

Efficacy

This has been a contentious issue for two principal reasons: first, contro-

Table 2.2   Comparison of thrombolytic agents

	Alteplase	Anistreplase	Streptokinase
Source	Tissue culture expression of human gene	Bacterial + human plasminogen	Bacterial
Mode of action	All work by activating plasminogen to plasmin		
Fibrin specificity	+	(+)	−
Plasma half-life	5–8 min	~ 90 min	20–30 min
Most common dose	100 mg over 3 h	30 units over 5 min	1 500 000 units over 60 min
Potentiated by aspirin	No data	No data	Yes
Potentiated by heparin	Yes	No data	Yes?
Antibody response	Minimal	Yes	Yes

versy over the extent to which observations on 'process' endpoints such as coronary patency could be extrapolated to 'outcome' endpoints such as function or survival; and second, the fact that efficacy as measured in clinical trials relates to the particular thrombolytic regimen as a whole rather than to any intrinsic property of the thrombolytic agent.

The working hypothesis that thrombolytic agents work principally by restoring and maintaining coronary patency, and that this is manifested both by better preservation of left ventricular function and by improved survival, still stands intact, despite the dense undergrowth of verbiage and special pleading that has grown up in the absence of adequate data. It is important to emphasize that early and sustained coronary patency is more important than patency at some arbitrarily chosen time interval, and that the relationship between coronary patency and, say, survival is not necessarily linear.

The earliest comparative trial of streptokinase and alteplase, the TIMI-1 trial,[15] showed *reperfusion* rates of 55% for streptokinase and 70% for alteplase. It has subsequently been suggested that the trial design, with the delay inherent in mandatory pre-treatment angiography, loaded the odds against streptokinase, which might be less effective at lysing older thrombus. In any event, subsequent studies have tended fairly consistently to show 90-minute coronary patency rates with streptokinase (usually without concomitant heparin) about 5–15% lower than with alteplase (usually given with heparin).[16]

Later patency rates with streptokinase or alteplase are very similar. Small-scale trials using left ventricular function as endpoint have failed to show consistent differences between streptokinase and alteplase[7,17] but had limited power to detect differences as small as 10–15%. The first large-scale trials to compare streptokinase and alteplase were GISSI-2 and its cousin the International Study Group Trial.[8,9] These showed no significant difference either on a combined endpoint of death/severe left ventricular dysfunction (GISSI-2) or on mortality alone between streptokinase and alteplase. These trials were criticized (in retrospect!) because alteplase was given without concomitant heparin (there was factorial randomization to late subcutaneous heparin starting at 12 hours). Smaller trials conducted whilst GISSI-2 and ISG were recruiting[18–20] have suggested that the administration of concomitant intravenous heparin can make a difference of between 15% and 30% in late coronary patency rates in patients receiving alteplase. It has been suggested, though not directly proven, that in the absence of heparin early patency rates in the alteplase and streptokinase arms of GISSI-2/ISG would have been rather similar.

Direct angiographic data are not available to assess the effect of combining heparin with streptokinase, but at least one study using non-invasive assessment of coronary patency has claimed that the efficacy of streptokinase is enhanced by concomitant heparin administration.[21] It has been suggested [22] that the administration of thrombolytic drugs in the absence of anticoagulants leads to thrombin activation, and thus to the promotion of rethrombosis.

Direct angiographic comparisons of streptokinase and anistreplase have given conflicting results: some show an advantage to anistreplase, whilst other studies were unable to document this.

The recently completed ISIS-3 trial, for which only preliminary results are currently available, attempted to compare streptokinase, duteplase (very similar to alteplase, but from a different manufacturer) and anistreplase, with further randomization to subcutaneous heparin starting at 4 hours after initiating thrombolysis.[23] Overall, there was no significant 35-day mortality difference between the three thrombolytic agents, irrespective of the use of heparin. It has been suggested, however, that the analysis of total mortality data might be diluted by patients with marginal or uncertain indications for thrombolysis. Subgroup analysis of patients with ST elevation on the electrocardiogram, treated within 6 hours of the onset of major symptoms, shows a just-significant mortality difference between duteplase plus heparin (9.0%) and streptokinase plus aspirin (10.3%). There was no significant difference between streptokinase and anistreplase, nor between any of the agents when each was combined with heparin. The most obvious way of interpreting the whole corpus of data is to say that better early and sustained coronary patency *is* probably reflected in better survival, but in practical terms the differences in efficacy between streptokinase, duteplase and anistreplase are small and may not be very important clinically.

Safety

Safety of thrombolytic therapy has to be seen in the context of therapeutic margins: an increased incidence of side effects will be tolerated if it is outweighed by greater efficacy. As with efficacy, clinical trials will give an estimate of the safety of a particular regimen rather than an individual agent. Mortality associated with haemorrhage in large clinical trials with different thrombolytic regimens has varied from 0.3% to 1%. Morbidity associated with bleeding has been between 5% and 10% in trials not involving arterial catheterization. There has been a trend towards higher cerebral haemorrhage rates with alteplase than with streptokinase. In the ISIS-3 trial cerebral haemorrhage was statistically more frequent with duteplase than with streptokinase (0.7% v. 0.3%, $p = 0.0001$), though the difference in total cerebrovascular event rate was smaller. Alteplase is the only agent for which a positive relationship between dose, thrombolytic efficacy and cerebral bleeding risk has been established.[24] Analysis of cerebral bleeding events in patients given alteplase indicates that patients with a low body weight are at increased risk when given a 'standard' dose of 100 mg, and dose reduction is advised in patients under 67 kg. Since elderly patients tend to have lower body weights, this helps to explain the increased haemorrhage risk in the elderly.

Addition of aspirin to the thrombolytic regimen has little effect on safety,[2] but this does not necessarily apply to other antithrombotic agents. Addition of subcutaneous heparin in the GISSI-2/ISG and ISIS-3 trials produced a modest increase in bleeding complications. A subgroup of patients in the ISIS-3 trial who were given intravenous heparin for non-protocol reasons had a much increased cerebral bleeding rate, but this must be interpreted with great caution. Similar bleeding rates were not experienced in the ECSG series of trials which combined alteplase with aspirin and intravenous heparin.

In summary, serious bleeding complications have been less of a problem than originally anticipated, and there is little to choose from between the available thrombolytic agents. There is evidence that bleeding complications with alteplase/duteplase may be dose related. Recent studies on the inhibition of thrombolysis-induced bleeding are discussed below.

Allergic complications are more common with streptokinase or anistreplase than with alteplase. Early allergic reactions include flushing, urticaria and hypotension, and very rarely an anaphylactic type reaction. Late allergic reactions include a serum-sickness type reaction with arthralgia, vasculitis and haematuria, and very rarely glomerulonephritis.[13] An early antibody response to streptokinase is very common, and high antibody titres may persist for six months or longer.[25] It is controversial whether these antibodies, which frequently fail to inhibit plasminogen activation in vitro, are of clinical relevance. There is some clinical evidence,[26] and much anecdote, to suggest that the risk both of allergic reactions and of unsuccessful recanalization is higher when streptokinase or anistreplase is given for a second time, and there may be a case for giving alteplase instead in this situation.

Ease of administration

Current 'standard' regimens for administering streptokinase, anistreplase and alteplase are detailed in Figure 2.1. Anistreplase has the advantage that it can be administered as a single intravenous injection over a period of 4 or 5 minutes, and this is a considerable potential advantage in casualty department or out-of-hospital use. There has been considerable interest in bolus or 'front-loaded' regimens of alteplase, and some of these are described below.

WHAT TO DO AFTER THROMBOLYSIS?

Early angiographic studies indicated that a substantial proportion of patients given thrombolysis were left with a major degree of residual coronary stenosis.[27] This conclusion has had to be modified in the light of subsequent experience. First, the quantitative cine-angiographic techniques used in some of these studies tended to overestimate residual stenosis; second, and more important, serial quantitative angiography has shown that vessel calibre shows a consistent trend to improve between 90-minute and 24-hour angiography, and between 24 hours and discharge.[28] This is presumably due largely to continuing lysis of thrombus both by activated plasminogen sequestered within the thrombus and by endogenous vascular thrombolysis. It remains true that patients with very poor perfusion of the distal vessel at early angiography have a greater chance of ending with an occluded vessel, but otherwise early angiographic appearances are poor at predicting the risk of late reinfarction: indeed the consequences of this are often most drastic in patients with the least residual stenosis and least stimulus to collateral formation.[29]

Against this background, it is perhaps not surprising that successive trials have failed to show that either immediate[5,30] or early elective angioplasty[6,31] improve prognosis in terms of mortality or infarct-free survival. A further complicating factor is the risk (8–10%) of occluding the vessel during early angioplasty. Reanalysis of the European cooperative study

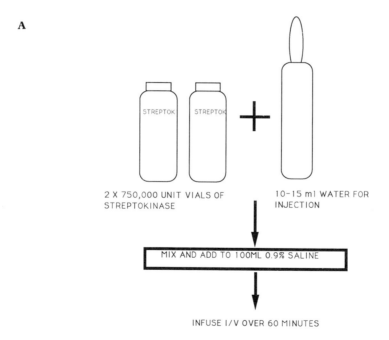

A

2 X 750,000 UNIT VIALS OF
STREPTOKINASE

10-15 ml WATER FOR
INJECTION

MIX AND ADD TO 100ML 0.9% SALINE

INFUSE I/V OVER 60 MINUTES

Notes: An alternative is to make up streptokinase as two injections of 750,000 units in 10 ml, each given over 5-10 minutes with a gap of 20 minutes

Fig. 2.1   Conventional dosage schedules for (**A**) streptokinase, (**B**) alteplase, and (**C**) anistreplase, in acute myocardial infarction. (Reproduced from de Bono DP, *Practical coronary thrombolysis*, Blackwells, Oxford, 1990.)

B

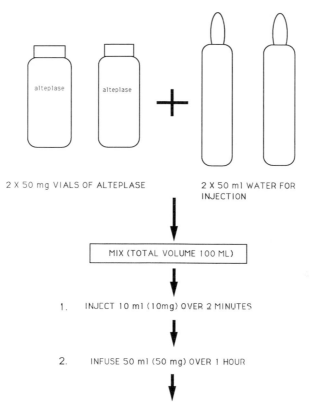

2 X 50 mg VIALS OF ALTEPLASE

2 X 50 ml WATER FOR
INJECTION

MIX (TOTAL VOLUME 100 ML)

1.   INJECT 10 ml (10mg) OVER 2 MINUTES

2.   INFUSE 50 ml (50 mg) OVER 1 HOUR

3.   INFUSE 40 ml (40 mg) OVER 2 HOURS

NOTE: If patient weighs less than 67 Kg adjust dose to 1.5 mg per Kg

C

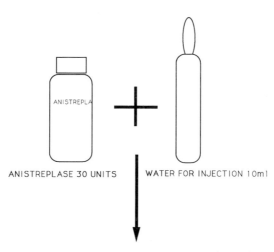

ANISTREPLASE 30 UNITS

WATER FOR INJECTION 10ml

MIX AND INJECT I/V OVER APPROXIMATELY 5 MINUTES

group data[32] on a trial of patients randomized to immediate angioplasty or conservative management indicated a small but significant benefit to left ventricular function if patients whose vessels reoccluded during angioplasty were excluded. This is obviously of academic interest only until angioplasty techniques improve.

In the SWIFT trial of early (48-hour) angiography with a view to angioplasty or bypass grafting after thrombolysis, there was no benefit to early intervention in terms of survival or reinfarction, and indeed the intervention group fared significantly worse in terms of the combined endpoint of reinfarction and mortality at three months.[6] Interestingly, between three and 12 months the event rate was higher in the conventional therapy group, although at 12 months there was still no overall benefit to early intervention. Similar results were obtained in the TIMI-IIb trial in the United States, although here the 'late intervention' rate in the conventionally treated group was much higher.[31] It is now generally accepted that patients with recurrent angina or a positive exercise test following myocardial infarction should be investigated with a view to revascularization.[32] The detection of silent ischaemia may identify a particularly high-risk group,[33] but there is currently little evidence that this is of benefit in asymptomatic patients with good exercise tolerance. Despite this, some 40% of patients undergoing revascularization after myocardial infarction have no symptoms at the time of the procedure.[10]

With regard to medical therapy, there is direct evidence that long-term beta-blockade[34] and long-term warfarin therapy[35] improve survival, and strong indirect evidence that aspirin is also effective. Angiotensin-converting enzyme inhibitors[36] are effective in limiting left ventricular dilatation. It is arguable whether every post-infarct (and thus usually post-thrombolysis) patient should receive a beta-blocker, aspirin or warfarin, and an angiotensin-converting enzyme inhibitor, or whether there should be some selectivity of medication. Unfortunately the clinical trials have not been helpful in this respect, and in default clinical judgment is needed!

PART 2

POTENTIAL NEW DEVELOPMENTS IN THROMBOLYSIS

New thrombolytic agents

New thrombolytic agents continue to be developed, although their potential commercial exploitation, in the light of the GISSI-2 and ISIS-3 trial results, remains problematical. Urokinase is scarcely a 'new' agent, but its use in Europe and the United States has been overshadowed by the cheaper streptokinase and the more fibrin-selective alteplase. It has been extensively used in Japan,[37] but not in the context of comparative trials against other agents. The German GAUS study showed similar patency rates in patients given intravenous alteplase (70 mg) or urokinase (3 million units).[38]

Early studies suggesting synergism between reduced doses of urokinase and alteplase have not been confirmed with respect to any beneficial effect on early coronary patency,[39] but there is some preliminary evidence that the addition of urokinase reduces the rate of reocclusion.[40] Urokinase's lack of antigenicity is an advantage over streptokinase, but its cost makes it non-competitive. It has a useful role in small doses as an aid to angioplasty in patients with unstable angina and intraluminal thrombus.

Saruplase (single-chain urokinase type plasminogen activator) is produced using recombinant DNA technology. Unlike low-molecular-weight urokinase, it has a lag period before reaching full thrombolytic activity in vitro, and (again unlike low-molecular-weight urokinase) it is relatively thrombus selective. Clinical trials using angiographic endpoints have shown it to be a highly effective thrombolytic agent with an attractive safety profile,[41] but large-scale 'outcome' comparisons with other thrombolytics are lacking.

The original hope that alteplase would be a 'safe' thrombolytic agent because it was fibrin specific has not been borne out by clinical experience, at least in coronary thrombolysis. However, the fibrin selectivity of alteplase is only relative, and it is still conceivable that a *very* fibrin-selective drug would have the advantages originally expected for alteplase. The tissue plasminogen activator from the vampire bat, *Desmodus rotundus*, appears to behave in this way, and initial trials are encouraging. An alternative approach is to use a monoclonal antibody with a very high affinity for fibrin, and link it either to urokinase or to a powerful but otherwise non-selective proteinase such as trypsin.[42,43]

Fibrin remains the most attractive 'target' for coronary thrombolysis, but different targets may be appropriate for other thrombolytic agents. We have explored the possibility of targeting thrombolytic agents to damaged segments of vessel wall using monoclonal antibodies which recognize damaged endothelium, with the aim of preventing local thrombosis after coronary artery surgery or angioplasty.[44]

The clinical evaluation of new thrombolytic agents is now problematical: angiographic patency studies are still the most 'efficient' way of evaluating a new agent in a small number of patients, but demonstration of the lack of benefit from immediate angioplasty makes early angiography hard to justify as a therapeutic procedure. It is possible, on a population basis, to distinguish fairly reliably between patients who reperfuse and those whose infarct-related vessel remains closed by using the rate of evolution of the ST segments[45,46] and the rate of change of plasma cardiac enzyme concentrations.[47] Although these techniques are less immediately convincing than patency studies, they are likely to be used increasingly.

New ways of using old agents

When efficacy and safety are equivalent, ways of administering a thrombo-

Table 2.3 Coronary patency results with 'newer' dosage regimens

Author/Acronym	Agent	Regimen	Patency
Neuhaus[48]	Alteplase	'Accelerated infusion' 15 mg bolus, 50 mg over 30 min, 35 mg over 60 min	70% at 60 min 90% at 90 min ($n = 74$) 8% reocclusion over 48 h
RAAMI[49]	Alteplase	15 mg bolus, 50 mg over 30 min, 35 mg over 60 min	76% at 60 min 82% at 90 min
TAMI-7[50]	Alteplase	1 mg/kg 30 min, 0.25 mg/kg 30 min, 1.25 mg/kg 90 min, 0.75 mg/kg 30 min, 0.5 mg/kg 60 min, 20 mg, wait 30 min, 80 mg/120 min	72% at 90 min ($n = 36$) 64% at 90 min ($n = 33$) 84% at 90 min ($n = 63$) 77% at 90 min ($n = 46$)
Kalbfleisch[51]	Duteplase	0.6 MU/kg over 60 min	58% at 60 min ($n = 72$) 76% at 90 min
Tranchesi[52]	Alteplase	'Single bolus' 70 mg bolus 60 mg bolus 50 mg bolus	72% at 60 min ($n = 25$) 32% at 60 min ($n = 29$) 45% at 60 min ($n = 28$)
Purvis[53]	Alteplase	'Double bolus' 20 mg, wait 30 min, then 50 mg 50 mg, wait 30 min then 20 mg 50 mg, wait 30 min, then 50 mg	75% at 90 min ($n = 20$) 70% at 90 min ($n = 20$) 90% at 90 min ($n = 19$)

lytic drug which save time and effort are an advantage. Anistreplase in particular benefits from a very simple dose regimen. Early studies on alteplase were heavily influenced by knowledge of its short plasma half-life and fear of reocclusion, and therefore involved prolonged administration over a period of 3 hours. There has been much recent interest both in 'compressed' administration schedules[48–51] and in bolus administration.[52,53] Results of recent studies are summarized in Table 2.3.

New antithrombotic agents to combine with thrombolysis

As discussed in Part 1, there has been belated recognition of the importance of concomitant antithrombotic therapy for the overall success of the thrombolytic 'package'. In addition to the conventional agents such as aspirin, heparin and warfarin, advances in understanding coagulation mechanisms have led to the development of a series of new antithrombotics (Table 2.4). In experimental models some of these agents, and in particular thrombin antagonists such as hirudin[54] and its derivatives, have shown great promise in enhancing the efficacy of thrombolysis and preventing reocclusion. It is

Table 2.4 New antithrombotic drugs as potential ancillary agents in coronary thrombolysis

Agent	Type	Mode of action
7E3	Monoclonal antibody	Blocks platelet IIb/IIIa receptor
Hirudin	Recombinant protein	Thrombin antagonist
BG8569 (Hirulog)	Synthetic peptide	Thrombin antagonist
Argatroban	Synthetic	Thrombin antagonist
Bitistatin	Peptide	Inhibits platelet adhesion to RGD binding site (?)
Echistatin	Peptide	Inhibits platelet adhesion to RGD binding site (?)

obviously difficult from small studies to know whether these advantages are combined with a satisfactory safety margin. The ultimate degree of advantage, if any, over aspirin and heparin will need to be evaluated by large-scale trials.

Prevention of reperfusion injury

Several years ago in vitro studies on the behaviour of isolated perfused hearts subjected to hypoxia and then normoxaemic reperfusion introduced the concept that actual irreversible myocardial damage, or at least a component of it, might be associated with reperfusion. The possible cellular basis of reperfusion injury has been discussed in two recent reviews.[55,56] Initial attention was focused on mechanisms of calcium transport, in that damaged myocytes rapidly accumulated calcium, and it appeared that irreversible damage could be reduced or at least deferred by reperfusing with calcium-free medium. It now seems clear that the calcium accumulation is not due to malfunction of 'physiological' calcium channels, but rather a non-specific response to severe membrane damage. Attention was next directed to a possible role of oxygen-derived free radicals. These highly reactive chemical species are continually being produced in tissues, but are capable of being scavenged by a variety of metabolic pathways. It has been suggested that under conditions of hypoxaemia the scavenging pathways become suppressed, and that unscavenged free radicals produced on reperfusion cause damage. There has been considerable controversy over whether or not excessive quantities of oxygen-derived free radicals are produced during ischaemia/reperfusion, and the possible mechanisms involved. Because free radicals are reactive species with a very short half-life, direct detection is not usually feasible, and reliance has to be placed on techniques such as spin trapping, whereby the free radical forms a more stable adduct with certain 'marker' molecules added to the system. Unfortunately there are very considerable possibilities for artefact: in particular, minute quantities of iron as a contaminant can catalyse the production of spurious free radicals in in vitro systems.

An alternative approach to attempting to detect free radicals during ischaemia/reperfusion is to reduce or prevent damage using some kind of radical scavenging system. The most convincing experiments so far are those of Bolli and collaborators[57] in the dog, where free radical scavenging agents prevented 'myocardial stunning' after coronary occlusion and release. The extent to which these observations are transferable to humans is uncertain, particularly as myocardial stunning is particularly difficult to show convincingly in patients.

Preliminary experiments with free radical scavenging agents in patients have given equivocal or disappointing results.

Treatment of thrombolysis-associated bleeding

The incidence and morbidity of, and risk factors for, thrombolysis-associated bleeding have already been discussed in Part 1. The actual treatment of thrombolysis-associated haemorrhage has so far largely rested on a priori reasoning and anecdote. In animal models plasmin inhibitors such as aprotinin and tranexamic acid are effective in reducing or preventing excessive bleeding associated with alteplase infusion.[58,59] There is increasing clinical experience with the use of high-dose aprotinin in preventing bleeding associated with cardiac surgery or hepatic transplantation,[60] and its use in reversing thrombolysis-associated bleeding in patients is logical, although clinical trials are for obvious reasons hard to organize.

Very early thrombolysis

There is general agreement that the earlier thrombolytic therapy is initiated after coronary thrombosis the better the likely outcome. Several studies have demonstrated the feasibility of out-of-hospital administration of thrombolytic drugs,[61] although whether or not this is of major benefit will depend on local geography.

Conclusions

The introduction of thrombolytic therapy has, in many ways, been a model for the rapid and convincing evaluation and establishment of a valuable treatment. Now that the dust is beginning to settle over the controversies about the most appropriate agents, there remain important questions to be resolved about concomitant therapy and the best strategy for myocardial preservation.

REFERENCES

1 Gruppo Italiano per lo Studio della Streptochinasi nell'Infarto Miocardico. Long term effects of intravenous thrombolysis in acute myocardial infarction: final report of the GISSI study. Lancet 1987; ii: 871–874

2 ISIS-2 (Second International Study of Infarct Survival) Collaborative Group. Randomised trial of intravenous streptokinase, oral aspirin, both or neither among 17,187 cases of suspected acute myocardial infarction. Lancet 1988; ii: 349–360

3 Wilcox RG, Von der Lippe G, Olsson CG, Jensen G, Skene AM, Hampton JR, for the Anglo-Scandinavian Study of Early Thrombolysis. Effects of alteplase in acute myocardial infarction: 6 month results from the ASSET study. Lancet 1990; 335: 1175–1178

4 AIMS Trial Study Group. Long term effects of intravenous anistreplase in acute myocardial infarction: final report of the AIMS study. Lancet 1990; 335; 427–431

5 Simoons ML, Arnold AER, Betriu A et al. Thrombolysis with tissue plasminogen activator in acute myocardial infarction: no additional benefit from immediate percutaneous coronary angioplasty. Lancet 1988; i: 197–203

6 SWIFT (Should We Intervene Following Thrombolysis) Trial Study Group. SWIFT trial of delayed elective intervention v. conservative treatment after thrombolysis with anistreplase in acute myocardial infarction. Br Med J 1991; 302: 555–560

7 White HD, Rivers JT, Maslowski AH et al. Effect of streptokinase as compared with that of tissue plasminogen activator on left ventricular function after first myocardial infarction. N Engl J Med 1989; 320: 817–821

8 Gruppo Italiano per lo Studio della Streptochinasi nell'Infarto Miocardico. GISSI-2. A factorial randomised trial of alteplase versus streptokinase and heparin versus no heparin among 12,490 patients with acute myocardial infarction. Lancet 1990; 336: 65–71

9 The International Study Group. In hospital mortality and clinical course of 20,891 patients with suspected acute myocardial infarction randomised between alteplase and streptokinase with or without heparin. Lancet 1990; 336: 71–75

10 Arnold AER. Benefits and risks of thrombolysis for acute myocardial infarction. Thesis, Erasmus University, Rotterdam, 1990

11 Vermeer F, Simoons M, Baer F et al. Which patients benefit most from early thrombolysis with intracoronary streptokinase? Circulation 1986; 74: 1379–1389

12 de Jaeghere P, Balk A, Simoons ML et al. Intracranial haemorrhage and thrombolytic therapy. Eur Heart J 1990; 11: 47 (abstr)

13 de Bono DP. Practical coronary thrombolysis. Blackwells, Oxford, 1990, pp 6–15

14 Collen D. In: Sobel BE, Collen D, Grossbard EB, eds. Tissue plasminogen activator in thrombolytic therapy. Marcel Dekker, New York, 1990, pp 3–24

15 Chesebro JH, Knatterud G, Roberts R et al. Thrombolysis in myocardial infarction (TIMI) trial, phase I: a comparison between intravenous tissue plasminogen activator and intravenous streptokinase. Circulation 1987; 76: 142–154

16 White HD. GISSI-2 and the heparin controversy. Lancet 1990; 336: 297–298

17 Magnani B. Plasminogen activator Italian Multicentre Study (PAIMS): comparison of intravenous recombinant single chain human tissue type plasminogen activator (rt-PA) with intravenous streptokinase in acute myocardial infarction. J Am Coll Cardiol 1989; 13: 19–26

18 Bleich SD, Nichols T, Schumacher R et al. Effect of heparin on coronary arterial patency after thrombolysis with tissue plasminogen activator in acute myocardial infarction. Am J Cardiol 1990; 66: 1412–1417

19 Hsia J, Hamilton WP, Kleiman N, Roberts R, Chaitman BR, Ross AM, for the Heparin–Aspirin Reperfusion Trial (HART) investigators. A comparison between heparin and low dose aspirin as adjunctive therapy with tissue plasminogen activator for acute myocardial infarction. N Engl J Med 1990; 323: 1433–1437

20 de Bono DP, Simoons ML, Tijssen J et al, for the European Cooperative Study Group. Early intravenous heparin enhances coronary patency after alteplase thrombolysis: results of a randomised double blind European Cooperative Study Group Trial. Br Heart J 1992; 67: 122–128

21 Melandri G, Branzi A, Semprini F, Cervi V, Galie N, Magnani B. Enhanced thrombolytic efficacy and reduction of infarct size by simultaneous infusion of streptokinase and heparin. Br Heart J 1990; 64: 118–120

22 Rapold HJ. Promotion of thrombin activity by thrombolytic therapy without simultaneous anticoagulation. Lancet 1990; 335: 481–482

23 Collins R, for the ISIS-3 (Third International Study of Infarct Survival) Collaborative group. Data presented at American College of Cardiology Meeting, Dallas, USA, March 1991

24 Mueller HS, Rao AK, Forman SA et al. Thrombolysis in myocardial infarction (TIMI): comparative studies of coronary reperfusion and systemic fibrinogenolysis with two forms of recombinant tissue type plasminogen activator. J Am Coll Cardiol 1987; 10: 479–490

25 Jalihal S, Morris GK. Antistreptokinase titres after intravenous streptokinase. Lancet 1990; 335: 184–185

26 White HD, Cross DB, Williams BF, Norris RM. Safety and efficacy of repeat thrombolytic treatment after acute myocardial infarction. Br Heart J 1990; 64: 177–184

27 Harrison DG, Ferguson DW, Collins SM et al. Rethrombosis after reperfusion with streptokinase: importance of geometry of residual lesions. Circulation 1984; 69: 991–999

28 Verstraete M, Arnold AER, Brower RW et al. Acute coronary thrombolysis with recombinant human tissue type plasminogen activator: initial patency and effect of prolonged infusion on patency rate. Am J Cardiol 1987; 60: 231–237

29 Hsia J, Kleiman NS, Aguiree F, Roberts R, Chaitman B, Ross AM. Angiographic predictors of reocclusion following initially successful thrombolysis. Circulation 1990; 82 (Suppl 3): 255 (abstr)

30 The TIMI Research Group. Immediate vs delayed catheterisation and angioplasty following thrombolytic therapy for acute myocardial infarction. TIMI 2A results. JAMA 1988; 260: 2849–2858

31 TIMI Study Group. Comparison of invasive and conservative strategies after treatment with intravenous tissue plasminogen activator in acute myocardial infarction: results of the thrombolysis in myocardial infarction (TIMI) phase II trial. N Engl J Med 1989; 320: 619–627

32 Arnold AER, Serruys PW, Rutsch W et al. Reasons for the lack of success of immediate angioplasty during recombinant tissue plasminogen activator treatment for acute myocardial infarction: a regional wall motion analysis. J Am Coll Cardiol 1991; 17: 11–22

33 Rogers WJ, Babb JD, Baim DS et al. Selective versus routine predischarge coronary arteriography after therapy with recombinant tissue type plasminogen activator, aspirin and heparin for acute myocardial infarction. J Am Coll Cardiol 1991; 17: 1007–1016

34 The Norwegian Multicentre study group. Timolol-induced reduction in mortality and reinfarction in patients surviving acute myocardial infarction. N Engl J Med 1981; 304: 801–807

35 Smith P, Arnesen H, Holme I. The effect of warfarin on mortality and reinfarction after myocardial infarction. N Engl J Med 1990; 323: 147–152

36 Sharpe N, Smith H, Murphy J, Greaves S, Hart H, Gamble J. Early prevention of left ventricular dysfunction after myocardial infarction with angiotensin converting enzyme inhibition. Lancet 1991; 337: 872–875

37 Kambara H, Kawai C, Kajiwara N et al. Randomised double blinded multicentre study: comparison of intracoronary single chain urokinase type plasminogen activator, pro-urokinase (GE-0943) and intracoronary urokinase in patients with acute myocardial infarction. Circulation 1988; 78: 899–905

38 Neuhaus KL, Tebbe U, Gottwik M et al. Intravenous recombinant tissue plasminogen activator (rt-PA) and urokinase in acute myocardial infarction: results of the German activator urokinase study (GAUS). J Am Coll Cardiol 1988; 12: 581–587

39 Tranchesi B, Bellotti G, Chamone DF, Verstraete M. Effect of combined administration of saruplase and single chain alteplase on coronary recanalisation in acute myocardial infarction. Am J Cardiol 1989; 64: 229–232

40 Califf RM, Topol EJ, Harrelson L et al., for the TAMI study group. In hospital clinical outcomes in the TAMI-5 study. J Am Coll Cardiol 1990; 15: 76a (abstr)

41 PRIMI trial study group. Randomised double blind trial of recombinant pro-urokinase against streptokinase in acute myocardial infarction. Lancet 1989; i: 863–867

42 Bode C, Matsueda GR, Hui KY, Haber E. Antibody directed urokinase: a specific fibrinolytic agent. Science 1985; 229: 765–767

43 Runge MS, Quetermous T, Bode C et al. A recombinant single chain urokinase plasminogen activator–antifibrin antibody molecule with increased thrombolytic efficacy in vitro. Circulation 1990; 82 (Suppl 3): 375 (abstr)

44 de Bono DP, Pringle S. Local inhibition of thrombosis using urokinase linked to a monoclonal antibody which recognises damaged endothelium. Thromb Res 1991; 61: 537–545

45 Hillis W S, Hogg KJ. ST segment changes as a surrogate end point in coronary thrombolysis. Br Heart J 1990; 64: 111–112

46 Saran RK, Been M, Furniss SS, Reid DS. Reduction of ST elevation after thrombolysis predicts either coronary reperfusion or preservation of left ventricular function. Br Heart J 1990; 64: 113–117

47 Puleo PR, Perryman MB. Noninvasive detection of reperfusion in acute myocardial infarction based on plasma activity of creatinine kinase MB subforms. J Am Coll Cardiol 1991; 17: 1047–1052

48 Neuhaus KL, Feuerer N, Jeep-Tebbe S, Niederer W, Vogt A, Tebbe U. Improved thrombolysis with a modified dose regimen of recombinant tissue-type plasminogen activator. J Am Coll Cardiol 1989; 14: 1566–1569

49 Carney R, Brandt, T, Daley P et al. Increased efficacy of rt-PA by more rapid administration: the RAAMI trial. Circulation 1990; 82 (Suppl III): 538 (abstr)

50 Wall TC, Topol EJ, George BS et al. The TAMI-7 trial of accelerated plasminogen activator dose regimens for coronary thrombolysis. Circulation 1990; 82 (Suppl III): 538 (abstr)

51 Kalbfleisch JM. Simplified short term administration of t-PA in patients with acute myocardiol infarction. Circulation 1990; 82 (Suppl III): 539 (abstr)

52 Tranchesi B, Verstraete M, Vanhove Ph et al. Intravenous bolus administration of recombinant tissue plasminogen activator to patients with acute myocardial infarction. Coronary Artery Dis 1990; 1: 83–88

53 Purvis JA, Trouton TG, Dalzell GWN et al. A dose ranging study of double bolus recombinant tissue plasminogen activator in acute myocardial infarction. J Am Coll Cardiol 1991; 17: 152A (abstr)

54 Mruk JS, Chesebro JH, Webster MWI, Hera M, Grill DE, Fuster V. Hirudin markedly enhances thrombolysis with rt-PA. Circulation 1990; 82 (Suppl 3): 135 (abstr)

55 Yellon DM, Downey JM. Current research views on myocardial reperfusion and reperfusion injury. Cardioscience 1990; 1: 89–98

56 Piper HM. Irreversible myocardial injury: definition of the problem. In: Piper HM, ed. Pathophysiology of severe ischemic myocardial injury. Kluwer, Dordrecht, 1990, pp 3–14

57 Bolli R, Patel BS, Jeroudi MO, Lai EK, McKay PB. Demonstration of free radical generation in 'stunned' myocardium of intact dogs with the use of the spin trap alpha phenyl N-tert-butyl nitrone. J Clin Invest 1988; 82: 476–485

58 Clozel JP, Banken L, Roux S. Aprotinin: an antidote for recombinant tissue-type plasminogen activator (rt-PA) active in vivo. J Am Coll Cardiol 1990; 16: 507–510

59 de Bono DP, Pringle S, Underwood I. Differential effects of aprotinin and tranexamic acid on cerebral bleeding and cutaneous bleeding time during rt-PA infusion. Thromb Res 1991; 61: 159–163

60 Royston D, Bidstrup BP, Taylor KM, Sapsford RN. Effect of aprotinin on need for blood transfusion after open heart surgery. Lancet 1987; ii: 1289–1291

61 Castaigne AD, Hervé C, Duval-Moulin A-M et al. Prehospital use of APSAC: results of a placebo controlled study. Am J Cardiol 1989; 64: 30A–33A

3

Hyperlipidaemia: should we treat patients? Should we treat populations? What treatment should we use?

P. N. Durrington

Few, if any, medical conditions have aroused such a clamour of debate and invective as hyperlipidaemia. The practising clinician, who is frequently harangued for inactivity in the management of hyperlipidaemia by enthusiasts with views, which are quite impractical, is justifiably perplexed by the admonishments of equally extreme would-be authorities, who take an entirely nihilistic view of the same evidence and whose approach if widely applied to other areas of medical practice would lead to the wholesale disintegration of virtually all medical services. It is, however, now possible to take a sensible view of the evidence and to absorb the management of hyperlipidaemia into mainstream clinical practice just as has been done with hypertension, which has many parallels.

THE CASE

Probably the greatest mistake in the analysis of the benefits of cholesterol-lowering in clinical trials has been a failure to consider the exact nature of the patient population studied. Thus, for example, the fact that when studies of lipid-lowering therapy have been conducted in people who do not have hypercholesterolaemia the findings are generally negative, would be of much less relevance to me as a clinician than if such trials had been conducted in the types of patient at high cardiovascular risk, in whom I might consider such therapy. Furthermore, the fact that a large number of people whose serum cholesterol was unaffected by lipid-lowering therapy did not appear to benefit in clinical trials, would assume an even greater lack of relevance to me as a clinician. Yet this is precisely the nature of the findings of many of the clinical trials over which the fiercest battles have been fought.

The full evidence supporting the hypothesis that serum cholesterol is causally linked to atheroma, particularly coronary atheroma, will not be reviewed here. It is important to remember, however, that in addition to that derived from clinical trials and a consideration of genetic hyperlipidaemias (see later), the case is also supported by the close association of

coronary heart disease (CHD) and serum cholesterol in different populations[1,2] and the influence of moving from one culture to another,[3] by studies
of the atheromatous lesions themselves and by evidence from cell biological
approaches, which establish that the cholesterol in the plaques is derived
from circulating low-density lipoprotein (LDL) and not synthesized in
situ, and that the LDL is intimately involved in the development of the
early fatty streak and in its progress to the mature plaque with its fibrous
cap,[4] by animal atheroma regression trials, particularly those in primates,
and by postmortem studies in man.

As a clinician I am not going to start this discussion with an examination
of clinical trial evidence, but by discussing patients with disorders of lipid
metabolism clearly linked with early-onset CHD morbidity and mortality.
I shall then go on to discuss how far, as clinicians, we should go in
converting people whose serum cholesterol is but a little raised into patients
and in the next section how far we should regard such people as the normal
population for whom nothing should be done apart from some rational-
ization of our national policies and attitudes to nutrition, which are presently an encouragement to coronary disease.

FAMILIAL HYPERCHOLESTEROLAEMIA

Familial hypercholesterolaemia (FH) in its heterozygous form affects about
1 in 500 people in the UK and USA and many other parts of the world.[5,6] It
is dominantly inherited and the majority of men and women with the
condition will have experienced some manifestation of CHD by the age of
60 years, with more than half of male and 15% of female untreated
heterozygotes dying before that age. The outlook in the rare homozygotes
is much worse, with myocardial infarction and angina developing during
childhood and survival beyond the third decade unusual. The serum
cholesterol in heterozygotes is usually between 9 and 11 mmol/l, but is
frequently somewhat lower in childhood and in younger women. Serum
triglycerides are generally in the normal range or only moderately elevated.
In adults the clinical diagnostic feature is the development of tendon
xanthomata, most evident in the tendons of the dorsum of the hand and the
Achilles tendons. FH results from delay in the catabolism of LDL (the
lipoprotein containing most of the serum cholesterol), which spends from
four to five days in the circulation in heterozygous FH and even longer in
homozygous FH, as opposed to two to three days in a normal person. This
is due to defective receptor-mediated LDL clearance. Usually this results
from one of a wide range of mutations in the LDL receptor gene on
chromosome 19, but occasionally is due to a defect in the gene of apolipoprotein B, which is located on chromosome 2.[7] Apolipoprotein B is the
protein component of LDL which is recognized by and binds to the LDL
receptor. With the elucidation of the molecular defect in FH, it was no
longer possible to question that LDL cholesterol was causally involved in

CHD.[4] FH is a classical inborn error of metabolism due to a single gene which produces a single defective protein. All its clinical manifestations (atheroma, xanthomata) must result either from the accumulation of metabolites (in this case LDL) proximal to the metabolic block.

The recognition and treatment of cases of FH at specialized centres is important not only because effective cholesterol-lowering medication is now available, but also because inexperienced physicians may deny them access to proper cardiological investigative and operative procedures out of ignorance of their poor prognosis, despite their apparent freedom from CHD risk factors other than hypercholesterolaemia.

TYPE III HYPERLIPOPROTEINAEMIA

This is generally an autosomal recessive condition with variable penetrance.[8] Its cardiac prognosis is probably similar to that of FH, but in addition peripheral arterial disease is a frequent manifestation. There is an increase in both serum triglycerides and cholesterol, both generally exceeding 8 mmol/l (320 mg/dl) in approximately equimolar proportion to one another. About half the patients have no other manifestation, but the rest have striate palmar xanthomata, tubero-eruptive xanthomata or both. The condition is rarer than FH, affecting between 1 in 1000 and 1 in 10 000 of the population. It results from a mutation in the gene of apolipoprotein E on chromosome 19, which decreases the binding of apolipoprotein E to the hepatic remnant receptor responsible for the clearance of chylomicron remnants and some of the lipoproteins derived from very-low-density lipoprotein (VLDL) at an intermediate stage before their conversion to LDL.[9] There can be no doubt that the accumulation of these lipoproteins is the cause of the arterial disease. The majority of patients with these apo E mutations experience no hyperlipidaemia or related problems until their system for remnant clearance becomes over-stretched, for example because of the development of obesity, diabetes or hypothyroidism. The condition is rare in women before the menopause, but occasionally lean, otherwise fit men as early as their second or third decade present with the condition and there is generally then another inherited tendency to hyperlipidaemia, usually to hypertriglyceridaemia, occurring coincidentally. Again, as with FH, effective lipid-lowering therapy is available.

FAMILIAL COMBINED HYPERLIPIDAEMIA

In addition to these well-defined genetic syndromes there is another hyperlipidaemia, commoner than either FH or type III hyperlipoproteinaemia, which seems to stand out from the broad mass of polygenic hyperlipidaemia, because it is associated with greater CHD risk, although its edges are in shadow.[10,11] Inheritance, either of the hyperlipidaemia itself, or perhaps of susceptibility to its effect, seems important. It often produces a combined increase in both serum cholesterol and triglycerides. The condition has been termed familial combined hyperlipidaemia, but it is doubtful that it represents a single disease entity. At one end of its spectrum insulin resistance is a closely related phenomenon, as also are obesity, hypertension and sometimes gout. At the other, insulin resistance is absent, and cholesterol and sometimes triglyceride levels may be relatively normal, but the serum LDL is nonetheless increased in concentration since the serum concentration of apolipoprotein B, the principal protein component of LDL, is raised (hyperapobetalipoproteinaemia). It seems likely that better diagnostic methods will gradually emerge to identify these other syndromes causing CHD in which modification of lipoproteins is an essential component of treatment. For the present they serve to emphasize that 'all cholesterol is not equal' and that there cannot be a single therapeutic response triggered by any particular level. The therapeutic response can only be determined by detailed consideration of the individual patient, leading to a clinical judgment of the likelihood of that individual developing CHD early in life.

CLINICAL TRIALS

Primary versus secondary

It is customary to divide lipid-lowering trials into primary and secondary prevention trials. The distinction has some relevance to the interpretation of their findings, but much less to clinical practice than some commentators have assumed. A substantial proportion of the people, whom we can identify on screening as destined to die prematurely from CHD, will already have some evidence of CHD. In the British Regional Heart Study evidence of pre-existing CHD was present in half or more of the middle-aged men in the upper quintile of CHD risk factors, of whom more than half were destined to have a major coronary event in the next five years.[12] Thus, in clinical practice when we select out a high-risk group from multiple risk factor screening, we will obtain a group of people, many of whom already have established CHD. Furthermore, the distinction between people in the multiple risk factor group who have coronary symptoms and those who do not might not be as great as we believe. A similar quantity of atheroma in one individual could produce stenosis in a critical part of the coronary tree, whereas in another it may not. However, in the asymptomatic patient the situation could rapidly change if a stenosis producing no previous symptoms were to ulcerate and subsequently thrombose. Conversely, someone with ECG changes and history of an earlier myocardial infarction whose coronary disease is confined to one artery may be less at risk than another person with triple-vessel disease, but who has not yet sustained a myocardial infarction. Thus, in clinical practice, unless the patient has had coronary angiography, when we treat hyperlipidaemia, frequently we cannot be sure to what extent we are engaged in primary or secondary prevention.

We should also consider carefully what a primary prevention trial actually involves in terms of coronary prevention. First, by excluding from a population of middle-aged men any who have symptomatic or ECG evidence of CHD, a trial group is being selected, whose CHD morbidity and mortality is less than that of the general population of middle-aged men. The other selection criterion, a modestly raised serum cholesterol concentration, is certainly not going to mean that in terms of CHD risk in the next few years these men are in any sense 'high risk': it cannot overcome the beneficial influence on prognosis of flushing out those with established CHD. Not only does this remove these trials further away from what we do in clinical practice, but it also means that it is quite unreasonable to expect such a trial to show an effect of cholesterol reduction on all-cause mortality, because CHD mortality even if favourably influenced will not make a sufficiently large contribution to the total death toll. Furthermore, if middle-aged men are selected for the trial in such a way that CHD (their usual major cause of mortality) is underrepresented as a cause of death, then the other major causes of premature mortality in middle age, namely malignancy and violence, will assume a higher proportion of the total deaths.

The second effect of removing the men with greatest likelihood of succumbing to CHD at the outset of the trial is that the benefit of cholesterol reduction will be delayed, since the number of CHD events which can be influenced will progressively increase during the trial as the influence of removing the high-risk group at the outset declines with the passage of time and age and the progress of previously occult coronary atheroma catches up with the men being studied. This effect will compound any delay in the influence of cholesterol reduction per se on the natural history of CHD. Thus, in prospective studies the placebo and active intervention group generally show progressively widening differences in CHD rates (Fig. 3.1). It is not until the primary prevention trials have essentially been allowed to become, at least in some respects, secondary preventive trials that maximum benefit of cholesterol reduction is seen. Thus, the overall effect of cholesterol-lowering over say five years of such a trial may be a less important indicator of benefit that its much bigger impact in the fifth year.

Clinical trial results

The results of the early clinical trials of lipid-lowering proved particularly difficult to interpret. In retrospect this was probably in large part because of their small size, which meant that they lacked statistical power and the play of chance would thus have had an undue influence on their results.[4] Within their confidence limits they generally showed benefit from cholesterol

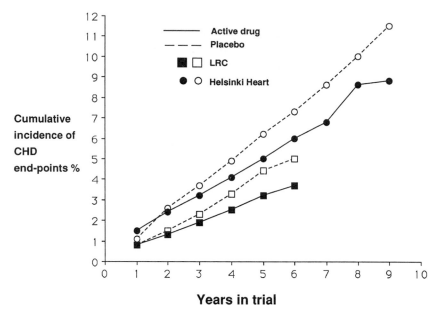

Fig. 3.1   Cumulative incidence (%) of cardiac endpoints in the Lipid Research Clinics (LRC) trial of cholestyramine versus placebo and the Helsinki Heart Study comparing gemfibrozil with placebo plotted as a function of the duration of the trial. (Redrawn from data in refs 18 and 20).

reduction.[13] Nonetheless, the publication in 1978 of the WHO cooperative trial[14] is generally hailed as the first clear indication that modifying serum lipid levels could affect the likelihood of CHD developing. In the trial 10 000 men from the top third of the serum cholesterol distribution of 30 000 screened in Edinburgh, Budapest and Prague were identified. Men with manifest CHD or other major diseases were excluded from the trial. The study group were randomized to receive clofibrate 800 mg b.d. or placebo capsules containing a similar quantity of olive oil. These men and another control group of 5000 from the lowest third of the cholesterol distribution were observed for an average of 5.3 years. The men receiving clofibrate on average had a serum cholesterol concentration 9% lower than those on placebo (Table 3.1). This resulted in an overall decrease in CHD events of 20%. This was mainly due to a 25% fall in the non-fatal myocardial infarction rate, whereas the incidence of fatal myocardial infarction, which was only 0.7% throughout the study, did not change significantly. In such a low-risk group, even with 10 000 men, it is doubtful that a significant decrease could have been expected. The age-standardized mortality rate did not differ significantly during the trial, although four years after its completion it was significantly increased in the men who had received clofibrate.[15] The increase was due to cholecystectomy, pancreatitis and neoplasms. The deaths due to gall bladder surgery and pancreatitis

Table 3.1 Main findings of the WHO,[14] LRC[18,19] and Helsinki[20,21] studies of primary prevention of ischaemic heart disease with lipid-modifying treatment

Trial	Number of men randomized	Age (y)	Treatment	Pre-treatment lipid levels (mg/dl; mmol/l)			Follow-up (y)	Average difference in lipid levels (%) (active minus placebo)			Change in ischaemic heart disease rates	
				Cholesterol	Triglycerides	HDL cholesterol		Cholesterol	Triglycerides	HDL cholesterol	Overall	Non-fatal myocardial infarction
WHO	10 627	30–59	Clofibrate 800 mg b.d.	248 (6.4)	–	–	5.3	–9	–	–	–20	–25
LRC	3806	35–59	Cholestyramine 8 g t.d.s.	280 (7.2)	155 (1.7)	44 (1.1)	7.4	–8.5	+3	+3	–19	–19
Helsinki	4081	40–55	Gemfibrozil 600 mg b.d.	270 (6.9)	176 (2.0)	47 (1.2)	5.4	–10	–35	+10	–34	–37

were related to cholelithiasis. Cholecystectomy was performed at rates of 2.1 per 1000 in the clofibrate-treated group and 0.9 per 1000 in the placebo group. Clofibrate-induced changes in the composition of bile would account for cholelithiasis and, it has been suggested, perhaps for neoplasms of the upper intestine, biliary tract and possibly large bowel.[16]

The main criticism of the WHO trial is not that it failed to show any benefit, but rather that it was designed so that any benefits, against which side effects could be set, were minimized. Drugs would not be used in practice in people whose serum cholesterol averaged only 6.4 mmol/l (248 mg/dl) (Table 3.1) and without any preliminary dietary treatment. The truth of this was demonstrated in the trial itself, since men with serum cholesterol levels which exceeded the median got most benefit, especially when other risk factors were present. Furthermore, whereas the benefits of cholesterol reduction were related to the initial cholesterol level and to the degree of cardiovascular risk, any ill effects were unrelated to cholesterol-lowering. Imagine the outcome of a trial of an antihypertensive drug or a hypoglycaemic agent carried out in people whose blood pressure or blood glucose was in the upper tercile of the population. Such a trial could only have revealed side effects and no benefits. Moreover (and this is not a criticism of the WHO trial in particular) it should be remembered that in clinical practice, unlike in a clinical trial, when a patient fails to respond to a drug it is discontinued. Thus, only patients who might derive some benefit from the drug are exposed to any possible long-term side effects. Almost certainly some high-risk patients did benefit from clofibrate therapy, but it was often prescribed before the WHO trial in patients with presumed CHD even when the serum cholesterol had not been measured. This latter practice was obviously to be discouraged as a result of the WHO trial, but the pendulum swung too far in the opposite direction. As Oliver wrote at the time: 'The results of this [the WHO] trial will be debated in many places. What is clear, at least, is that reduction of serum cholesterol concentration is relevant to the prevention of coronary heart disease'.[17] Fortunately we now have other clinical trial evidence and drugs which are emerging with better safety records than clofibrate.

The Lipid Research Clinics (LRC) trial was run from a series of special clinics throughout North America created for the purpose.[18,19] Almost 4000 middle-aged men with no evidence of CHD, whose serum cholesterol persisted above the 95th percentile for the US population after the intro-duction of a fairly unrestrictive lipid-lowering diet, participated. Their average cholesterol was 7.2 mol/l (280 mg/dl) (Table 3.1). Men whose serum triglycerides exceeded 300 mg/dl (3.4 mmol/l) were excluded. The trial group were randomized to receive either cholestyramine 6 sachets daily or placebo. After an average of just over seven years treatment the trial was analysed on an 'intention-to-treat' basis. This means that participants allocated to a particular group were analysed as part of that group even if they did not comply with the treatment. Again this would underestimate the benefits of lipid-lowering therapy in clinical practice, but obviously is a rigorous test of the cholesterol hypothesis, which avoids the possibility of selection bias. (Selection bias is, of course, what we aim for in clinical practice by trying to find a therapeutic option which suits a particular patient rather than always offering the same therapeutic response regardless of individual requirements.) There was therefore only a small average difference in cholesterol of 8.5% between the placebo and active treatment groups. A decrease of 8.5% in serum cholesterol is easily achievable in clinical practice by relatively moderate dietary restriction and incidentally would not be readily appreciable in practice given the biological variation in cholesterol and the laboratory error in many hospitals. Nevertheless, in the LRC trial there was a dramatic response in CHD, there being an approximately 20% decrease in fatal myocardial infarction, in non-fatal myocardial infarction, in development of positive exercise ECG, in new angina and in coronary bypass surgery. The consistent change in all these endpoints is important, because some authorities argued that the result lacked statistical significance because a one-tailed test had been used to analyse the results rather than a two-tailed test (disallowing the hypothesis that lowering cholesterol might increase CHD risk). The consistency of the effect on so many endpoints makes it only remotely possible that their improvement occurred by chance, and also strongly in support of that conclusion was the almost 50% decrease in coronary morbidity and mortality in men who took the full dose of cholestyramine, achieving a 25% decrease in their serum

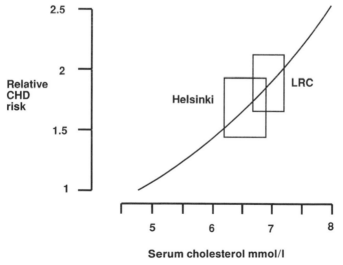

Fig. 3.2   The average serum cholesterol concentration in the placebo and intervention groups in the Lipid Research Clinics (LRC)[18] and Helsinki Heart Study[20] are shown by the two boxes and are superimposed on the relationship between cholesterol and coronary risk in the Framingham Study[40] for men aged 50 with systolic blood pressure of 135 mmHg, of whom 40% were smokers.

cholesterol concentration. Again as in the WHO trial there was about a 2% reduction in CHD rates for a 1% decrease in serum cholesterol as would be predicted from the relationship between CHD risk and serum cholesterol in prospective studies such as Framingham (Fig. 3.2).

The Helsinki Heart Study[20,21] was conducted in several clinics in Finland beginning in 1981. In many respects it was of similar design to the LRC trial and also involved about 4000 middle-aged men. They were asked to participate if the difference between their total serum cholesterol and their HDL cholesterol values exceeded 5.2 mmol/l (200 mg/dl). Men with hyper-triglyceridaemia were included. The average serum cholesterol of the participants after the introduction of a lipid-lowering diet was 6.9 mmol/l (270 mg/dl). They were randomly assigned to receive either gemfibrozil 600 mg b.d. or placebo. After five years the study was analysed on an 'intention-to-treat' basis, but as compliance with therapy was better than in the LRC study and the lipid responses were closer to those which might be encountered in clinical practice (Table 3.1). A 10% difference in choles-terol was associated with a 34% decrease in cardiac events in the drug-treated group and 37% fewer non-fatal cardiac deaths than in the placebo group. The differences were significant by two-tailed testing.

The Helsinki Heart Study raises important questions about whether modification of serum levels of lipoproteins other than LDL cholesterol is important. The reason is that the decrease in CHD was closer to 3% rather than 2% predicted for every 1% reduction in cholesterol. Was this due to the additional effect of decreasing triglycerides or of increasing HDL due to gemfibrozil as opposed to cholestyramine (Table 3.1)? The men who achieved the greatest improvement in their CHD risk were those with combined raised cholesterol and triglycerides (type IIb hyperlipoprotein-aemia).[22] These men, however, also had the lowest serum HDL cholesterol levels. One analysis suggests that their particularly favourable response was because of the gemfibrozil-induced increase in HDL rather than its undoubted triglyceride-lowering action.[21] This may, however, be an arte-fact of multivariate analysis in which variables, such as triglycerides with their high biological variability, fare badly[23] and this issue requires further elucidation. However, the issue is not whether there was benefit: the study as a whole is a remarkable demonstration of the value of cholesterol-lowering in the prevention of CHD. The safety record of gemfibrozil during the trial was also good and laid to rest concern that the side effects of clofibrate encountered in the WHO trial might apply generally to other lipid-lowering agents, particularly other fibric acid derivatives, such as gemfibrozil.

One other feature of both the Helsinki Heart Study and LRC trial was that the benefit of treatment in reducing CHD events was first evident within two years (Fig. 3.1). This is encouraging for patients whose hyper-lipidaemia is not discovered until middle age or later and this relatively rapid improvement is consistent with the rather rapid decline in CHD mortality in countries such as the UK during the years of fat restriction and increased unrefined carbohydrate consumption imposed by the dietary policies during and immediately following the Second World War.[24]

Neither the LRC nor the Helsinki Heart Study demonstrated a decrease in all-cause mortality between drug- and placebo-treated men. Much has been made of this by the traditional detractors of the 'cholesterol hypothesis'. Their argument is somewhat specious. As has already been discussed, the men in both studies, because they had been specifically selected for their lack of evidence of pre-existing CHD, were fitter in cardiovascular terms than middle-aged men in general. Neither study was equipped, therefore, to show an effect on all-cause mortality, since cardiovascular mortality would be underrepresented. The men in the studies would not, by and large, have been at sufficiently high risk to justify lipid-lowering drug therapy on the basis of current recommendations. What the trials show us is that we can influence CHD morbidity and mortality by lowering cholesterol, but that if we wish to influence total mortality we had better reserve our efforts for patients in whom the risk of dying prematurely of CHD is rather greater than from one of the other common causes of premature death, namely accidents and malignancy. If we were to consider just the Helsinki and LRC trials and ignore all other evidence (the onus would, of course, be on us to justify such a position, which would be difficult), we should have to agree that they provide strong evidence that coronary morbidity is decreased by cholesterol-lowering. Even such an effect is impressive. To delay the onset of angina, non-fatal myocardial infarction or coronary surgery may be of great importance both in terms of human suffering and in economic terms; death from CHD is cheap, whereas the cost of relieving the suffering it produces is expensive. It should also be remembered that, even if we were able to totally abolish CHD deaths in a country such as the UK (the world leader in this respect), we should extend the life expectancy of the average man by only two or three years. Of course, mortality is important and such figures hide the importance of preventing premature death from CHD, but they do serve to emphasize that for a great number of people coronary morbidity may be a more important consideration.

If we take a slightly less conservative view of the LRC and Helsinki Heart Trials, we can conclude that, if we were to use lipid-lowering medication in people at higher risk of CHD death, we should decrease total mortality. Such a view would be supported by data from other trials, which will be reviewed next. First, however, it is necessary to consider the argument in the Helsinki and LRC trials that non-cardiovascular causes of death were increased by cholesterol-lowering medication, thus counteracting the decrease in coronary deaths. Such a view would lack statistical significance. Also, as has already been discussed, the removal of a large proportion of men who would die from CHD must influence the proportion of total mortality due to malignancy and accidents. Furthermore, since neither study was designed to test the effect of cholesterol-lowering on malignancy or accidents the play of chance influenced whether these were more prolific in the placebo or intervention group: the men were not matched in the two groups with respect to risk factors for malignancy or violent death. No consistent relationship between cholesterol reduction and mortality from cancer has been found in trials,[25] but an effect of increasing the deaths 'not related to illness' has been claimed.[26] Such deaths are a ragbag: accidental, suicide and violence (is there any reason to suppose that being run down by a truck, shot by an intruder or taking one's own life have a single cause?). Also to achieve such a relationship careful selection of only six cholesterol-lowering trials is required,[27-30] including two which ran for less than two years. Clearly there was no randomization in any of these for risk factors such as driving ability, aggressive or depressive personality, predilection for having affairs with the wives of gangsters, etc. Elaborate arguments involving loss of cholesterol from brain cell membranes leading to mental instability have been proposed,[31] but in reality serum cholesterol levels must drop below the first percentile before any change in cell membrane composition could occur.[32] Nothing even approaching this was achieved (Fig. 3.2).

Again we can distance ourselves from all these arguments, if, as clinicians, we choose to treat patients whose greatest chance of premature death is from CHD. In the Stockholm Secondary Prevention study, 555 patients (20% women) who had survived myocardial infarction were randomly assigned to receive lipid-lowering medication (clofibrate and niacin) or placebo.[33] There was a 13% decrease in serum cholesterol and a 19% reduction in serum triglyceride levels. In this high-risk group a 26% decline in all-cause mortality stemming from a 36% fall in CHD mortality was evident over the five years of the study. This seems to support the view that, if we choose patients whose likelihood of dying from CHD is substantially greater than from any other cause we can influence all-cause mortality.

Some studies of cholesterol-lowering therapy, which may provide additional mortality data in high-risk patients, are in progress and have yet to be reported. However, the strength of existing evidence from many sources and logical argument that high-risk patients stand to gain most from cholesterol-lowering means that new trials in high-risk patients, as in familial hypercholesterolaemia for example, which are left to run until significant numbers of untreated patients are dead, cannot ethically be undertaken. Clinicians who stand back in the hope of having the results of such trials are missing the point: they will have to make up their minds to a large extent on present evidence. Another difficulty in trying to find effects on all-cause mortality in future investigations is that patients with CHD cannot reasonably be denied the benefits of new cardiovascular drugs and of myocardial revascularization by surgery or angioplasty. This means that the CHD mortality in any closely scrutinized group of patients will be kept low and such deaths as do occur are likely to be related as much to other failures of other treatments as to unsuccessful cholesterol reduction, although other endpoints such as new coronary events and need for coronary artery surgery will, of course, remain pertinent indicators of the success of lipid-lowering therapy. This is well illustrated by the recent results from the Program on the Surgical Control of the Hyperlipidaemias (POSCH).[34] This involved 838 middle-aged people (more than 90% men) who had previously had a myocardial infarction. They were randomized either to have partial ileal bypass (PIB) surgery to lower their serum cholesterol or not. Their serum cholesterol was on average 6.5 mmol/l (250 mg/dl) at the onset and it was 23% lower in the PIB group than in the unoperated group during the 9.7 years of the trial. There was an increase in serum triglycerides of 20–30%. Unlike the Stockholm Secondary Prevention trial, which was successful in reducing all-cause mortality, the POSCH study did not achieve statistical significance in this respect, although there were fewer deaths in the PIB group. The major reason for this was that the overall mortality in the Stockholm study was 26% over five years, whereas the total mortality in POSCH – over almost twice as long – was only 13%. There are several reasons for the low mortality in POSCH. Men in Stockholm were recruited between 1972 and 1976, whereas in POSCH this was done between 1975 and 1983. All the patients in POSCH had coronary angiography and those with left mainstem disease were excluded. Furthermore, advances in medical, angioplastic and surgical treatment for CHD by the time of POSCH may have considerably reduced the risks for myocardial infarction survivors attending major cardiological centres. For example, in POSCH 189 coronary artery bypass operations were performed (interestingly only 52 of these were in the PIB and 137 in the other group – a highly significant difference). So there were too few CHD deaths even in a secondary prevention study for lipid-lowering management to affect all-cause mortality significantly. The combined endpoint of CHD mortality and morbidity, which is the one used in the primary prevention studies, was convincingly significantly influenced in POSCH (82 in the PIB group versus 125 in the other group), as would be expected.

Thus, cholesterol-lowering trials, which attempt to look at all-cause mortality as an endpoint, may not be possible either on grounds of cost or size (if they are low-risk primary prevention trials), and also in high-risk patients advances in medical and surgical care mean that it is no longer ethical or reasonable to allow trials in high-risk patients to run beyond significant differences in morbidity, to the point where bodies are piled high enough in the non-intervention group to satisfy the pundits of the 'all-cause-mortality cause'. What we do need is more information from clinical trials, which will allow us to be more confident about the treatment of the elderly and of women, since most of the evidence so far relates to middle-aged men. Future developments may well centre on coronary angiographic studies.

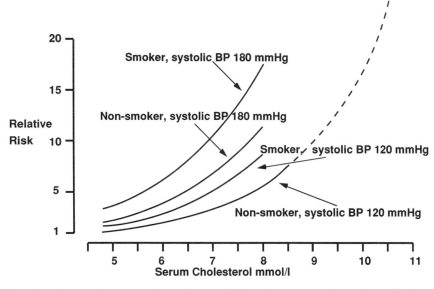

Fig. 3.3   The relative coronary heart disease risk (1 = risk of non-smoker with systolic blood pressure 120 mmHg) relative to the serum cholesterol of men aged 35. The solid lines are from the results of the 16-year follow-up in Framingham.[40] The dotted line is predicted from the relationship at lower cholesterol levels, but is compatible with a greater than 50% mortality by the age of 60 years in male heterozygous for familial hypercholesterolaemia in clinical studies[5] and with the death of all the people with tendon xanthomata in the early years of the Framingham study.

The results of angiographic studies to date have been encouraging. The three early studies using cholestyramine,[35] clofibrate and nicotinic acid[36] or diet [37] all showed decreased progression of coronary disease. The two most recent ones employing the combination of niacin and colestipol[38] and the combined effects of colestipol with either niacin or lovastatin[39] have in addition shown evidence for regression.

THE DENOUEMENT

Should we treat patients?

The case is made by the trials that lowering cholesterol decreases the likelihood of CHD mortality and morbidity. If we also wish to influence all-cause mortality, they tell us that we had better choose to intervene in higher-risk individuals than many of those included in the trials. The curve relating cholesterol to CHD risk is exponential;[40] the benefit therefore from lowering cholesterol will be greater the higher it is initially (Fig. 3.3). The slope of the curve relating cholesterol to CHD risk also becomes progressively steeper if it is combined with other risk factors (Fig. 3.3). Thus the risk of any given cholesterol level will depend on the presence or absence of other risk factors. These facts and the results of intervention trials have been weighed by many consensus panels in many nations, the best known being the US National Cholesterol Education Program Expert Panel,[41] the European Atherosclerosis Society,[42] the British Cardiac Society[43] and the British Hyperlipidaemia Association.[44] Consensus has to be viewed with some caution as has been pointed out by Oliver,[45] himself a member of two of these panels.[42,43] There is, however, remarkable agreement in certain areas between these various reports. First there is agreement that for middle-aged men the optimal serum cholesterol should be around 5.2 mmol/l (200 mg/dl). There is no good evidence to suggest that lower levels when they occur spontaneously are harmful,[25] but only exceptionally, perhaps after coronary artery surgery, should lower levels be a therapeutic target. Indeed, although no clear threshold below which the risk of CHD becomes non-existent is evident from the curve relating CHD risk to serum cholesterol concentration,[46] it is, nonetheless, the case that the curve is fairly flat up to 6.5 mmol/l (250 mg/dl). There is general agreement that this is a level which should be considered more critically in terms of future monitoring, clinical evaluation and therapy.[47] In the UK, however, it should be remembered that one-quarter of the adult population have cholesterol levels which exceed 6.5 mmol/l.[48,49] Unless it is particularly high, say greater than 7.8 mmol/l (300 mg/dl), serum cholesterol alone seldom justifies lipid-lowering drug therapy.

It is important to remember, particularly in establishing individual risk, that CHD is a multifactorial disease. The clinician can identify patients who are at risk by looking for combinations of such factors as pre-existing CHD or other atherosclerotic disease, diabetes mellitus, smoking history, hypertension[12] and adverse family history.[50-52] In such patients moderate elevations of serum cholesterol above 6.5 mmol/l may be important in coronary prevention, because many of these factors are immutable (past medical history, family history) or their treatment has not been conspicuously associated with a decline in CHD risk (treatment of glycaemia in diabetes, treatment of high blood pressure). Only two – stopping cigarette-smoking[53] and cholesterol reduction – have reliably been shown to decrease CHD risk. The importance of stopping cigarette-smoking cannot be overstated in this context and, furthermore, it is another reason why coronary prevention in clinical practice is potentially more effective than in cholesterol-lowering trials. In the Oslo study 1232 men with cholesterol between 7.5 and 9.8 mmol/l (290–380 mg/dl) were randomly allocated to receive advice about stopping smoking and a lipid-lowering diet or neither of these.[54] There was a 47% decrease in CHD mortality and morbidity in the intervention group compared to non-intervention during the subsequent five years, associated with differences of 13% in serum cholesterol, 20% in serum triglycerides and 8% in the number of men stopping smoking.

For people whose serum cholesterol is between 5.2 and 6.5 mmol/l

(200–250 mg/dl) advice about general health measures to prevent coronary disease, and dietary advice to avoid obesity and to modify fat intake according to the recommendations of the Committee on the Medical Aspects of Food Policy,[55] perhaps in the form of a printed pamphlet, is appropriate in most cases (see next section). For most, repeat serum cholesterol should be undertaken within five years, but this must depend on availability of resources. Some patients with established CHD, particularly those who have had coronary surgery, justify more intensive management. This is because in the two coronary angiographic trials of lipid-lowering therapy which showed regression of atheroma serum cholesterol values in the intervention groups were on average 4.7 mmol/l (210 mg/dl), compared to 6.00 mmol/l (230 mg/dl) and 6.6 mmol/l (255 mg/dl) in the non-intervention groups.[38,39] Serum lipids have been consistently shown to be the most important variables (apart from surgical technique) in determining the rate of occlusion of coronary bypass grafts.[56–58] This is not the case for restenosis after coronary angioplasty,[59] but there is also the rate of progress of atheroma in the rest of the coronary circulation to consider in such patients, and they too should thus receive more intensive management of serum lipids.

Above 6.5 mmol/l (250 mg/dl) there should be further lipid monitoring after advice about diet, perhaps in the form of a diet sheet. People whose cholesterol persists above 6.5 mmol/l should ideally be referred to a dietician.[60] For some, whose cholesterol persists above 6.5 mmol/l and who are deemed to be at increased CHD risk, lipid-lowering drugs are indicated (see later). Factors which militate in favour of the introduction of lipid-lowering drugs are shown in Table 3.2. At the present time evidence does not generally justify the introduction of drug treatment for hypertriglyceridaemia[61] or for low high-density lipoprotein (HDL) cholesterol[64] when

Table 3.2   Factors which favour the introduction of lipid-lowering therapy in a patient whose serum cholesterol exceeds 6.5 mmol/l, despite diet

1. *Genetic*
   a. Genetic hyperlipidaemia, e.g. familial hypercholesterolaemia, type III hyperlipoproteinaemia
   b. Adverse family history of coronary artery disease
   c. Cholesterol persistently > 7.8 mmol/l (300 mg/dl)
   d. Serum triglycerides raised as well as cholesterol and/or low HDL cholesterol

2. *Personal susceptibility*
   a. Previous history of myocardial infarction, angina of effort or peripheral arterial disease
   b. Coronary artery bypass surgery

3. *Other risk factors*
   a. Diabetes mellitus
   b. Hypertension
   c. Past history of cigarette-smoking

4. *Age and gender*
   Raised cholesterol is a better indicator of risk in men, particularly young men

these occur in the absence of an elevated total serum on LDL cholesterol level. These are, however, factors which will increase the risk from any given level of cholesterol and will therefore make the decision to prescribe lipid-modifying drug therapy more likely in borderline hypercholesterolaemia.[63]

At the present time it is not possible to have as clear a view of how to manage hyperlipidaemia in women, in children and in the older age range as we do in young and middle-aged men. It seems reasonable to manage women at particularly high risk in the same way as men; for example, those with some manifestation of CHD, genetic hyperlipidaemia or diabetes mellitus (which erodes much of their natural protection against CHD)[64] or who have multiple risk factors, particularly if combined with an adverse family history or a premature menopause. In general, however, women may have different cardiovascular risk factors to men and different optimal cholesterol levels.[65] Hormone replacement therapy is also a treatment option in women with hypercholesterolaemia,[66] particularly if they have had hysterectomy so that oestrogen can be used without a progestogen. It should not be overlooked, however, that despite encouraging findings in population studies there are still worries about thrombotic effects of oestrogens in individual women with established CHD. In younger women when there is the possibility of pregnancy the choice of lipid-lowering drugs is limited (see later).

Familial hypercholesterolaemia can be diagnosed in childhood, since other causes of hypercholesterolaemia are rare then. It seems reasonable to start dietary therapy in boys from the age of 5 or younger, if the parents wish it.[6] Bile acid sequestrating agents may be added later, say around 9 or 10 years old in boys when there is a particularly adverse family history, such as father developing CHD in his twenties or mother before the menopause. Inhibitors of 3,hydroxy-3,methylglutaryl-CoA (HMG-CoA) reductase should probably be reserved until the late teens for those particularly at risk.

The benefits of lipid-lowering therapy have yet to be established in the elderly. In terms of relative risk, cholesterol loses its ability to discriminate with age. Thus, the chance of dying from CHD are 5.5 times greater in a 35-year-old man whose serum cholesterol is 8.00 mmol/l (310 mg/dl) as opposed to one whose cholesterol is 4.8 mmol/l (185 mg/dl). On the other hand, at 60 the chances of the man with the cholesterol of 8.00 mmol/l dying of CHD are 1.5 times greater than a man of similar age with low cholesterol.[40] However, because the absolute risk of CHD increases steeply with age it is likely that even small differences in relative risk are important in terms of absolute numbers.[67] Furthermore, even if cholesterol loses its predictive power in old age when CHD is at its most prevalent, decreasing its level might still be beneficial. We must await clinical trial evidence. In the meantime screening programmes in the elderly can have little justification, but there are certain situations where clinicians should exercise their judgment; for example, after coronary bypass surgery, evident biological youth despite chronological old age, or where there are clear differences in longevity even after the age of 60 within a family dependent on inherited hyperlipidaemia. It is also not the case that lipid-lowering medication commenced earlier in life should be stopped in old age unless some contraindication develops.

Should we treat populations?

There is a great dichotomy of thought about how we should reduce the level of cholesterol within the community. There can be no doubt that decreasing its average level would decrease CHD rates.[68] One option is to identify by screening all the people with high levels and then to give them dietary and sometimes drug therapy. The argument against this strategy is that most CHD occurs in people who come from the middle range of the cholesterol distribution, and by simply intervening in those in the higher range we would not make as much impact on CHD rates as we might, if the whole frequency distribution of cholesterol was shifted downwards, taking the middle range with it. There are several problems associated with this viewpoint. First, this debate has been going on for many years, during which time very little has been done to help those people at the top end of the distribution, when we have excellent evidence that they can be helped. FH is about as frequent as insulin-dependent diabetes. Why are patients with FH specially selected for medical neglect? Clinical medicine is not intended to affect the cause of death in the community as a whole, but is a service which doctors provide to individual patients. Second, although there is strong evidence for benefit from intervention in high-risk patients, it is clear from the earlier part of this chapter that the case for 'lifestyle intervention' is largely circumstantial. Third, there is no reason to believe that an elected government in the UK will have any coherent policy about a national diet, in which health is the prime consideration: this has only proved possible previously during the coalition of the years of the Second World War. The Committee on Medical Aspects of Food Policy[55] made very sensible recommendations in 1984, but there has been nothing official done to decrease either obesity or the total amount of energy derived from fat in the diet of the average Briton since then. Fourth, there is no reason to believe that dietary advice intended to reduce serum cholesterol, when given to people who have no knowledge of their serum cholesterol, will be effective.[69]

Fifth, most of the advice about CHD prevention has already been heeded by the professional classes and both the risk of the disease and its prevalence is increasingly focused in socio-economic classes 4 and 5, in whom public policy is likely to be least effective.[70] Sixth, it is often said that a high-risk screening policy is too expensive. However, this view is often based on the cost of the clinical trials and the assumption that the same indications for drug therapy would be used in clinical practice. In fact, the cost of screening for high cholesterol using non-fasting cholesterol[71] and instituting dietary treatment is cheap and, if only a small proportion of people receive lipid-lowering drugs, highly cost effective.[69,72] Furthermore, even these estimates are likely to underestimate rather than overestimate the benefits, since they do not take into account the effects of advice against smoking, which would also be given in practice, or the favourable effects on other members of the family and of market forces it would generate on the food and farming industries.

Finally, there may be hidden dangers in lowering cholesterol in those people whose cholesterol is already less than 5.2 mmol/l. Although it is largely possible to discount this possibility,[25] it nonetheless does raise the issue as to why people whose chances of premature death from CHD are low should be given advice about coronary prevention when they might be better focusing their attention on some other health issue more relevant to them. It seems that at both ends of the cholesterol spectrum the individual is to be made to suffer. Of course, ideally opposition to the tobacco industry and rationalizing food subsidies to the farming industry, the food industry, recommendations to the catering industry and the educational authorities (yes, even the medical schools)[73] should receive official and governmental support, if coronary prevention is to be successful. However, this cannot be alloyed to a screening programme which omits the measurement of cholesterol, which apart from smoking is the only other proven mutable risk factor for CHD and must therefore be the other major focus of attention in the population. This is the view behind the National Cholesterol Education Program in the USA. In the UK the opportunities for health promotion provided by the NHS reforms could readily provide the basis for a national CHD prevention programme by general practitioners. They are the only section of the profession able to make a substantial impact on CHD. They deserve the full support of their colleagues in chemical pathology in providing ready access to cholesterol analysis and from the Regional Health Authorities in providing community dietetic services and referral centres for patients at particularly high cardiovascular risk. Ideally preventive cardiology clinics should be established rather than the present piecemeal arrangement of lipid clinics, hypertension clinics, anti-smoking clinics, etc. It has been suggested that cholesterol measurement in a screening programme might be reserved for those people found to have other cardiovascular risk factors.[74] There is considerable logic to this case, but in practice it has been found not to reduce the number of cholesterol measurements to the point where the saving in cost and time justifies the increased complexity it imposes.[75]

What treatment should we use?

The treatment of hyperlipidaemia was covered in detail by Dr Illingworth in the previous edition of *Recent advances in cardiology*[76] and again even more recently.[77] Diet is the cornerstone of the management of hyperlipidaemia. Regardless of the type of hyperlipidaemia in an obese person it will improve or resolve entirely with weight reduction.[78] The most effective weight-reducing diet is one which is low in fat of any description. In the non-obese the majority of hyperlipidaemias will respond to the removal of saturated fat from the diet. Previously the energy defect thus created was replaced with carbohydrate or polyunsaturated fat. Increasingly, however, attention is being focused on mono-unsaturated fats, which may have advantages over both of these.[79,80] Olive oil, which is a rich source of mono-unsaturates, is a major dietary component in many Mediterranean European countries, where there are much lower CHD rates than their northern counterparts. However, it is expensive and it is unlikely that its production will ever be increased to supply cheaply countries other than those where it originates. New mutants of the sunflower and rapeseed can, however, provide other commercial sources of mono-unsaturates, which can be produced in large quantities economically. The cholesterol-lowering diet should not be portrayed as self-denial, but the positive and attractive aspects of essentially changing to a more southern European cuisine should be emphasized.

It cannot be overstated that a failure of the serum cholesterol to fall below 6.5 mmol/l on dietary treatment is not in itself an indication for lipid-lowering drug therapy.[81] Such therapy is reserved for patients who, on clinical grounds, are deemed to be at genuinely high CHD risk.

For patients with hypercholesterolaemia, but no associated hypertriglyceridaemia, bile acid sequestrating agents (cholestyramine, colestipol) remain the drugs of first choice. Bile acid sequestrating agents tend to increase serum triglycerides and should not be used when hypertriglyceridaemia is the dominant abnormality. They are best taken in a dose of two sachets before breakfast. In larger, more frequent doses they often cause nausea, heartburn and constipation. However, in patients with only moderate elevation of cholesterol their use as monotherapy in the small doses suggested should not be overlooked. Some patients with more severe hypercholesterolaemia will tolerate larger doses and, particularly in children and women of child-bearing potential, the author is reluctant to turn to other agents. For other groups of patients, other agents either alone or in combination with bile acid sequestrating agents may be employed. In patients whose hypercholesterolaemia is combined with hypertriglyceridaemia, the fibrate drugs (bezafibrate, fenofibrate, gemfibrozil) are first-line therapy. Fibrate drugs may be tried as a sole therapy in patients with moderate hypercholesterolaemia who do not respond or cannot tolerate bile acid sequestrating agents. They are also often highly effective in primary type III and V hyperlipoproteinaemia and in diabetes. Their cholesterol-lowering effect is not usually great enough in more marked hypercholesterolaemia when it is due to raised LDL, as in FH. They may then be used in combination with bile acid sequestrating agents, but increasing use of HMG-CoA reductase inhibitor (statin) drugs (lovastatin, pravastatin, simvastatin) is being made. These agents are often effective even in marked hypercholesterolaemia as monotherapy, although advantage may be taken of their synergism with bile acid sequestrating agents, by prescribing two sachets of bile acid sequestrating agent in the morning with an evening dose of the statin. Statins have a small triglyceride-lowering effect as well as their potent cholesterol-lowering properties. They are generally the only agents likely to bring the cholesterol level below 5 mmol/l (200 mg/dl). Fibrate drugs when used in patients with cholesterol levels of less than 6.5 mmol/l, particularly if hypertriglyceridaemia is present, may actually raise LDL cholesterol.[81,82] This should not detract from their use at higher cholesterol levels, particularly when triglycerides are raised, since they also raise HDL cholesterol and were highly effective in reducing CHD risk in the Helsinki Heart Study, particularly in patients with combined hypercholesterolaemia and hypertriglyceridaemia.

Patients on statins should be monitored for evidence of myositis or hepatotoxicity. The risk of myositis is increased if they are used in combination with fibrates or with cyclosporin. In some patients after cardiac transplantation this latter combination may be justified. Fibrate therapy will also cause myositis in patients with diminished renal function, in whom they should not be used, and care should be taken if they are introduced in patients receiving anticoagulant therapy, which they potentiate.

Nicotinic acid features highly in recommendations from the USA. Few European centres, however, have found patients prepared to tolerate the unpleasant flushing it produces in the doses required for it to be effective, quite apart from its more serious side effects that require frequent monitoring. Various analogues or slow-release forms which produce less flushing have not gained much popularity, although the most recent of these, Acipimox, may have potential. Probucol is a cholesterol-lowering drug, which lowers HDL cholesterol more markedly than LDL. Despite its undoubted antioxidant properties it requires further clinical evaluation before it can be regarded as beneficial in its overall action. Fish oil in fish may be important in the dietary treatment of hyperlipidaemia, but as a pharmacological agent, despite its triglyceride-lowering properties, it frequently exacerbates primary hypercholesterolaemia, diabetic hyperlipidaemia and type III hyperlipoproteinaemia. There is some evidence that it is beneficial after coronary surgery or myocardial infarction, but this may not relate to its effects on lipid metabolism.[83]

KEY POINTS FOR CLINICAL PRACTICE

Screening programmes for coronary heart disease (CHD) should include the measurement of non-fasting cholesterol and should be widely available. Many factors (personal history of CHD, abnormal ECG, adverse family history, cigarette-smoking, high blood pressure, diabetes) allow high-risk individuals to be identified, but for only two – cholesterol and cigarette-smoking – has intervention been reliably shown to decrease CHD risk. Cholesterol-lowering dietary advice should be given to people found to have undesirably high levels of cholesterol. There can be no justification for withholding lipid-lowering drug therapy when undesirably high levels of cholesterol persist despite diet in those who, on clinical grounds, are considered to be at substantially increased CHD risk.

REFERENCES

1 Keys A. Coronary heart disease: the global picture. Atherosclerosis 1975; 22: 149–192
2 Simons LA. Interrelations of lipids and lipoproteins with coronary artery disease mortality in 19 countries. Am J Cardiol 1986; 57: 5G–10G
3 Marmot MG, Syme SL, Kagan A, Kato H, Cohen JB, Glesky J. Epidemiologic studies of coronary heart disease and stroke in Japanese men living in Japan, Hawaii and California: prevalence of coronary and hypertensive heart disease and associated risk factors. Am J Epidemiol 1975; 102: 514–525
4 Steinberg D. The cholesterol controversy is over: why did it take so long? Circulation 1989; 80: 1070–1078
5 Goldstein JL, Brown MS. Familial hypercholesterolaemia. In: Stanbury JB, Wyngaorden JB, Fredrickson DS, Goldstein JL, Brown MS, eds. Metabolic basis of inherited diseases, 5th edn. New York: McGraw-Hill, 1983, pp 672–712
6 Durrington PN (ed) Familial hypercholesterolaemia. In: Hyperlipidaemia diagnosis and management. London: Wright, 1989, pp 91–113
7 Myant NB, Gallagher JJ, Knight BL et al Clinical signs of familial hypercholesterolaemia in patients with familial defective apolipoprotein B-100 and normal low density lipoprotein receptor function. Arteriosclerosis 1991; 11: 691–703
8 Durrington PN (ed) Type III hyperlipoproteinaemia. In: Hyperlipidaemia diagnosis and management. London: Wright, 1989, pp 157–165
9 Mahley RW, Weigraber KH, Innerarity TL, Rall SC. Genetic defects in lipoprotein metabolism: elevation of atherogenic lipoproteins caused by impaired catabolism. JAMA 1991; 265: 78–83
10 Grundy SM, Chait A, Brunzell JD. Familial combined hyperlipidaemia workshop. Arteriosclerosis 1987; 7: 203–207
11 Durrington PN (ed) Common hypercholesterolaemia: polygenic hypercholesterolaemia and familial combined hyperlipidaemia. In: Hyperlipidaemia diagnosis and management. London: Wright, 1989, pp 114–134
12 Shaper AG, Pocock SJ, Phillips AN, Walker M. Identifying men at high risk of heart attacks: strategy for use in general practice. Br Med J 1986; 293: 474–479
13 Peto R, Yusuf S, Collins R. Cholesterol-lowering trial results in their epidemiologic context. Circulation 1985; 72 (Suppl III): III–451
14 Committee of Principal Investigators. Report on a cooperative trial in the primary prevention of ischaemic heart disease using clofibrate. Br Heart J 1978; 40: 1069–1118
15 Report of the Committee of Principal Investigations. WHO cooperative trial on primary prevention of ischaemic heart disease using clofibrate to lower serum cholesterol: mortality follow-up. Lancet 1980; ii: 379–385
16 Hill H, Aries VC. Faecal steroid composition and its relationship to cancer of large bowel. J Pathol 1971; 104: 129–139
17 Oliver MF. Cholesterol, coronaries, clofibrate and death. N Engl J Med 1978; 299: 1361
18 Lipid Research Clinics Program. The lipid clinics coronary primary prevention trial results. I. Reduction in incidence of coronary heart disease. JAMA 1984; 251: 351–364
19 Lipid Research Clinics Program. The lipid research clinics coronary primary prevention trial results. II. The relationship of reduction in incidence of coronary heart disease to cholesterol lowering. JAMA 1984; 251: 365–374

20 Frick MH, Elo O, Haapa K et al. Helsinki Heart Study: primary-prevention trial with gemfibrozil in middle-aged men with dyslipidemia. Safety of treatment, changes in risk factors, and incidence of coronary heart disease. N Engl J Med 1987; 317: 1237–1245

21 Manninen V, Elo O, Frick MH et al. Lipid alterations and decline in the incidence of coronary heart disease in the Helsinki Heart Study. JAMA 1988; 260: 641–651

22 Huttunen JK, Manninen V, Tenkanen L, Heinonen OP, Koskinen P, Frick MH. Drug-induced changes in high-density lipoprotein cholesterol and coronary heart disease: experiences from the Helsinki Heart Study. In: Miller NE, ed. Second international symposium on high density lipoproteins and atherosclerosis. Amsterdam: Elsevier, 1989, pp 85–92

23 Durrington PN. Biological variation in serum lipid concentrations. Scand J Clin Lab Invest 1990; 50 (Suppl 198): 86–91

24 Trowell HC. Dietary fibre: metabolic and vascular diseases. Monograph 7 in the series The Present State of Knowledge. London: Norgina, 1975

25 Editorial. Low cholesterol and increased risk. Lancet 1989; i: 1423–1425

26 Muldoon MF, Manuck SB, Matthews KA. Lowering cholesterol concentrations and mortality: a quantitative review of primary prevention trials. Br Med J 1990; 301: 309–314

27 Canter D. Lowering cholesterol concentrations and mortality. Br Med J 1990; 301: 814

28 Rossouw JE, Rifkind BM. Lowering cholesterol concentrations and mortality. Br Med J 1990; 301: 814

29 Smith GD, Shipley MJ, Marmot MG, Patel C. Lowering cholesterol concentrations and mortality. Br Med J 1990; 301: 552

30 Ravnskov U. Lowering cholesterol concentrations and mortality. Br Med J 1990; 301: 814

31 Mann FD. The dynamics of free cholesterol exchange may be critical for endothelial cell membranes in the brain. Perspect Biol Med 1990; 33: 531–534

32 Marenah CB, Lewis B, Hassall D et al. Hypocholesterolaemia and non-cardiovascular disease: metabolic studies on subjects with low plasma cholesterol concentrations. Br Med J 1983; 286: 1603–1606

33 Carlson LA, Rosenhamer G. Reduction of mortality in the Stockholm ischaemic heart disease secondary prevention study by combined treatment with clofibrate and nicotinic acid. Acta Med Scand 1988; 223: 405–418

34 Buchwald H, Varco RL, Matts JP et al. Effects of partial ileal bypass surgery on mortality and morbidity from coronary heart disease in patients with hypercholesterolaemia. N Engl J Med 1990; 323: 946–955

35 Brensike JF, Levy RI, Kelsey SF et al. Effects of therapy with cholestyramine on progression of coronary arteriosclerosis: results of the NHLBI type II coronary intervention study. Circulation 1984; 64: 313–324

36 Nikkila EA, Viikinkoski P, Valle M, Frick MH. Prevention of progression of coronary atherosclerosis by treatment of hyperlipidaemia: a seven year prospective angiographic study. Br Med J 1984; 289: 220–223

37 Arntzenius AC, Komhout D, Barth JD et al. Diet, lipoproteins and the progression of coronary atherosclerosis. The Leiden intervention trial. N Engl J Med 1985; 312: 805–811

38 Blackenhorn DH, Nessim SA, Johnson RL, Sanmarco ME, Azen SP, Cashin-Hemphill L. Beneficial effects of combined colestipol–niacin therapy on coronary atherosclerosis and coronary venous bypass grafts. JAMA 1987; 257: 3233–3240

39 Brown G, Albers JJ, Fisher LD et al. Regression of coronary artery disease as a result of intensive lipid-lowering therapy in men with high levels of apolipoprotein B. N Engl J Med 1990; 323: 1289–1298

40 Dawber TR. The Framingham study: the epidemiology of atherosclerotic disease. Cambridge, MA: Harvard University Press, 1980

41 Report of the national cholesterol education program expert panel on detection, evaluation and treatment of high blood cholesterol in adults. Arch Intern Med 1988; 148: 36–69

42 Study Group. European Atherosclerosis Society strategies for the prevention of coronary heart disease. I. A policy statement of the European Atherosclerosis Society. Eur Heart J 1987; 8: 77–88

43 Report of the British Cardiac Society Working Group on Coronary Disease Prevention. London: British Cardiac Society, 1987, pp 1–31
44 Shepherd J, Betteridge DJ, Durrington PN et al. Strategies for reducing coronary heart disease and desirable limits for blood lipid concentrations: guidelines of the British Hyperlipidaemia Association. Br Med J 1987; 295: 1245–1246
45 Oliver MF. Consensus or nonsensus conferences on coronary heart disease. Lancet 1985; i: 1081
46 Stamler J, Wentworth D, Neaton JD. Is relationship between serum cholesterol and risk of premature death from coronary heart disease continuous and graded? Findings in 356,222 primary screens of the multiple risk factor intervention trial (MRFIT). JAMA 1986; 256: 2823–2828
47 Lewis B. Plasma lipid concentrations: the concept of 'normality' and its implications for detection of high cardiovascular risk. J Clin Pathol 1987; 40: 1118–1127
48 Thelle DS, Shaper AG, Whitehead TP, Bullock DG, Ashby D, Patel I. Blood lipids in middle-aged British men. Br Heart J 1983; 49: 205–213
49 Mann JI, Lewis B, Shepherd J et al. Blood lipid concentrations and other cardiovascular risk factors: distribution, prevalence and detection in Britain. Br Med J 1988; 296: 1702–1706
50 Colditz GA, Stampfer MJ, Willett WC, Rosner B, Speizer FE, Hennekens CH. A prospective study of parental history of myocardial infarction and coronary heart disease in women. Am J Epidemiol 1986; 123: 48–58
51 Hopkins PN, Williams RR, Kuida H et al. Family history as an independent risk factor for incident coronary artery disease in a high-risk cohort in Utah. Am J Cardiol 1988; 62: 703–707
52 Jorde LB, Williams RR. Relation between family history of coronary artery disease and coronary risk variables. Am J Cardiol 1988; 62: 708–713
53 Royal College of Physicians. Health or smoking? London: Pitman, 1983
54 Hjermann I, Velve Byre K, Holme I, Leren P. Effect of diet and smoking intervention on the incidence of coronary heart disease: report from the Oslo study group of a randomised trial in healthy men. Lancet 1981; ii: 1304–1310
55 Committee on Medical Aspects of Food Policy, Department of Health and Social Security. Diet and cardiovascular disease (report on health and Sound Subjects No. 28). London: HMSO, 1984
56 Palac RT, Meadows WR, Hwang MH, Loeb HS, Pifarre R, Gunnar RM. Risk factors related to progressive narrowing in aortocoronary vein grafts studied 1 and 5 years after surgery. Circulation 1982; 66: (Suppl I): 40–44
57 Campeau L, Enjalbert M, Lesperance J et al. The relation of risk factors to the development of atherosclerosis in saphenous-vein bypass grafts and the progression of disease in the native circulation: a study 10 years after aortocoronary bypass surgery. N Engl J Med 1984; 311: 1329–1332
58 Fox MH, Gruchow HW, Barboriak JJ et al. Risk factors among patients undergoing repeat aorto-coronary bypass procedures. J Thorac Cardiovasc Surg 1987; 93: 56–61
59 McBride W, Lange RA, Hillis LD. Restenosis after successful coronary angioplasty: pathophysiology and prevention. N Engl J Med 1988; 318: 1734–1737
60 Bhatnagar D, Durrington PN. Coronary risk factors: value of screening and preventive strategies in general practice. Fam Pract 1990; 7: 295–300
61 Consensus Conference Treatment of Hypertriglyceridaemia. JAMA 1984; 251: 1196–1200
62 Rifkind BM. High-density lipoprotein cholesterol and coronary artery disease: survey of the evidence. Am J Cardiol 1990; 66: 3A–6A
63 Bhatnagar D, Durrington PN. Borderline hypercholesterolaemia: when to introduce drugs. Postgrad Med J 1989; 65: 543–552
64 Barrett-Connor EL, Cohn BA, Wingard DL, Edelstein SL. Why is diabetes mellitus a stronger risk factor for fatal ischaemic heart disease in women than in men? The Rancho Bernardo study. JAMA 1991; 265: 627–631
65 Crouse JR. Gender, lipoproteins, diet, and cardiovascular risk: sauce for the goose may not be sauce for the gander. Lancet 1989; i: 318–320
66 Godsland IF, Wynn V, Crook D, Miller NE. Sex, plasma lipoproteins and atherosclerosis: prevailing assumptions and outstanding questions. Am Heart J 1987; 114: 1467–1503

67 Benfante R, Reed D. Is elevated serum cholesterol level a risk factor for coronary heart disease in the elderly? JAMA 1990; 263: 393–396

68 Lewis B, Mann J, Mancini M. Reducing the risk of coronary heart disease in individuals and in the population. Lancet 1986; i: 956–959

69 Report by the Standing Medical Advisory Committee to the Secretary of State for Health. Blood cholesterol testing: the cost-effectiveness of opportunistic cholesterol testing. London: Ministry of Health, 1991

70 Blater M. Health and lifestyles. London: Tavistock/Routledge, 1990

71 Neil HAW, Mant D, Jones L, Morgan B, Mann JI. Lipid screening: is it enough to measure total cholesterol concentration? Br Med J 1990; 301: 584–587

72 Reckless JPD. The economics of cholesterol lowering. Baillière's Clin Endocrinol Metab 1990; 4: 947–972

73 Crimlisk S. Teaching prevention of heart disease. Br Med J 1990; 301: 115

74 The Sixth King's Fund Forum Consensus Statement. Blood cholesterol measurements in the prevention of coronary heart disease. London: King Edward's Hospital Fund for London

75 Imperial Cancer Research Fund OXCHECK Study Group. Prevalence of risk factors for heart disease in OXCHECK trial: implications for screening in primary care. Br Med J 1991; 302: 1057–1060

76 Illingworth DR. Management of lipoprotein abnormalities. In: Rowlands DJ, ed. Recent advances in cardiology 10. Edinburgh: Churchill Livingstone, 1987, pp 71–100

77 Illingworth DR. Treatment of hyperlipidaemia. Br Med Bull 1990; 46: 1025–1058

78 Durrington PN (ed) Diet. In: Hyperlipidaemia diagnosis and management. London: Wright, 1989, pp 166–194

79 Grundy SM. Dietary therapy of hyperlipidaemia. Bailliere's Clin Endocrinol Metab 1987; 1: 667–698

80 Mensink RP, Katan MB. Effect of monounsaturated fatty acids versus complex carbohydrates on high-density lipoproteins in healthy men and women. Lancet 1987; i: 122–125

81 Durrington PN (ed) Drug therapy of hyperlipidaemias. In: Hyperlipidaemia diagnosis and management. London: Wright, 1989, pp 195–218

82 Vega GL, Grundy SM. Primary hypertriglyceridaemia with borderline high cholesterol and elevated apolipoprotein B concentrations. JAMA 1990; 264: 2759–2763

83 Dehmer GJ, Popma JJ, van den Berg EK et al. Reduction in the rate of early stenosis after coronary angioplasty by a diet supplemented with n-3 fatty acids. N Engl J Med 1988; 319: 733–740

4

Chronic heart failure: epidemiology, aetiology, pathophysiology and treatment

H. J. Dargie   J. McMurray

DEFINITIONS

In pathophysiological terms, heart failure can be defined as an inability of the heart to deliver blood (oxygen) at a rate commensurate with the requirements of the metabolizing tissues despite normal or increased ventricular filling pressures (or can only do so at the expense of increased ventricular filling pressures – 'diastolic dysfunction'). This standard definition implies a defect only in the heart (the pump) whereas recent evidence suggests that an abnormality of the arterial tree (albeit a secondary one) also contributes to the failure to deliver oxygen to the metabolizing tissues. Clinically, heart failure is the familiar syndrome of dyspnea, fatigue and oedema arising as a consequence of this inadequate delivery of oxygen.

EPIDEMIOLOGY

Aetiology

In the Framingham study, initiated in 1949, hypertension was the major aetiological factor in 75% of cases of chronic heart failure (CHF), with coronary heart disease (CHD) accounting for only 10% of cases.[1,2] Recent data from the USA, in particular from the very large SOLVD registry and treatment groups, show that coronary artery disease is now the major cause of CHF.[1-3] In the registry ($n = 6300$) coronary disease accounts for three-quarters of CHF in white male patients. Hypertension is a much more common cause in blacks (36% of cases) and hypertension and dilated cardiomyopathy are more common in females. Coronary disease accounts for 71% of cases of CHF in the SOLVD treatment arm ($n = 2524$) and 81% of cases in the prevention arm ($n = 4000$). In a recent UK study, all admissions with CHF to a single district (community) hospital in London were prospectively studied. One hundred and forty cases were identified and the underlying diagnoses are shown in Table 4.1.[4] That only 41% of cases were definitely attributable to CHD probably reflects the difficulty in diagnosis of CHD without full investigation.

Table 4.1   Causes of CHF in the London community hospital study (140 patients)[4]

Coronary artery disease	57	(41%)
Acute MI	15	
Old MI	28	
Prior angina	14	
Uncertain	51	(36%)
Echo-global hypokinesia	14	
Echo-regional hypokinesia	2	
Echo-hypertrophy	1	
No echo	34	
Valve disease	13	(9%)
Hypertension	9	(6%)
Cor pulmonale (COPD)	4	(3%)
Thyrotoxicosis	2	(15%)
Congenital heart disease	2	(1%)
Dilated cardiomyopathy (normal coronaries)	2	(1%)

MI, myocardial infarction; COPD, chronic obstructive pulmonary disease.

Prevalence and incidence

The Framingham study estimated an annual incidence rate of CHF of 3.7 new cases per 1000 men and 2.5 per 1000 women.[1] For both sexes aged 35–64 years, the incidence rate was 3 per 1000, but this rose sharply to 10 per 1000 for those aged 65–94 years. For 1983 this led to a calculated incidence in the USA of 400 000 cases. In the same year a prevalence of 2.3 million cases in the USA population was given. In a recent survey of three family doctor practices serving a population of 30 204 in London, 117 patients (0.4%) were determined to have heart failure. For those under 65 years the prevalence was 0.06%, whereas it was 2.8% in those over 65 years (the mean age of those with CHF was 73 years and 61% were female).[4] Extrapolated to the UK as a whole, this would give an overall prevalence rate considerably lower (about half) that estimated for the USA.

Hospital discharge rates

Hospital discharge rates reflect both the prevalence of CHF and its morbidity (i.e. patients may be admitted more than once because of CHF). Two recent surveys from the·USA and one from the UK have examined hospital admission/discharge figures for CHF.[4–6]

In 1985, CHF as the first principal diagnosis accounted for 585 000 discharges and CHF as one of up to seven discharge diagnoses was mentioned in 1 731 000 cases. For those between 45 and 64 years of age, this gave a rate of 228/100 000 and for those over 65 years a rate of 1634/100 000 (the corresponding rates for CHF as one of seven diagnoses were 670/100 000 and 4851/100 000). Discharge rates over the 15 years studied had been rising steadily for all race, sex and age groups (except those aged 35–54 years) and were higher for non-whites compared to whites, men compared to women and the elderly compared to the non-elderly.

In the London district (community) hospital study CHF accounted for 4.9% of all admissions over a six-month period. There were an equal number of male and female admissions. Only 29 patients were under 65 years of age, and the mean age of admissions was 73 years. Extrapolated to the UK as a whole, this gives an estimated yearly admission rate of 100 000–120 000 which, proportionately, is comparable with the USA hospital discharge rates.

Morbidity

The SOLVD registry and treatment groups also provide interesting information on morbidity for CHF.[3] In patients with overt CHF the annual hospitalization rate approached 45% (Table 4.2). Some of the factors leading to hospitalization, e.g. thromboembolic events, respiratory infection, should be amenable to preventive treatment. The recently published SOLVD (treatment arm) report shows that angiotensin-converting enzyme (ACE) inhibitors can substantially reduce the rate of hospitalization in patients with CHF.[7]

Mortality

The probability of dying within five years of onset of CHF was found to be 62% for men and 48% for women in the Framingham study.[1] Many studies have since confirmed this dismal prognosis. Gillum estimated that, in the USA community as a whole, CHF was the primary cause of death in 30 657 patients in 1982 and was mentioned on 200 000 death certificates.[5] For white males of all ages, CHF accounted for 11 449 deaths in 1981, giving a mortality rate of 13/100 000 for those aged 35–74 years and 210/100 000 in those over 75 years. Population rates were lower in white females but higher in blacks of both sexes.

Table 4.2   Annual event/hospitalization rates in SOLVD treatment/prevention groups (all patients with LVEF ≤ 35%)

	CHF present (%)	No CHF (%)
Death	12	5
Hospitalization for CHF	15	5
Recurrent MI	4	3
Non-fatal cardiac arrest	2	1
Thrombo-embolic event	2	1
Pulmonary infection	4	2
Hospitalization for cardiovascular reason	30	20
Hospitalization for non-cardiovascular cause	15	7

Hospital case fatality rates have recently been reported to be between 9% (males aged 35–64 years) and 16% (males aged greater than 75 years) in the USA (rates were lower for females).[5,6] In the UK, however, the London community hospital study reported a 30% in-hospital mortality, with a further 14% mortality in the first year following discharge.[4]

Treatment trials have also provided information on mortality in CHF and show a clear increment in rate with increasing clinical severity. The SOLVD registry and treatment groups reported a one-year mortality of 5% in those with left ventricular dysfunction without overt CHF. In patients with overt CHF, annual mortality was 12% (amongst white males 11% 21–44 years, 12.5% 45–64 years and 22% older than 65 years; mortality was higher in females). In the first Veterans Administration Cooperative Vasodilator Heart Failure Trial (V-HeFTI) study of mild–moderate CHF, the one-year mortality rate was 19.5% in the placebo group.[7a] In studies of patients with severe CHF, the one-year mortality may be as high as 40–60%.[8,9]

CAUSES OF HEART FAILURE

Many pathological processes can cause heart failure (Table 4.3). Primary myocardial damage may occur due to myocardial infarction or idiopathic dilated cardiomyopathy. Valvular regurgitation may lead to secondary myocardial damage, as may chronic hypertension and aortic stenosis. Rarely the myocardium may be injured by inflammatory or infiltrative processes (Table 4.3). Pericardial disease, endocardial disease and mitral stenosis may also lead to the heart failure syndrome,.though ventricular systolic function is usually normal. This chapter will mainly refer to the CHF due to systolic dysfunction arising as a consequence of coronary artery disease or dilated cardiomyopathy.

INVESTIGATION (Fig. 4.1)

The diverse aetiology of the heart failure syndrome makes firm establishment of a precise diagnosis of paramount importance. Non-cardiac causes of dyspnea, fatigue and ankle oedema are common but difficult to differentiate by clinical examination.[10–12] Definitive diagnosis ensures (a) appropriate treatment (medical and/or surgical) and (b) the avoidance of inappropriate and potentially hazardous treatment. Despite this need for precise diagnosis, many patients are not referred for expert assessment (20% in the London community hospital study).[4] Furthermore, those patients that are referred from their family doctor may have been misdiagnosed,[12] and it is now well appreciated that it is difficult to make an accurate diagnosis only on the basis of symptoms and signs.[10,11,11a]

Investigations are therefore necessary and are aimed mainly at (a) confirming the presence of left ventricular systolic dysfunction, (b) excluding

Table 4.3 Causes of CHF

A. Mechanical abnormalities
1. Increased pressure load
(a) Central (aortic stenosis, hypertrophic obstructive cardiomyopathy, etc.)
(b) Peripheral (systemic arterial hypertension, etc.)
2. Increased volume load (valvular regurgitation, shunts, increased venous return, etc.)
3. Obstruction to ventricular filling (mitral or tricuspid stenosis)
4. Pericardial constriction, tamponade
5. Endocardial or myocardial restriction
6. Ventricular aneurysm
7. Ventricular dyssynergy
B. Myocardial (muscular) abnormalities or loss of myocytes
1. Primary abnormalities or loss of myocytes
(a) Idiopathic dilated cardiomyopathy
(b) Neuromuscular disorders
(c) Myocarditis
(d) Metabolic (diabetes mellitus, etc.)
(e) Toxic (alcohol, cobalt, etc.)
(f) Presbycardia
2. Secondary myocardial abnormalities or loss of myocytes
(a) Dysdynamic (secondary to mechanical abnormalities)
(b) Ischaemia (coronary heart disease)
(c) Metabolic
(d) Inflammation
(e) Infiltrative diseases (e.g. sarcoidosis)
(f) Systemic diseases
(g) Chronic obstructive lung disease
(h) Myocardial depression due to drugs (e.g. beta-blockers, Ca^{2+} antagonists)
C. Altered cardiac rhythm or conduction disturbances
1. Standstill
2. Fibrillation
3. Extreme tachycardia or bradycardia
4. Electrical asynchrony, conduction disturbances

Adapted from Hurst JW, Schlant RC, Rackley CE, Sonnenblick EH, Wenger NK. The Heart 78th ed. New York: McGraw Hill

operable valvular disease (particularly obstructive valvular disease and significant mitral regurgitation which may be silent) and (c) excluding coronary artery disease where surgery would be appropriate. Doppler echocardiography is thus an investigation of fundamental importance (Fig. 4.1) yet many patients presenting with CHF still do not have this investigation, at least in the UK (42% did not have echocardiography in the London community hospital study).[4]

Rarer but important diagnoses not to be missed are adult congenital heart disease and infective endocarditis (echocardiography also assists in making both these diagnoses). Also important is the identification of coexisting pathology (e.g. anaemia, thyrotoxicosis, myeloma, renal failure, Paget's disease) and medication (e.g. calcium channel blockers,[14] beta-blockers, antidepressants, chlorpropamide, antiarrhythmics, steroid hormones and non-steroidal anti-inflammatory drugs (NSAIDs) that may precipitate or aggravate the syndrome.

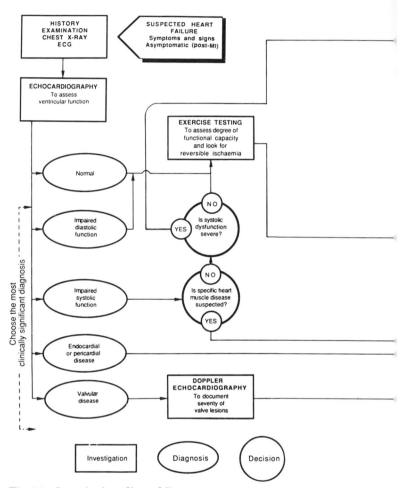

Fig. 4.1   Investigation of heart failure.

PATHOPHYSIOLOGY

This section discusses the pathophysiology of CHF due to systolic dysfunction and how this pathophysiological understanding forms the basis of
treatment.

Central haemodynamics

Traditionally the haemodynamic derangement in heart failure has been

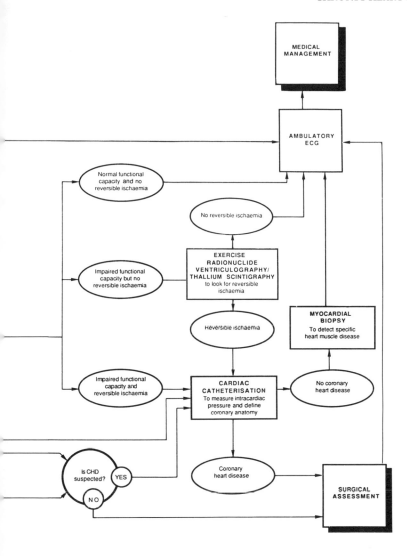

considered in terms of the three major determinants of stroke volume, i.e. contractility, preload and afterload. The heart, however, cannot be considered completely in isolation from the vasculature (ventriculovascular coupling is a crucial consideration) or from the neural and hormonal influences working upon it. Heart rate is obviously a major determinant of cardiac output, though often little considered, and the normal force–frequency relationship may be reversed in CHF.

Contractility

Physiologically contractility refers to a muscle's ability to shorten independently of its end-diastolic length and the load opposing shortening (and, in vivo, heart rate). Until recently loss of contractility has been equated with loss of functioning muscle through infarction or a cardiomyopathic process. It is now apparent, however, that surviving muscle may show abnormal contractile responsiveness. For example, the normal inotropic response to catecholamines may be reduced, due to β-adrenoreceptor (first messenger) down-regulation and G-protein (second messenger) changes.[15–18]

Abnormally high concentrations of circulating hormones, neurotransmitters and other toxins may also injure or even destroy remaining muscle, giving rise to the concept of a self-perpetuating vicious cycle of deteriorating cardiac function.[15–19] Alterations of calcium homeostasis, sarcoplasmic reticulum function, myocardial metabolism (LDH isoenzymes), mitochondrial function and myosin isoforms have also been described in CHF.[20] The extracellular matrix of the myocardium – the collagen interstitium – has many functions. It ensures myocyte alignment and coordinates delivery of force. Abnormalities of the collagen interstitium and myocyte alignment may also occur in CHF.

Inotropic agents are given to increase contractility.

Preload

Preload describes the relation of end-diastolic fibre stretch to muscle function whereby an increase in stretch causes an increase in function (the Frank–Starling mechanism); this relationship is often illustrated in the form of a ventricular function curve (Fig. 4.2). In the intact heart preload is usually equated to end-diastolic volume, which is related to ventricular

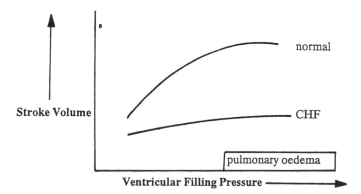

Fig. 4.2 Relationship between stroke volume and ventricular filling pressure in the normal heart and the failing heart (CHF). The ventricular function curve ('Starling Curve') is depressed in chronic heart failure (CHF).

compliance (often overlooked) and end-diastolic pressure (EDP). Preload is increased in CHF due to extracellular fluid volume expansion, veno-constriction, a reduction in venous capacitance and, in many cases, a decrease in ventricular compliance. Because the left ventricular function curve is depressed in CHF, an increase in preload leads to little increase in cardiac output and, when the EDP reaches a critical level, pulmonary oedema will occur (Fig. 4.2). Coronary perfusion pressure (aortic diastolic pressure − left ventricular EDP) is also reduced by a high preload (the subendocardium may, in particular, become ischaemic). Preload reduction by venodilatation/diuretic treatment reduces the risk of pulmonary oedema, reduces the preload contribution to afterload, and increases coronary perfusion. By decreasing ventricular radius, functional atrio-ventricular (AV) valve regurgitation and, perhaps through improved mechano-electrical feedback, arrhythmias, may also be reduced.[23,24]

Afterload

Afterload refers to the load applied after the onset of muscle contraction. In the intact organism this equates to the wall tension that must be developed to eject the ventricular contents. This can be derived from the law of Laplace (simplified to wall stress $= p \times r/2T$, where $p =$ intraventricular pressure, $r =$ radius of endocardial surface of ventricle and $T =$ wall thickness).

Left ventricular volume is thus a determinant of preload and afterload. Left ventricular systolic pressure is governed by aortic impedance. Aortic impedance is largely determined by systemic vascular resistance (SVR) though large artery compliance, blood viscosity and intra-arterial blood volume make contributions that are rarely considered (see below).[14,25,25a]

Myocyte hypertrophy reduces the load per fibre and this compensatory mechanism is initially successful in normalizing wall stress (though leads to other problems such as impaired subendocardial blood flow). Systemic and local neurohumoral mediators probably contribute to the process of hypertrophy. Eventually the increase in ventricular radius outstrips wall thickness and afterload increases. In contrast to the normal ventricle, the falling ventricle is exquisitely sensitive to changes in afterload (Fig. 4.3). A small increase in SVR can result in a serious decrease in cardiac output; conversely, a small decrease in afterload can substantially increase cardiac output. This principle underlies the use of vasodilators (particularly arterial dilators) in CHF.

Systemic vascular resistance and vasoconstriction

Numerous factors operate to increase SVR and therefore afterload (the same factors act on the venous circulation to increase preload). Vascular stiffness is increased by vessel wall sodium content.[26,27] Heightened sym-

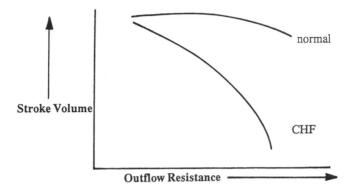

Fig. 4.3 Relationship between stroke volume and outflow resistance ('afterload') in the normal heart and the failing heart (CHF). The failing heart is particularly sensitive to increases in outflow resistance.

pathetic neural traffic and circulating catecholamines were one of the first and most important neuroendocrine abnormalities to be described in CHF.[28] It is widely believed that this and the other neurohumoral systems mentioned below are activated in CHF in an attempt to restore the reduced arterial pressure and organ perfusion typifying the syndrome.[27,29-35] Increased circulating concentrations of angiotensin II, arginine vasopressin (AVP) and neuropeptide Y also act to cause smooth muscle vasoconstriction.[28-35] Vascular autocrine/paracrine abnormalities have also been suggested, e.g. activation of a tissue renin–angiotensin system. Some of these endocrine/paracrine influences may also act as growth factors leading to structural remodelling of arterioles.

Endothelial (as well as smooth muscle) function may also be abnormal in CHF. Increased levels of endothelin, a powerful endothelial-derived vasoconstrictor, have been demonstrated in CHF and impaired endothelial-mediated vasorelaxation has been shown in this syndrome.[36,37]

Not only arterial resistance is altered in CHF; it also seems that arterial compliance is reduced in this syndrome, and this may be a potential therapeutic target in the future.[16,25]

Peripheral haemodynamics and regional blood flow

As already described, the arterial tree in CHF is subject to numerous neural and circulating vasoconstrictor influences. These influences lead to redistribution of the limited cardiac output away from non-critical tissues (e.g. the skin) to crucial organ beds (e.g. the brain). Two major organ/tissue beds do not receive an adequate blood flow, i.e. the kidney and skeletal muscle. These deficiencies may ultimately lead to the cardinal manifestations of CHF, i.e. fluid retention, dyspnea, muscle fatigue and exercise intolerance (see below).

NEUROENDOCRINE ABNORMALITIES

Many of the neurohormonal disturbances that occur in CHF and their haemodynamic consequences have already been discussed above. The sympathetic nervous system, renin–angiotensin–aldosterone system (RAAS), AVP and endothelin all also have potent renal effects leading to sodium and water retention and renal vasoconstriction. Aldosterone causes potassium and magnesium wasting. At least some of these hormones (e.g. angiotensin II and AVP) probably contribute to the intense thirst found in so many patients with CHF. In high concentrations, angiotensin II and catecholamines may be directly cardiotoxic in their own right.

Many other hormonal abnormalities have been described in CHF (Table 4.4).[38–41] The increased levels of the vasodilator–natriuretic substances, prostaglandins, atrial natriuretic factor (ANF), dopamine and calcitonin gene-related peptide (CGRP), are of most interest as these may counter some of the vasoconstrictor-antinatriuretic influences already described;[38–41,42] further augmentation of the concentrations and effects of the former hormones has also formed the basis of a new therapeutic approach in CHF (see Treatment).[43,44]

The hormonal abnormalities described above are frequently present in the early or even asymptomatic stages of CHF.[27,29,32] They become more marked as the severity of the syndrome increases and some (e.g. the RAAS) may be further stimulated by diuretic therapy.[45] Many hormonal abnormalities have individually been related to the risk of ventricular arrhythmias and death in CHF.[30,31,33,38] Indeed, as already pointed out, there is

Table 4.4 Hormonal and related abnormalities in CHF

Vasoconstrictor hormones
- ↑ noradrenaline
- ↑ angiotensin II
- ↑ AVP
- ↑ neuropeptide Y
- ↑ endothelin

Vasodilator hormones
- ↑ ANF
- ↑ blood pressure
- ↑ prostaglandins
- ↑ dopamine
- ↑ CGRP
- ↑ substance P
- ↓ endothelium derived relaxing factor-like activity

Other circulatory factors
- ↑ opioid peptides
- ↑ TNF
- ↑ neopterin
- ↑ erythropoietin
- ↑ digitalis-like factor

good reason to believe that neurohumoral derangements once initiated by the haemodynamic changes in CHF then contribute to its pathophysiology and progression (i.e. they are not just 'markers' of illness). It is this belief that has led to the use of neurohumoral modulators in the treatment of CHF. The successful prototype of neurohumoral modulators has been the RAAS antagonists, the ACE inhibitors, and it is of interest to note that these drugs appear to improve prognosis most in those patients with RAAS activation (see Treatment).[33]

Cardiovascular reflexes

Much of the neurohumoral activation found in CHF may arise from abnormal baroreflex function.[46-48] The arterial and cardiopulmonary mechanoreceptors appear to be less able to inhibit the vasomotor centres in CHF; this leads to enhanced sympathetic nervous system outflow (and indirectly RAAS stimulation). Parasympathetic autonomic function is also abnormal in CHF and diminished vagal tone (parasympathetic outflow) is thought to contribute to the loss of heart rate variability in CHF. Abnormal autonomic activity of this kind is considered to be a risk factor for ventricular arrhythmias. The cause of abnormal baroreceptor function in CHF is not known for certain though increased circulating vasopressin levels may play a role.

Cardiac transplantation may restore normal baroreceptor function in CHF patients. Certain drugs, e.g. ACE inhibitors and digoxin, have been shown to improve baroreceptor function in CHF.[47,48] Exercise may have a similar benefit.

Electrolyte abnormalities

CHF is also characterized by plasma and cellular electrolyte abnormalities partly as a result of neurohormonal stimulation and partly as a consequence of diuretic treatment.[27,49,50] Plasma and, more importantly, cellular potassium and magnesium deficiency are common and relate to the risk of arrhythmias and prognosis in CHF.[31,51] Whether these relationships are causal or not is unknown, though there are theoretical reasons why this might be the case.

Muscle [^{3}H]ouabain binding sites (labelling sodium–potassium pumps) and muscle calcium concentration have also been reported to be decreased in CHF and these changes could contribute to the muscle dysfunction found in CHF (see below).[52]

Potassium and magnesium deficiency also increase the risk of digoxin toxicity (see below).

Intracellular sodium may be increased in CHF and this has been suggested to cause vascular wall 'stiffness' and contribute to impaired vasodilatation in CHF.[26]

Finally, plasma sodium may be low in CHF. This may indicate severe CHF with intense renin–angiotensin system and vasopressin activation and reduced renal water excretion (water excess); it may also occur with thiazide diuretic use (causing impaired free water excretion) and due to excessive diuresis (leading to sodium depletion).

Renal changes in CHF

Chronic heart failure is characterized by a reduction in renal blood flow (RBF).[27,53–55] RBF falls in CHF due to a reduction in cardiac output and probably due to the effects of neurohumoral systems on the renal vasculature (afferent renal arterioles and renal papillary vessels). Glomerular filtration rate (GFR) is preserved, at least until the syndrome is advanced. GFR is preserved in the face of a fall in RBF by an increase in filtration fraction (FF). FF is believed to be increased as a consequence of the preferential vasoconstrictor effect of angiotensin II on glomerular efferent arteriolar tone and probably also by the effect of ANF on glomerular ultrafiltration and the renal efferent arterioles. Removal of this effect of angiotensin II and ANF (e.g. by an ACE inhibitor) can cause a fall in GFR (see below).[56] In other words, the kidney behaves in a similar way as in renal artery stenosis (see below).

One consequence of an increase in FF is that proximal tubular sodium reabsorption will be increased in CHF and this will also occur because of the direct effect of angiotensin II and the sympathetic nervous system on this part of the nephron. Aldosterone and reduced renal papillary blood flow have a similar effect on the distal nephron while aldosterone encourages potassium (and magnesium) loss. Other abnormalities of glomerular and tubular function and their interdependence have been described in CHF.

The renal circulation in CHF may be affected in one other important way. Several groups have now described a relatively high incidence of renal artery stenosis in patients with CHF (especially if intermittent claudication is present) – perhaps not a surprising finding in patients with vascular disease.[57] This observation has implications for the prescribing of ACE inhibitors.

Muscle abnormalities

Impaired muscle blood flow and muscle electrolyte depletion have already been referred to.[58,59] A much wider array of skeletal muscle abnormalities has recently been described in CHF.[50,60–62] Alterations in fibre type, muscle enzymatic activity, muscle metabolism and muscle strength have been reported. Skeletal muscle fatigue is a cardinal symptom of CHF. Reduced muscle protein synthesis occurs relatively early in CHF and frank wasting (protein breakdown) occurs in advanced CHF.[63] Tumour necrosis factor also may contribute.[64]

Not only skeletal muscle is affected. Diaphragmatic and intercostal muscle fatigue has also been described in CHF.[65]

Pulmonary and ventilatory abnormalities

Numerous pulmonary abnormalities in addition to respiratory muscle weakness have been reported in CHF.[58]

Patients with CHF ventilate more than healthy controls at the same external workload and metabolic rate (most readily described by the relationship of minute ventilation to minute production of carbon dioxide, VE/VCO_2).[66,67] This primary abnormality in CHF has recently been related to increased ventilation of physiological dead space; the reason is not known.

Reversible airways obstruction has been found in CHF.[68] Abnormal sleep respiration with arterial desaturation has also been reported in CHF.

Finally, cough is common in CHF (and can be drug induced; see below). Coughing represents a metabolically demanding form of exercise and the diaphragm and other respiratory muscles involved use a significant proportion of resting cardiac output in the patient with CHF.

Cause of symptoms

The major symptoms of CHF are breathlessness and fatigue, especially during exercise. Despite a massive investigative effort and the numerous abnormalities outlined above, it is not known what causes the symptoms of CHF.

In CHF (unlike acute heart failure) there is no clear relationship between left atrial pressure (or other haemodynamic variables) and dyspnea. Lung stiffness, increased physiological dead space, circulating metabolites and abnormalities of skeletal muscle blood flow and metabolism have been suggested to contribute to dyspnea. Muscle fatigue and exercise intolerance similarly do not correlate with indices of left ventricular pump function such as ejection fraction and cardiac output. Muscle fatigue has been attributed to impaired muscle blood flow, and where exercise time increases with a drug there is usually an accompanying increase in muscle blood flow.[58,59] The other complex histological and metabolic changes found in skeletal muscle in CHF may also contribute to exercise intolerance.

DRUGS USED IN THE TREATMENT OF CHF

DIURETICS

Diuretics remain the mainstay of treatment of CHF. In the oedematous patient diuretics also enhance vasodilator responsiveness.[26] They remain the single most effective symptomatic treatment for CHF though their effect on mortality has never been tested.[69,70] They also remain first-line treatment for CHF. Three groups of diuretics are used to treat CHF: (a) loop diuretics, (b) thiazide diuretics and (c) potassium-conserving diuretics.

Loop diuretics

These are usually the preferred class of diuretic in CHF. Frusemide and bumetanide are the two best-established agents of this type. The effective dose of frusemide is usually 40 mg (equivalent to 1 mg of bumetanide) though, as there is often reduced diuretic efficiency in CHF, a dose as high as 80–120 mg may be necessary. If a greater diuretic response is needed, repeated rather than larger doses should be used. Very high-dose (up to 4000 mg per day) frusemide may be needed in refractory CHF if there is significant renal dysfunction.[71] It is our preferred approach to add another diuretic with a different nephron site of action before increasing the dose of frusemide above 120 mg b.d.

Thiazide diuretics

These agents are less effective than loop diuretics (they lead to excretion of up to 5–10% of the filtered load of sodium compared to up to 35% with loop diuretics) and have a more prolonged action (up to 72 hours). In our practice, thiazides (e.g. bendrofluazide 10 mg) are usually used in addition to loop diuretics in the treatment of 'resistant' CHF (i.e. following the principle of 'sequential nephron blockade') though others use these agents as first-line treatment of mild CHF.[71]

Metolazone

Metolazone is a potent quinazoline sulphonamide diuretic which can be used instead of a conventional thiazide diuretic in resistant CHF. Metolazone 2–10 mg is very effective in combination with frusemide and may only be required for a limited period (often only a few days).[72]

With both metolazone and thiazides careful monitoring of hydration status, blood chemistry and renal function is essential (see below).

Potassium-conserving diuretics

Spironolactone is a competitive aldosterone inhibitor. Amiloride and triamterene act independently of aldosterone to prevent Na/K exchange in the distal nephron (all three agents also prevent H^+ loss, which also reduces K^+ loss). These drugs are, by themselves, weak natriuretics and enhance the sodium-losing effects of other diuretics when given in combination;

there is also a report that spironolactone and captopril in combination may induce natriuresis in resistant CHF.[73]

Both loop diuretics and thiazides cause potassium depletion, which patients with CHF are already predisposed to due to neuroendocrine activation. Potassium deficiency increases the risk of digitalis toxicity (and toxicity from other potentially arrhythmogenic drugs such as tricyclic antidepressents, phenothiazines and antiarrhythmic agents). There is also evidence that hypokalaemia predisposes to serious ventricular arrhythmias in patients with ischaemic heart disease. There is thus a strong case for careful avoidance of potassium depletion in patients with CHF. This can best be achieved (in terms of efficacy and compliance) by prescription of potassium-conserving diuretics.

Magnesium depletion is also common in diuretic-treated CHF patients and has similar adverse effects to potassium depletion. It may also be impossible to correct potassium deficiency unless magnesium deficiency is corrected first. Potassium-conserving diuretics also conserve magnesium.

Hyperkalaemia can also occur with the use of potassium-sparing diuretics, especially in the elderly. This is primarily a risk in patients with impaired renal function or diabetes mellitus and in patients taking other drugs such as potassium supplements, ACE inhibitors and NSAIDs (see Drug interactions).

In addition to electrolyte abnormalities, diuretics cause neuroendocrine stimulation.[45, 69] Frusemide has been shown to stimulate the RAAS both acutely and chronically. Acutely frusemide also increases sympathetic nervous system (SNS) activity and SNS and RAAS activation in these circumstances is associated with a sharp increase in systemic vascular resistance. These potentially adverse neuroendocrine and haemodynamic changes can be countered by treatment with ACE inhibitor.[45] Potassium-conserving diuretics (including spironolactone) may also activate the RAAS.

Drug interactions with diuretics

The potential interactions between diuretic drugs and NSAIDs are of particular concern in the elderly. Most NSAIDs blunt the natriuretic effect of diuretics by poorly understood and possibly different mechanisms. Sulindac may not have this effect. NSAIDs may also cause worsening renal dysfunction and hyperkalaemia in patients treated with potassium supplements and ACE inhibitors. Nephrotoxicity may be particularly common when NSAIDs and potassium-conserving diuretics, especially triamterene, are combined.

Hyperkalaemia due to combination of an ACE inhibitor and a potassium-sparing diuretic may occur, though in our practice appears much less common than expected, and an ACE inhibitor alone may be insufficient to prevent electrolyte depletion.

DIGOXIN

Digoxin is the most frequently used of the cardiac glycosides. Classically digoxin is considered as an inotrope due to its ability to inhibit the sarcolemmal sodium pump (Na/K-ATPase) leading to intracellular sodium influx and an increase in intracellular calcium (interestingly this effect is still preserved in myocardium from patients with severe CHF when that of phosphodiesterase inhibitors is lost).[74] However, digoxin also improves baroreceptor function and decreases SNS activity, leading to increased limb blood flow.[75] In addition, digitalis glycosides have complex direct and indirect electrophysiological effects (these slow the ventricular rate in atrial fibrillation).

After years of controversy, three large double-blind randomized placebo-controlled trials, and several smaller studies, have shown digoxin to be of benefit in patients in sinus rhythm with mild, moderate and severe CHF.[74, 76] Digoxin reduces the need for additional diuretic therapy, reduces the rate of hospitalization, decreases the symptoms and signs of CHF, increases ejection fraction (LVEF) and improves exercise tolerance. The magnitude of this benefit is, however, probably smaller than that of ACE inhibitors and the latter are to be preferred for their effect on prognosis (though a study of the effect of digoxin on mortality is under way). The practical question about digoxin is really whether it confers benefit when given in addition to (rather than instead of) an ACE inhibitor. In terms of acute haemodynamic and neuroendocrine responses, such additional benefit is seen.[74] Only one chronic dosing study has addressed this potential interaction.[77] No additional benefit (other than an increase in LVEF) from digoxin was seen, though the design of this study was unsatisfactory and low serum digoxin levels (0.81 ± 0.03 ng/ml) were achieved (see below). In addition this was a study of patients with *mild* CHF (receiving the ACE inhibitor quinapril).[77] Recently there has been a preliminary report of a digoxin withdrawal study (RADIANCE Study). In patients with moderately severe CHF treated with diuretics and ACE inhibitors. Compared to continuation of digoxin, placebo substitution lead to a substantial deterioration in wellbeing, exercise tolerance and ventricular function.[77a]

Use of digoxin

Many complicated nomograms and other dose-selecting systems have been devised, but none have proved more effective than physicians' 'intuitive' prescribing. Depending on age, weight, renal function and concomitant therapy, a loading dose of 0.375–0.75 mg may be given in four divided portions over 24 hours. If a loading dose is omitted, a daily maintenance dose (usually 0.125 or 0.25 mg) will not give steady-state plasma concentrations for at least seven days and for possibly up to three weeks if there is marked renal dysfunction. In patients with atrial fibrillation, ventricular rate can be used as a guide to dose adequacy. In patients in sinus rhythm, plasma digoxin concentration is a useful but inexact guide to prescribing. The generally accepted therapeutic range is 0.9–3.2 nmol/l (0.7–2.5 mg/ml). Levels below 0.9 nmol/l are almost always subtherapeutic; toxicity may be present at any level above this but is increasingly likely above 3.2 nmol/l. For beneficial clinical effect, plasma levels of digoxin at the upper end of the therapeutic range seem to be needed.[74] This frequently requires doses of 0.375–0.5 mg. Even amongst the elderly up to 20% of patients will require a daily dose of 0.25 mg or more to achieve adequate plasma digoxin concentrations. The tendency is very much to prescribe doses that may be too low for fear of toxicity.

Toxicity

Digoxin toxicity affects the gastrointestinal (anorexia, nausea, vomiting), neurological (fatigue, confusion, xanthopsia) and cardiovascular (cardiac arrhythmias) systems. Digoxin has gained a certain notoriety for producing adverse effects particularly in the elderly, and toxicity rates of up to 20% have been reported in hospitalized elderly patients. However, the incidence of digoxin toxicity in outpatient populations appears to be low, averaging about one episode per 20 years of treatment, and recent large heart failure studies with digoxin support the latter findings, with the incidence of adverse effects no greater with digoxin than placebo.[74, 78] Furthermore, with the development of new treatments, the mortality from digoxin toxicity has dropped to 1% or less.[78] This suggests that appropriate use of digoxin in adequate dosage with careful clinical follow-up and biochemical monitoring of drug levels is not associated with undue toxicity.

Drug interactions

The major interactions with digoxin are shown in Table 4.5. The quinidine–digoxin interaction is well recognized and plasma levels may double as a consequence of reduced renal and extrarenal clearance. A similar interaction is believed to occur with quinine, a drug frequently prescribed in the elderly for leg cramps. Digoxin dosage should be halved if quinine is prescribed, and plasma level checked after five days. Erythromycin and tetracycline may result in 50–120% increases in plasma digoxin concentrations in the 10–15% of patients who harbour *Eubacterium lentum* in their bowel.

XAMOTEROL

Xamoterol is a partial β_1-adrenoreceptor agonist licensed in certain countries for the treatment of mild CHF.[79, 80] When endogenous adrenergic

Table 4.5 Drug interactions with digoxin

Enhanced effect		
Increased digoxin concentrations	Pharmacokinetic interaction	Quinidine
		Quinine
		Captopril
		Amiodarone
		Spironolactone
		Ibuprofen
		Verapamil
	Increased absorption	
Increased sensitivity		Antibiotics
		Diuretics
		Laxatives
		Corticosteroids
		Carbenoxolone
		β_2-Adrenoceptor agonists
Reduced effect		
Decreased digoxin concentrations	Decreased absorption	Cholestyramine
		Colestipol
		Antacids
		Neomycin
		Bran
		Cathartics
	Increased excretion	
Decreased inotropic effect		Hydralazine
		Disopyramide
		Procainamide
		Amiloride

activity is low, xamoterol activates the β_1-adrenoreceptor, causing moderate inotropic and chronotropic stimulation, but when SNS activity is high (e.g. during exercise) it behaves mainly as a β-adrenoreceptor antagonist. In theory, in the presence of xamoterol, the cardiac β-adrenoreceptor is thus exposed to a relatively constant level of adrenergic stimulation. Several studies have shown that xamoterol improves the symptoms and signs of mild CHF and increases exercise tolerance (the drug has also an anti-anginal effect; see below).[79, 80] Recently, however, a large placebo-controlled study in patients with severe CHF treated with diuretics and ACE inhibitors showed a significantly increased mortality on xamoterol (this adverse outcome has not been detected in a large follow-up of patients with mild to moderate CHF treated with xamoterol).[80] Differentiation of mild from moderate CHF is difficult and full evaluation including functional assessment (i.e. ECG, chest radiograph, echocardiograph and exercise test) is advised before xamoterol is used. Treatment (200 mg b.d. or 200 mg once daily if serum creatinine $> 250\,\mu mol/l$ or creatinine $< 35\,ml/min$ per $1.73\,m^2$) should be started in hospital under supervision. At the moment, the precise place for xamoterol in the treatment of CHF is unclear; its anti-ischaemic properties may make it useful for the large subgroup of patients with heart failure and angina.

ACE INHIBITORS

The prototype ACE inhibitors, captopril and enalapril, have been convincingly shown to improve the symptoms and signs of CHF, to increase exercise tolerance and to reduce mortality.[7, 9, 56, 81] Initially these effects were demonstrated in severe (NYHA class III/IV CHF) but are also obtained in patients with less severe (NYHA class II/III CHF).[7, 9] There is reason to believe that all ACE inhibitors share these properties.

How do ACE inhibitors work: symptoms, exercise tolerance?

The effects of ACE inhibitors in CHF are protean.[56, 81]

The primary effect of ACE inhibitors is to inhibit the production of the hormone angiotensin II. Angiotensin II is a potent vasoconstrictor, antinatriuretic, stimulant of aldosterone, stimulant of AVP and facilitator of sympathetic neural transmission. Probably the main effect of ACE inhibitors, therefore, is to cause vasodilatation; initially arterial dilatation was emphasized but lately it has become clear that venodilatation also follows ACE inhibition, i.e. ACE inhibitors are 'balanced vasodilators'.[82] This may be very important in terms of peripheral as well as central haemodynamics as 'driving pressure' (arterial minus venous pressure) is one determinant of muscle perfusion.[83] It has also been suggested that ACE inhibitors may also cause vasodilatation by increasing prostaglandin/kinin production; there is some evidence to support this, though early work with angiotensin II antagonists and renin inhibitors in humans suggests that this effect may not be a major one.

The most important net effect of vasodilatation in CHF seems to be an increase in blood flow at rest and particularly during exercise to skeletal muscle; this is believed to lead to an increase in exercise capacity. Interestingly, this effect is a delayed one, appearing only after many weeks of therapy.[58, 59, 83, 84] Other beneficial effects improving muscle function and exercise capacity may be normalization of muscle electrolytes and metabolism.[49, 50]

How do ACE inhibitors work: mortality?

ACE inhibitors improve survival in moderate and severe CHF. Amelioration of progressive contractile dysfunction and reduction of arrhythmias may both contribute.[7, 9, 85, 86, 93] Both the CONSENSUS and SOLVD studies, however, found only a reduction in deaths due to pump failure (though it is widely accepted that it is difficult to differentiate between these two outcomes in clinical practice).

ACE inhibitors seem to cause only a modest increase in myocardial contractile function and cardiac output or ejection fraction compared to other vasodilators. This is partly because, though stroke volume increases, heart rate usually falls, leading to little change in cardiac output; 'forward ejection' may be improved through a reduction in mitral regurgitation, though overall LVEF may not change.[23] There is, however, growing evidence that these drugs can prevent progressive pump failure, particularly if given in the earlier stages of CHF (see below). Ventricular cavity size is reduced and true remodelling occurs.[87] This presumably reflects preservation of myocardial function through reduction in haemodynamic load and potentially toxic neuroendocrine exposure.

Some studies suggest that ACE inhibitors reduce ventricular arrhythmias, presumably through reduction in neuroendocrine stimulation, correction of autonomic and baroreceptor dysfunction, correction of electrolytic abnormalities and improvement in myocardial mechano-electrical status,[56, 81, 81a] though this has not been confirmed by the SOLVD investigators.

Do ACE inhibitors work in mild CHF?

As already stated, there is no doubt that ACE inhibitors are beneficial in moderately severe and severe (i.e. NYHA class III and IV) CHF. Is this also the case for milder (NYHA class II) CHF?

Recent studies with captopril, quinapril and perindopril have shown that ACE inhibitors significantly improve symptoms and exercise time in patients with NYHA class II and III CHF.[84, 88] The Munich Mild Heart Failure Trial (MMHFT) is particularly notable in also examining the effect of an ACE inhibitor on progression of CHF (to NYHA class IV) and death over a three-year follow-up period.[89] The results of this double-blind placebo-controlled study of captopril 25 mg b.d. in predominantly NYHA class II patients are shown in Table 4.6. In this study the most ill patients (e.g. older patients and those in class III, with an enlarged heart on chest X-ray/echocardiogram and requiring loop diuretics) had the greatest risk of progression (41% on placebo, 28% on captopril). Patients with fewer risk factors showed less progression of CHF (13% on placebo, 0% on captopril). The SOLVD treatment arm and V-HeFT II studies also included many patients with class II CHF who seemed to benefit symptomatically and prognostically from treatment with enalapril.[7, 93]

At the time of writing, the SOLVD prevention arm has also just reported. In patients with impaired ventricular function (LVEF < 35%), but

Table 4.6 Munich mild heart failure trial

Endpoint	Captopril ($n = 83$)	Placebo ($n = 87$)	
Death—pump failure	4	11	$p < 0.1$
Death—sudden	11	10	$p = $ n.s.
Progression of CHF	9	23	$p < 0.01$

without heart failure (i.e. fluid retention), enalapril significantly reduced progression to overt heart failure (37% reduction in risk over the four years of study). The survival and ventricular enlargement (SAVE) study has also recently reported. In this study captopril, started within 2 weeks of myocardial infarction, reduced mortality and the development of heart failure by 15–20% over the subsequent 3–4 years.

ACE inhibitors or other drugs?

ACE inhibitors are superior to the alternative vasodilators hydralazine and prazosin in terms of symptom relief and reduction in mortality.[90, 93] In fact, the symptomatic and mortality benefits of ACE inhibitors are seen regardless of whether patients are taking concomitant cardioactive medications such as digoxin or conventional vasodilators.[7, 9] In terms of symptoms and exercise tolerance, ACE inhibitors are at least as efficacious as the inodilator enoximone[91] and the vasodilator flosequinan;[92] the latter drugs, however, cause more side-effects and enoximone may increase mortality in CHF (see below). ACE inhibitors may, however, have no advantage over the dopaminergic drug ibopamine in terms of exercise tolerance and have yet to be tested against the neutral endopeptidase inhibitors; these latter two types of agent may prove to be the first real competition for ACE inhibitors (see below).

ACE inhibitors and other drugs?

From a clinical viewpoint, the real question to be answered is probably not whether ACE inhibitors are better than other drugs but whether combination therapy has any additional advantage for the patient.

ACE inhibitors are probably more effective than digoxin but both drugs together might have extra benefit. One study supports this view and another does not (but is a small, poorly designed study in patients with mild CHF; see above).[74, 77 77a]

Combining enoximone with captopril has been studied (see below).[94] A similar study with flosequinan and hydralazine ± isosorbide dinitrate is merited.

PROBLEMS STILL TO BE ADDRESSED

Can ACE inhibitors replace diuretics as the sole therapy for CHF?

The answer to this question is still 'no'. Heart failure (i.e. LV dysfunction associated with fluid retention) does not adequately respond to ACE inhibitors without the addition of diuretic therapy, and the substitution of ACE inhibitors for diuretics does not keep CHF under control (whether ACE inhibitors can prevent fluid retaining CHF is a different question).[69, 70] The results of the prevention limb of SOLVD and the SAVE study suggest that progression to a fluid-retaining state might indeed be avoided or delayed by treatment with ACE inhibitors. The emergence of new truly diuretic–vasodilator agents (dopamine and ANF analogues) makes this an even more interesting area for investigation.

Do ACE inhibitors benefit or harm particular groups of patients?

CHF is usually addressed as if it were a single homogeneous entity, which it is not. Some time ago Packer reported that a high serum creatinine and a high right atrial pressure are predictive of a poor response to ACE inhibitor treatment.[55] The SOLVD treatment and prevention limbs and the SAVE study have recently shown a significant reduction in unstable angina and myocardial infarction with enalapril treatment (another recent report, however, suggests that captopril may aggravate angina in patients with CHF[95]). ACE inhibitors may thus have additional effects in certain patient subsets and patient heterogeneity will have to be considered more carefully in future studies.

Do ACE inhibitors improve or worsen diastolic dysfunction?

CHF due to systolic dysfunction has been the subject of this chapter. 'Diastolic heart failure' is a subject of much interest. It is not clear what the effects of ACE inhibitors are on diastolic function.

What is the correct dose of ACE inhibitor?

Perhaps the biggest omission in the development of ACE inhibitor therapy has been the failure to undertake dose–response studies. Recently quinapril has been shown to have a dose–response relationship for exercise tolerance.[84] High-dose ACE inhibitor therapy is no more effective than low-dose therapy in suppressing resting neuroendocrine activity but is better at inhibiting the neurohumoral activation occurring on exercise.[96]

Are there clinically significant differences between ACE inhibitors?

There is no doubt that there are chemical and pharmacological differences between agents but whether these have any clinical significance is still unknown.

Possible areas of difference that could be of importance include:

1. Long/short acting: more clinical evidence is available regarding this pharmacological difference than any other.[53, 54, 97] Initially the major difference identified between long (e.g. enalapril, lisinopril) and short (e.g.

captopril) ACE inhibitors was effect on renal function. In two studies long-acting agents were found to cause a greater rise in blood urea and/or creatinine. Though not confirmed in all subsequent studies,[54] this difference is plausible and predictable especially where large, fixed doses (i.e. leading to a longer duration of action) of ACE inhibitor are given without adjustment of diuretic dose. This is clearly not what happens in clinical practice and, in any case, the small rise in urea/creatinine that may occur is not of any clinical significance.

Much more intriguing differences have been reported between lisinopril and captopril in a recent study.[97] In a parallel group comparison, Giles et al found a greater improvement in symptoms, ejection fraction and exercise time in the lisinopril-treated group. It is not clear whether there is a difference between 'long-acting' agents and 'high-dose' therapy, and the previously cited report by Kirlin et al,[96] showing similar suppression of the RAAS by high and low-dose ACE inhibition at rest but superior inhibition by high-dose therapy on exercise, may be relevant to the findings of Giles et al.[97] Even more intriguingly, Pouleur et al recently reported that the mortality in captopril-treated patients in the Xamoterol Severe Heart Failure Study was 9.7%, whereas it was 4.3% in enalapril/lisinopril-treated patients ($p < 0.02$);[98] because this was a retrospective subgroup analysis, this finding must be treated cautiously.

2.   — SH group: this could be relevant to free radical scavenging,[99] prostanoid production and nitrate tolerance.

3.   Tissue ACE inhibition: this could be relevant to renal, vascular and cardiac effects.

Prodrug versus non-prodrug does not seem to have mattered in practice. Hepatic versus renal excretion may have to be addressed with the development of new agents such as fosenopril which undergo significant biliary excretion.

Guidelines for use

When ACE inhibitors are prescribed for heart failure, the first dose should ideally be given in hospital. Certain precautions should be taken before treatment is started (see Table 4.7). A low dose should be given initially, e.g. 6.25 mg of captopril, 2.5 mg of lisinopril, 2.5 mg of enalapril (1.25 mg in the very elderly) and 2.5 mg of quinapril. The patient should remain seated or preferably supine until the peak haemodynamic effect of the drug has been observed; it is important to remember that this can be delayed in the elderly up to (and even beyond) 3–4 hours with captopril, 4–6 hours with lisinopril, 6–8 hours with enalapril and 2–3 hours with quinapril. To reduce the inconvenience of prolonged monitoring and the danger of an extended period of hypotension, should it occur, there is an argument for initiating treatment with captopril in all patients and switching to another

Table 4.7 Precautions to take prior to use of ACE inhibitors in chronic heart failure

Exclude significant obstructive valvular disease
Exclude significant carotid artery stenosis
Check for renal artery bruits
Check for evidence of volume depletion (jugular venous pressure, postural BP)
Check blood chemistry (Na^+, K^+, urea, creatinine)
Perform urinalysis (blood, protein)
If patient on $\geqslant 80$ mg of frusemide (or equivalent), reduce dose of diuretic by half 48–72 hours prior to introduction of ACE inhibitor, if possible
Withhold potassium supplements/potassium-conserving diuretics

ACE inhibitor later as preferred. First-dose hypotension, if symptomatic, can usually be corrected by head-down tilt (if tolerated) and by infusion of saline; angiotensin II is rarely needed. Atropine can be given for bradycardia. Once therapy has been successfully introduced, the dose can be increased to achieve maximum symptomatic benefit, though this is often delayed for weeks or months. Symptomatic hypotension and renal dysfunction are the main limiting factors to dose titration and must be checked for (see below).

Adverse effects

These are well known and some have already been mentioned. Side effects may be dose related; this is important as higher serum concentrations for any given dose may be obtained in the elderly. Hypotension is the most common adverse event. In practice, however, this is rarely troublesome. In SOLVD 7402 patients were given enalapril 2.5 mg b.d. for two to seven days and only 2.2% developed symptomatic hypotension.[7] Other large studies have confirmed these findings.[93, 100] Apart from hypotension, deterioration in renal function is the most commonly seen adverse effect, and patients with occult renovascular disease, hyponatraemia, diabetes mellitus and volume depletion are at increased risk. Though a high proportion of patients with severe heart failure will experience some increase in urea and creatinine when started on an ACE inhibitor, this is generally unimportant. In the SOLVD treatment arm urea rose by only 8.8 μmol/l and potassium by 0.2 mmol/l. In the two to seven-day run-in, only 0.2% of the 7402 patients treated with enalapril 2.5 mg b.d. were withdrawn because of worsening renal function. If a serious deterioration in renal function does occur, reduction in the dose of diuretic (if possible), ACE inhibitor or substitution of a shorter-acting ACE inhibitor (if appropriate) may help. Other adverse effects include taste disturbance, skin rash, proteinuria, leucopenia and angioedema; these are very uncommon. It has recently been suggested that dry cough is one of the most common ACE inhibitor adverse effects and that this association is not yet sufficiently recognized in clinical practice. In the V-HeFT II study, however, only 1%

of enalapril-treated patients and 1% of hydralazine–ISDN-treated patients had treatment withdrawn because of cough.[93]

CONVENTIONAL VASODILATORS

Nitrates

Nitrates cause vascular smooth muscle relaxation by increasing intracellular cyclic guanine monophosphate (cGMP). This effect is seen predominantly in the capacitance and pulmonary vessels, resulting acutely in a reduction in preload (though some reduction in arteriolar tone is seen). Up to half of patients with CHF are prescribed nitrates, though in many cases this may be for coexisting myocardial ischaemia. In CHF per se, the evidence of sustained symptomatic benefit and improvement in exercise tolerance with nitrates alone is equivocal. Currently nitrates can only be recommended in CHF when optimal doses of diuretics, digoxin and ACE inhibitors have failed to give adequate symptomatic control. Nitrates can, however, be used earlier for their anti-anginal properties where appropriate.

Of the two main oral nitrate preparations, ISDN undergoes presystemic metabolism with considerable inter-individual variability in the final plasma concentrations achieved, whereas isosorbide mononitrate (ISMN) does not. It has been suggested that the bioavailability of ISDN may be reduced by the hepatic congestion and reduction in liver blood flow that characterizes severe CHF. In contrast to ISDN, there is a predictable dose–response relationship of ISMN and the pharmacokinetics of this preparation are not affected by CHF. ISDN 20–40 mg t.d.s. or ISMN 10–40 mg t.d.s. (or once-daily slow-release ISMN) should initially be used in an asymmetrical dosing schedule to avoid tolerance. In the V-HeFT I and II studies (see below) ISDN was titrated to a daily dose of 160 mg.[7, 93, 100a, 101] Alternatively, transcutaneous glyceryl trinitrate 5–10 mg, which bypasses the portal circulation (i.e. enters the systemic circulation directly), can be given (remembering to remove the patch to allow a nitrate-free interval). This expensive form of therapy is probably only warranted where there is severe hepatic congestion. The side effects of nitrates are headache, flushing, hypotension and tachycardia.

Hydralazine

Hydralazine is a direct acting vasodilator with a predominantly arterial effect. There is little evidence that treatment with hydralazine alone leads to sustained symptomatic improvement in CHF and it is certainly not as effective as an ACE inhibitor.[90] Certain authorities feel that hydralazine is, however, a useful adjunct to conventional therapy (diuretic, ACE inhibitor, digoxin) in patients with resistant CHF, at least for haemodynamic stabilization. In these patients, larger than conventional doses may be needed (usually 300–600 mg and often up to 900 mg daily). Unfortunately hydralazine is not well tolerated: in the V-HeFT I study, 22% of patients discontinued treatment and only 55% were titrated to the predetermined target dose of 300 mg per day.[7] The most common side effects were headache, dizziness, nausea and vomiting. Rarely a lupus-like syndrome may develop and myocardial and cerebral ischaemia may be exacerbated (hydralazine is metabolized by acetylation in the liver at a rate that is genetically determined; fast acetylators may need a higher dose and slow acetylators are at greater risk of toxicity).

Hydralazine and ISDN in combination

Hydralazine and ISDN in combination cause 'balanced vasodilatation' (see Pathophysiology). This combination (up to 300 mg and 160 mg daily dose, respectively) was found to reduce mortality compared to placebo in patients with mild to moderate CHF.[7, 101] In the first Veterans Trial (V-HeFT I) first-year mortality was reduced from 19.5% to 12.1%. Though LVEF was increased there was no consistent increase in exercise tolerance. The results of the V-HeFT II study have recently been reported.[93] In this trial over 800 male patients were randomized to treatment with either hydralazine–ISDN or enalapril. Enalapril was associated with a better survival (mortality 9% at one year, 18% at two years, 31% at three years and 42% at four years compared to 13% at one year, 25% at two years, 36% at three years and 47% at four years, $p = 0.03$ for first and second year). Surprisingly, the combination of hydralazine–ISDN gave a greater improvement in exercise tolerance and LVEF than enalapril (the greater number of survivors in the enalapril group may have influenced these results). Treatment with hydralazine–ISDN was discontinued more often than that with enalapril (headache, palpitations and nasal congestion were more common with the former). Hydralazine–ISDN must, therefore, be considered only as an alternative for patients who cannot tolerate ACE inhibitors; there may, however, be merit in combining both forms of treatment, though this requires further study.

α-Adrenoceptor antagonists

It is widely held that while α-adrenoceptor antagonists may result in early improvement, they have no long-term efficacy, in terms of symptoms or prognosis, in CHF. Two studies, one old and one new, however, contradict this consensus (mostly derived from investigation of prazosin). Weber et al (1980) found trimazosin to be of benefit in CHF (improved symptoms and exercise capacity compared to placebo).[102] DiBianco et al (1991)[103] discovered doxazosin to be superior to placebo in a number of ways (rate of cardiac events, rate of hospitalization, ventricular arrhythmia suppression and improvement in daily activity measured by pedometry).

While the most generous conclusion might be that the jury is still out on α-antagonists, these agents, like the other conventional vasodilators, can only be recommended in the patient refractory to treatment with diuretics, digoxin and ACE inhibitors (indeed hydralazine and/or ISDN are to be preferred to α-antagonists).

ANTIARRHYTHMIC DRUGS

Symptomatic arrhythmias in CHF should obviously be treated. What of asymptomatic arrhythmias? Approximately 50% of patients with advanced CHF die suddenly. It is widely believed that most of these deaths are due to ventricular tachyarrhythmias, and up to half of patients with NYHA Class III/IV CHF have non-sustained ventricular tachycardia (VT) on ambulatory ECG monitoring; patients with ECG evidence of VT have a worse prognosis.[104] The apparently obvious link between the presence of ventricular arrhythmias and the occurrence of sudden death was, however, weakened by the Cardiac Arrhythmia Suppression Trial (CAST) study (and a subsequent overview of a number of other post-myocardial infarction (MI) studies).[105] Though CAST was a post-MI study, about half of the patients entered had an LVEF < 40%. In this study mortality was actually increased by treatment with the Class Ic antiarrhythmics flecainide and encainide. In the light of this finding, the use of antiarrhythmic drugs in CHF patients with asymptomatic ventricular arrhythmias has to be considered carefully.[104, 106] One antiarrhythmic, amiodarone, used carefully, appears safe and effective in CHF (interestingly this drug was also shown significantly to reduce the incidence of cardiac arrest and mortality in a post-MI population similar to that in CAST).[107] For these reasons, we do not believe the findings of CAST can be applied to all antiarrhythmic agents. We would thus consider using amiodarone in patients with very frequent complex ventricular premature beats (VPBs) and frequent non-sustained VT that is present despite correction of electrolyte disturbance, ischaemia, etc. This may result in surprising symptomatic benefit[108] and may also improve prognosis, though this still needs to be definitely shown (see below).[109]

Amiodarone

Amiodarone is a Class III antiarrhythmic agent with little or no negative inotropic effect (an almost unique property in this group of drugs). Amiodarone also has Class I activity, blocks β-adrenoreceptors, has peripheral vasodilator effects and exhibits anti-anginal properties.[109a] Amiodarone is slowly absorbed from the gastrointestinal tract and has a very long elimination half-life. A large loading dose (1200–1600 mg for one to two weeks) is

Table 4.8   Side effects of amiodarone

1.	Pulmonary	Pneumonitis
2.	Cardiac	Pro-arrhythmia
		Sinus node dysfunction
		AV nodal dysfunction
3.	Neuromuscular	Tremor
		Vivid dreams
		Gait ataxia
		Sensory/motor neuropathy
		Myopathy
4.	Cutaneous	Photosensitivity
		Blue-grey pigmentation
5.	Thyroid*	Hyperthyroidism
		Hypothyroidism
6.	Ocular	Corneal microdeposits
7.	Gastrointestinal	Nausea/vomiting/anorexia
		Elevated liver enzymes
8.	Other	Epididymitis

* The diagnosis of hyperthyroidism is difficult and should not be based on serum T_4 level. Clinical symptoms of weight loss etc. or recurrence of arrhythmias are important pointers. A high serum T_3 and flat TRH test are also useful.

A progressive fall in T_4 and rise in TSH point to the development of hypothyroidism.

required to achieve full steady-state drug effect as quickly as possible (and even then the effect may be delayed for hours if given intravenously, or days to weeks if given orally). The dose can be reduced to 600–800 mg per day for a further one to three weeks and then to 200–400 mg per day maintenance therapy. Amiodarone is extremely effective in abolishing/controlling both supraventricular (e.g. atrial fibrillation) and ventricular tachyarrhythmias. In patients with CHF, low-dose treatment (200 mg per day) has also been shown to increase LVEF and exercise tolerance.[108] In another study, amiodarone has been shown to reduce mortality in patients with CHF, though further confirmation of this effect is awaited.[109]

For these reasons, we use amiodarone in CHF for the control of symptomatic ventricular arrhythmias, for atrial fibrillation not controlled by digoxin, for angina not responding to conventional therapy and in patients with frequent non-sustained ventricular tachycardia not responding to optimization of anti-failure therapy and correction of electrolyte abnormalities.

Adverse effects

Apart from the general concern about the long-term efficacy of antiarrhythmic agents, there has been a particular concern over the specific adverse effects of amiodarone. These are listed in Table 4.8. The most common side effect reported is nausea, and the most serious side effect is pneumonitis.

Skin pigmentation, disturbance of liver enzymes and thyroid dysfunction are not uncommon. Photosensitivity can be countered with a high–UVB sun protection factor sunscreen. Most of these complications regress over weeks to months following drug withdrawal (though pneumonitis may require steroid treatment and can progress to pulmonary fibrosis). Chest radiographs, thyroid function tests and pulmonary function tests should be serially monitored.

Drug interactions

Amiodarone may also exert a pro-arrhythmic effect especially if given with other drugs that prolong the QT interval, e.g. Class IA antiarrhythmics (should be avoided in CHF), tricyclic antidepressants, phenothiazines, erythromycin and diuretics (causing electrolyte disturbances). Amiodarone increases warfarin effect and plasma digoxin concentration (reduce dose by approximately one-third and one-half, respectively). Amiodarone also interacts with drugs contraindicated in CHF such as sotalol and calcium antagonists.

INVESTIGATIONAL AGENTS

PHOSPHODIESTERASE INHIBITORS

These drugs act as inotropes and vasodilators (inodilators); their pharmacological effect is to inhibit breakdown of cyclic AMP.

Two agents in this class have been studied extensively.

Enoximone

In two single-centre studies, enoximone has been found to have similar effects to captopril on exercise tolerance in patients with moderate to severe CHF (no placebo control was included in these studies).[91, 94] Yet in two recently reported American multi-centre studies, enoximone was found to have no sustained benefit over placebo in similar groups of patients.[110, 111] In another carefully designed and conducted study, enoximone was found to significantly improve cardiac output, limb blood flow and exercise tolerance in patients with severe CHF uncontrolled by diuretics and captopril.[94] One American multi-centre study reported a significant excess of deaths in the enoximone group.[110] A recent UK multicentre mortality study showed enoximone significantly reduced survival in patients with severe CHF.

Milrinone

Milrinone was compared to digoxin withdrawal (placebo), continued digoxin and the combination of both drugs in a study of 230 patients with moderate to severe CHF (Milrinone Multicenter Trial Group).[76] Milrinone improved exercise tolerance to the same extent as digoxin but was not as effective as digoxin in other respects. Milrinone increased ventricular arrhythmias. The PROMISE (Prospective Randomized Milrinone Survival Evaluation) study has reported recently.[76a] In this trial 1088 patients with NYHA Class III/IV CHF treated with diuretics, digoxin and ACE inhibitors were randomized to milrinone or placebo. The study was discontinued prematurely because of a significant excess mortality in the milrinone group (intention to treat mortality 24% on placebo, 30% on milrinone; 'on treatment' mortality 19% on placebo and 25% on milrinone); the increase in mortality was most marked in Class IV patients.

Though not entirely consistent, the data on these two phosphodiesterase inhibitors do suggest there may be a beneficial effect on symptoms and exercise tolerance. The magnitude of this benefit is not greater than that of ACE inhibitors or even digoxin; importantly, however, enoximone at least can have benefit in addition to that of diuretics and ACE inhibitors. In contradistinction to conventional treatments milrinone and possibly enoximone appear to worsen mortality (a mortality study of the latter agent is currently under way). The ethics of prescribing a treatment that may improve the quality of life but reduce its quantity have yet to be fully considered.

FLOSEQUINAN

Flosequinan is currently described as a balanced vasodilator of unknown action. Flosequinan is superior to placebo in patients with mild, moderate and severe CHF, improving haemodynamics (including limb blood flow), symptoms, signs and exercise tolerance.[92, 112, 113] In another study, flosequinan was as efficacious as captopril in terms of exercise tolerance, though captopril was better tolerated.[92] At this stage, flosequinan appears a promising alternative to ACE inhibitors in CHF. A mortality study with flosequinan is planned. A study to investigate the possible advantage of adding flosequinan to ACE inhibitors will also be needed.

IBOPAMINE

Ibopamine is a dopaminergic agent. It represents a new approach in neuroendocrine modulation in CHF, i.e. augmentation of the concentration of an endogenous hormone believed to have beneficial effects (see also Neutral endopeptidase inhibitors). Ibopamine has vasodilator, inotropic and natriuretic effects in patients with CHF (though the latter are less marked than those of frusemide). It improves symptoms and signs and increases exercise capacity in patients with moderately severe CHF treated with diuretics and digoxin.[43] Ibopamine increases calf blood flow. In a comparative study, ibopamine has been found to be as efficacious as captopril. The preliminary data available on this drug make it an attractive therapeutic option in CHF, either as an alternative or an addition to ACE inhibitors, especially in mild CHF; ibopamine with its mild natriuretic activity might act as a diuretic sparing agent.

NEUTRAL ENDOPEPTIDASE (NEP) INHIBITORS

These agents inhibit the breakdown of the vasodilator–natriuretic peptide ANF (ANF also suppresses the RAAS and SNS). Two groups have reported favourable acute haemodynamic responses to these agents in CHF. Northridge et al[44] have also found that candoxatril (UK 79 300) has comparable natriuretic and diuretic effects to frusemide, a more favourable haemodynamic profile and preferable neuroendocrine effects (i.e. augmentation rather than reduction in ANF levels and no stimulation of the RAAS). The effects of candoxatril are sustained on chronic dosing for up to a month (unpublished data). Studies to evaluate the efficacy of candoxatril in terms of exercise tolerance are under way. NEP inhibitors may be an alternative to diuretics for patients with mild CHF and may also represent alternative or additional treatments to ACE inhibitors.

RENIN INHIBITORS

ACE is a non-specific metalloendopeptidase. Consequently ACE inhibition has effects other than blockade of angiotensin I to II conversion. ACE is identical to kininase, for example, and ACE inhibition may lead directly to an increase in kinin production and indirectly to an increase in prostaglandin production. These non-angiotensin effects of ACE inhibitors have been suggested to account for some of the side effects of ACE inhibitors such as cough and taste disturbance. This has led to the search for more specific RAAS inhibitors, such as inhibitors of the specific enzyme renin. Renin inhibitors may also display different tissue penetration profiles (relevant to 'tissue RAAS' inhibition) and may circumvent the angiotensin II/aldosterone 'escape' seen with chronic ACE inhibition. One peptide renin inhibitor, enalkiren, has been tested acutely in CHF.[114, 115] Enalkiren has predictable and favourable haemodynamic effects and, in a comparative study, these were similar to those seen with captopril.[115] Enalkiren has to be given intravenously but non-peptide orally active renin inhibitors (e.g. RO 42–5892 and CGP 38560A) are available and have shown promise in hypertension; to our knowledge, studies of these agents in CHF have not been reported.

ANGIOTENSIN II ANTAGONISTS

These agents have been developed even more recently than the renin inhibitors and for similar reasons. Angiotensin II receptor (receptor type 1,

AT_1) antagonists may thus have the advantages of specificity and may also exhibit different tissue penetration. These agents should also antagonize all angiotensin II, even that generated through non-ACE pathways. In addition, AT_1 antagonists have good oral bioavailability and are long acting, in contradistinction to renin inhibitors. The leading compounds in this area are DUP-753 and its active metabolite EXP3174. DUP-753 has a comparable blood pressure-lowering effect to enalapril in hypertensive subjects. Studies in CHF are under way.

WHERE TO TREAT CHF

There is recent evidence that 'heart failure clinics' with dedicated staff and special expertise may obtain better treatment results in CHF in terms of quality of life and survival.[116] The growing complexity of treatments available for CHF suggests that such clinics are a worthwhile development.

HOW TO TREAT CHF

Routine treatment

First, a precise diagnosis must be made. Valvular disease, major recurrent myocardial ischaemia, rhythm disturbances and diastolic dysfunction require specific therapies. Most patients, however, will have systolic dysfunction arising from coronary artery disease or dilated cardiomyopathy. In them, contributing factors such as anaemia, thyroid disease, hypertension, alcohol abuse, excessive intake of salt and fluids, drugs (e.g. negative inotropes and NSAIDs) and arrhythmias (e.g. atrial fibrillation) should be corrected where possible. Thereafter, initial drug therapy should be with a diuretic and an ACE inhibitor. For the mildly symptomatic patient, a thiazide diuretic may suffice. In the patient with pulmonary oedema, a loop diuretic is usually required. Normally frusemide will suffice, though in patients with recurrent gout, diabetes that is difficult to control, hearing impairment or allergic reactions to frusemide, bumetanide may be preferred. The initial dose of frusemide and bumetanide should be 40 mg and 1 mg, respectively. An ACE inhibitor should also be added at the time of commencing the diuretic, observing the contraindications and precautions alluded to above (if an ACE inhibitor is not tolerated, other vasodilators or digoxin may be given instead). The majority of patients will be controlled with this therapy. If the patient remains symptomatic, the dose of diuretic should be doubled (if there is renal impairment it may be trebled). Thereafter digoxin may be added (if not already given) and nitrates may be tried. Electrolytes should be monitored carefully, and it is our experience that hypokalaemia is often not prevented by concomitant use of an ACE inhibitor.

Digoxin and nitrates may be indicated at a much earlier stage for their ancillary properties, e.g. in patients with atrial fibrillation and myocardial ischaemia. Similarly, xamoterol may be used in patients with mild to moderate heart failure who also have angina or atrial fibrillation that is difficult to control with digoxin alone. ACE inhibitors should be the treatment of choice for hypertension in patients with heart failure. In patients with AF, or with evidence of atrial or ventricular thrombus, anticoagulation should be considered (some might broaden this recommendation).[116a]

Other measures

Where possible, regular exercise should be encouraged as this has been shown to be associated with an improved sense of well-being, more efficient cardiopulmonary performance and, possibly a better survival.[117, 118] Due to a relatively high rate of hospitalization for respiratory infection (4% in SOLVD), influenza and pneumococcal vaccinations are recommended. Attention to diet (avoid excess sodium intake and obesity) and alcohol intake have been mentioned. Care in co-prescribing cannot be over-emphasized. Smoking should be prohibited, not least because it has a vasoconstrictor effect in CHF.[119]

RESISTANT HEART FAILURE

This usually requires hospital admission. Careful reassessment of the original diagnosis and a further search for contributing factors is indicated. A 1.5-litre fluid restriction with careful monitoring of fluid balance and daily weight is employed. In the oedematous patient with tricuspid incompetence, a period of intravenous diuretic therapy is often helpful. Where renal function is normal or only moderately impaired a thiazide diuretic, such as bendrofluazide or chlorothiazide, can be added to therapy with a loop diuretic (e.g. after a ceiling dose of frusemide 120 mg b.d. or equivalent has been reached). If renal function is significantly impaired, metolazone can be used instead of a thiazide. With both these regimes, fluid-volume status and blood chemistry must be carefully followed. In rare cases, high-dose (1–4 g) intravenous frusemide (or bumetanide equivalent) may be required to initiate and maintain diuresis. Occasionally the patient with refractory oedema may diurese when spironolactone is added to an ACE inhibitor but this combination demands special monitoring of serum potassium.[73] In the oedematous, uraemic patient, dopamine 2.5–5 μg kg^{-1} min^{-1} can result in a dramatic diuresis. Occasionally ultrafiltration or haemofiltration may be required to correct very resistant fluid overload.

If a patient remains resistant to diuretics, ACE inhibition (if tolerated) and digoxin, a period of temporary intravenous inotropic or vasodilator therapy may be considered. Invasive haemodynamic monitoring is often useful as undertreatment (i.e. where pulmonary artery occlusion pressure

[PAOP] remains excessively high) and overtreatment (i.e. excessive reduction in PAOP) and cannot be accurately diagnosed clinically or by radiographic appearances in the patient with chronic severe heart failure.[10, 11]

Dobutamine may restore arterial pressure and thus be particularly useful in patients too hypotensive to benefit from treatment with an ACE inhibitor. Some units use the short-acting intravenous vasodilator sodium nitroprusside (SNP) to improve haemodynamics (the response to SNP may show what haemodynamic goals are achievable and whether there is undertreatment with oral vasodilators, i.e. should the dose be increased or another agent added?). The 'inodilators' enoximone and milrinone may also have a role in this situation, though there is relatively little experience with these agents. Because of their powerful vasodilator properties, they are best reserved for patients with raised filling pressures and a systolic arterial pressure $\geqslant 80$ mmHg.

With all of these measures, the majority of patients with CHF can be offered at least temporary remission.

INTRACTABLE CHF

Cardiac transplantation

Heart transplantation is an extremely effective treatment for advanced CHF. The difficulty is in knowing who to choose for this form of therapy.[120, 121] Donor organ supply currently falls far short of demand for surgery in most countries. Consequently all who could benefit cannot be considered for transplantation and some form of rationing has to be applied. Most cardiologists and transplant surgeons would agree that the basic criteria for transplantation are advanced (NYHA Class III and IV) CHF due to irreversible cardiac disease associated with an unacceptable quality of life and/or a very high risk of early mortality. A low LVEF

Table 4.9 Contraindications to cardiac transplantation

Advanced age
Fixed pulmonary hypertension (> 4 Wood units)
Poor renal function (GFR < 30 ml/min)
Parenchymal lung disease
Pulmonary infarction
Hepatic disease
Continuing peptic ulceration
Peripheral and cerebrovascular disease
Malignant disease
Insulin-treated diabetes mellitus
Other severe disease likely to limit rehabilitation
Drug or alcohol addiction
Severe psychiatric disease
Likely non-compliance with treatment

Table 4.10   Questions to be asked in apparently intractable CHF

---

1. Is CHF the correct explanation for deterioration (e.g. has lung cancer developed)?
2. Is there a role for conventional surgery (e.g. coronary artery bypass grafting, aneurysmectomy, pericardectomy)?
3. Is there *over*treatment (e.g. overdiuresis with uraemia and electrolyte disturbance or digoxin toxicity)?
4. Is there *under*treatment (e.g. is there any treatment that could be added or increased)?
5. Is there non-compliance (e.g. with drugs, diet, alcohol intake)?
6. Is there a co-prescribed or 'over-the-counter' medication with adverse effects?
7. Is there thyroid disease?
8. Is there infective endocarditis?
9. Is there pulmonary infection?
10. Is there inappropriate bradycardia (i.e. might pacing help)?
11. Is pulmonary thromboembolism occurring?

($< 15\%$), a low VO_2 ($< 14\,\mathrm{ml\,kg^{-1}\,min^{-1}}$) and a high PAOP/low cardiac index (CI) ($> 20\,\mathrm{mmHg}/ <2.5\,1\,\mathrm{min^{-1}\,m^{-2}}$) despite maximum medical therapy (see below) are predictive of a high mortality within a year. The stability of the patient's condition should also be considered. Stevenson has shown that patients with advanced stable CHF have less potential gain in terms of quality of life but more to gain in terms of prognosis; these patients form a relatively large population.[121] Patients with unstable, progressive advanced ('intractable') CHF are a smaller group who gain both in terms of quality of life and survival.[121] Because of donor organ limitation, most transplants are, therefore, performed in the latter group. Further rationing criteria are applied, most notably age (Table 4.9).

To diagnose intractable CHF and the need for transplantation, a 'checklist' of questions (Table 4.10) must first be considered.[120] Thereafter aggressive inotropic and vasodilator therapy monitored invasively[10–11a] and aimed at haemodynamic goals such as a PAOP of $\leqslant 15\,\mathrm{mmHg}$ and systemic vascular resistance (SVR) of $\leqslant 1200\,\mathrm{dynes\,s^{-1}\,cm^{-5}}$ has been advocated.[121] Patients who fail to respond (and apparently many will respond) to this treatment or those who respond but show subsequent instability (e.g. increasing fluid retention despite diuretic adjustment, worsening renal function, systolic blood pressure falling below 80 mmHg, falling serum sodium, frequent angina, recurrent dangerous arrhythmias) should be referred for transplantation unless there is a contraindication (Table 4.9).[120, 121]

In very specialized centres, some of these patients may require a period of temporary mechanical support until a donor organ becomes available.[122]

Alternatives to transplantation

Total artificial hearts and permanent implantable ventricular support devices continue to undergo evaluation in specialist centres.[122] Dynamic cardiomyoplasty has been reported to be of benefit in a number of small studies.[123] The long-term place of these therapies in ordinary practice has yet to be defined.

REFERENCES

1 McKee PA, Castelli WP, McNamara PM, Kannel WB. The natural history of congestive heart failure. N Engl J Med 1971; 285: 781–787

2 Teerlink JR, Goldhaber SZ, Pfeffer MA. An overview of contemporary etiologies of congestive heart failure. Am Heart J 1991; 121: 1852–1853

3 SOLVD Investigators. Studies of left ventricular dysfunction (SOLVD). Rationale, design and methods: two trials that evaluate the effects of enalapril in patients with reduced ejection fraction. Am J Cardiol 1990; 66: 315–322

4 Sutton GC. Epidemiologic aspects of heart failure. Am Heart J 1990; 120 (6 part 2): 1539–1540

5 Gillum RF. Heart failure in the United States 1970–1985. Am Heart J 1987; 113: 1043–1045

6 Ghali JK, Cooper R, Ford E. Trends in hospitalisation rates for heart failure in the United States, 1973–1986. Arch Int Med 1990; 150: 769–773

7 SOLVD Investigators. Effect of enalapril on survival in patients with reduced left ventricular ejection fractions and congestive heart failure. N Engl J Med 1991; 325: 293–302

7a Cohn JN, Archibald DG, Ziesche S et al. Effect of vasodilator therapy on mortality in chronic congestive heart failure. N Engl J Med 1986; 314: 1547–1552

8 Massie BM, Conway M. Survival of patients with congestive heart failure: past, present and future prospects. Circulation 1987; 75(Suppl IV): IV. 11–IV. 19

9 CONSENSUS Trial Study Group. Effects of enalapril on mortality in severe congestive heart failure. N Engl J Med 1987; 316: 1429–1435

10 Editorial. Clinical signs in heart failure. Lancet 1989; ii: 309–310

11 Stevenson LW, Perloff JK. The limited reliability of physical signs for estimating haemodynamics in chronic heart failure. JAMA 1989; 261: 884–888

11a Chakko S, Woska D, Martinez H et al. Clinical, radiographic and hemodynamic correlations in chronic congestive heart failure: conflicting results may lead to inappropriate care. Am J Med 1991; 90: 353–359

12 Remes J, Miettinen H, Reunanen A, Pyorala K. Validity of clinical diagnosis in primary health care. Eur Heart J 1991; 12: 315–321

13 Schreiber TL, Fisher J, Mangla A, Miller D. Severe 'silent' mitral regurgitation: a potentially reversible cause of refractory heart failure. Chest 1989; 96: 242–246

14 Editorial. Calcium antagonist caution. Lancet 1991; i: 885–886

15 Parmley WW. Pathophysiology and current therapy of congestive heart failure. J Am Coll Cardiol 1989; 18: 771–785

16 Francis GS, Cohn JN. Heart failure: mechanisms of cardiac and vascular dysfunction and the rationale for pharmacologic intervention. FASEB J 1990; 4: 3068–3075

17 Poole-Wilson PA. The management and treatment of chronic heart failure. In: Dawson AM, Besser GM, eds. Recent advances in medicine, no. 20. Edinburgh: Churchill Livingstone, 1987, pp 161–175

18 McMurray J, McLay J, Chopra M et al. Evidence for enhanced free radical activity in chronic congestive heart failure secondary to coronary artery disease. Am J Cardiol 1990; 65: 1261–1263

19 Braunwald E. 'The pathogenesis of congestive heart failure': then and now. Medicine 1991; 70: 68–81.

20 Schultheiss HP. Effect on the myocardial energy metabolism of angiotensin-converting enzyme inhibition in chronic heart failure. Am J Cardiol 1990; 65: 74G–81G

21 Buchwald A, Till H, Unterberg C, Oberschmidt R et al. Alterations in the mitochondrial respiratory chain in human dilated cardiomyopathy. Eur Heart J 1990; 11: 509–516

22 Hisatome I, Ishiko R, Miyakoda H et al. Excess purine degradation caused by an imbalance in the supply of adenosine triphosphate in patients with congestive heart failure. Br Heart J 1990; 64: 359–361

23 Stevenson LW, Brunken RC, Belil D et al. Afterload reduction with vasodilators and diuretics decreases mitral regurgitation during upright exercise in advanced heart failure. J Am Coll Cardiol 1990; 15: 174–180

24 Dean JW, Lab MJ. Arrhythmia in heart failure: role of mechanically induced changes in electrophysiology. Lancet 1989; i: 1309–1312

25 Cohn JN. Future directions in vasodilator therapy for heart failure. Am Heart J 1991; 121: 969–974

25a Herrlin B, Sylven C. Increased arterial oxygen content: an important compensatory mechanism in chronic moderate heart failure. Cardiovasc Res 1991; 25: 384–390

26 Sinoway L, Minotti J, Musch T et al. Enhanced metabolic vasodilation secondary to diuretic therapy in decompensated congestive heart failure secondary to coronary artery disease. Am J Cardiol 1987; 60: 107–111

27 Anand IS, Ferrari R, Kalra GS et al. Edema of cardiac origin, studies of body water and sodium, renal function, haemodynamic indexes and plasma hormones in untreated congestive heart failure. Circulation 1989; 80: 299–305

28 Ferguson DW, Berg WJ, Sanders JS, Kempf JS. Clinical and hemodynamic correlates of sympathetic nerve activity in normal humans and patients with heart failure: evidence from direct micro-neurographic recordings. J Am Coll Cardiol 1990; 16: 1125–1134

29 Remes J, Tikkanen I, Fyhrquist F, Pyorala K. Neuroendocrine activity in untreated heart failure. Br Heart J 1991; 65: 249–255

30 Cohn J, Levine TB, Olivari MT et al. Plasma norepinephrine as a guide to prognosis in patients with chronic congestive heart failure. N Engl J Med 1984; 311: 819–823

31 Cleland JGF, Dargie HJ, Ford I. Mortality in heart failure: clinical variables of prognostic value. Br Heart J 1987; 58: 572–582

32 Francis GS, Benedict C, Johnstone DE et al. Comparison of neuroendocrine activation in patients with left ventricular dysfunction with and without congestive heart failure: a substudy of the studies of left ventricular dysfunction (SOLVD). Circulation 1990; 82: 1724–1729

33 Swedberg K, Eneroth P, Kjekshus J, Wilhelmsen L. Hormones regulating cardiovascular function in patients with severe congestive heart failure and their relation to mortality. Circulation 1990; 82: 1730–1736

34 Maisel AS, Scott NA, Motulsky HJ et al. Elevation of plasma neuropeptide Y levels in congestive heart failure. Am J Med 1989; 86: 43–48

35 Anand IS, Ferrari R, Karla GS et al. Edema of cardiac origin: studies of body water and sodium, renal function, haemodynamic indexes, and plasma hormones in untreated congestive cardiac failure. Circulation 1989; 80: 299–305

36 McMurray J, Ray SG, Morton JJ, Dargie HJ. Endothelin may be a circulating vasoconstrictor in chronic heart failure. Br Heart J 1991; 66: 76

37 Kubo SH, Rector TS, Williams RE et al. Vasodilatation mediated by endothelial derived relaxing factor is reduced in patients with heart failure. Circulation 1990; 82 (Suppl III): 111-592

38 Gottlieb SS, Kukin ML, Ahern D, Packer M. Prognostic importance of atrial natriuretic peptide in patients with chronic heart failure. J Am Coll Cardiol 1989; 13: 1534–1539

39 Mukoyama M, Nakao K, Hosada K et al. Brain natriuretic peptide as a novel cardiac hormone in humans. J Clin Invest 1991; 87: 1402–1412

40 Kawashima S, Fukutake N, Nishian K et al. Elevated plasma beta-endorphin levels in patients with congestive heart failure. J Am Coll Cardiol 1991; 17: 53–58

41 Edvinsson L, Ekman R, Hedner P, Valdemarsson S. Congestive heart failure: involvement of perivascular peptides reflecting activity in sympathetic, parasympathetic and afferent fibres. Eur J Clin Invest 1990; 20: 85–89

42 McMurray J, Dargie HJ. Neurohumoral aspects of heart failure. Curr Opinion Cardiol 1989; 4: 355–359

43 Conderelli M, Bonaduce A, Montemurro A et al. The long term efficacy of ibopamine in treating patients with severe heart failure: a multicenter investigation. J Cardiovasc Pharmacol 1989; 14 (Suppl 8): 583–592

44 Northridge DB, Jardine A, Samuels GMR et al. Preliminary studies with a novel atriopeptidase inhibitor in animals, normal volunteers and heart failure patients. Lancet 1989; ii: 591–593

45 Goldsmith SR, Francis G, Cohn JN. Attenuation of the pressor response to intravenous furosemide by angiotensin converting enzyme inhibition in congestive heart failure.
46 Rea RF, Berg WJ. Abnormal baroreflex mechanisms in congestive heart failure: recent insights. Circulation 1990; 81: 2026–2027
47 Osterziel KJ, Dietz R, Schmid W et al. ACE inhibition improves vagal reactivity in patients with heart failure. Am Heart J 1990; 120: 1120–1129
48 Marin-Neto JA, Pintya AO, Gallo L, Maciel BC. Abnormal baroreflex control of heart rate in decompensated congestive heart failure and reversal after compensation. Am J Cardiol 1991; 67: 604–610
49 Cleland JGF, Dargie HJ, East BW et al. Total body and serum electrolyte composition in heart failure: the effects of captopril. Eur Heart J 1985; 6: 681–688
50 Sylven C, Hanssen E, Cederholm T et al. Skeletal muscle depressed calcium and phosphofructokinase in chronic heart failure and upregulated by captopril: a double blind placebo controlled study. J Int Med 1991; 229: 171–174
51 Gottlieb SS, Baruch L, Kukin ML et al. Prognostic importance of serum magnesium concentration in patients with congestive heart failure. J Am Coll Cardiol 1990; 16: 827–831
52 Dorup I, Skajaa K, Clausen T, Kheldsen K. Reduced concentrations of potassium, magnesium and sodium–potassium pumps in human skeletal muscle during treatment with diuretics. Br Med J 1988; 296: 455–458
53 Packer M, Lee WH, Yushak M, Medina N. Comparison of captopril and enalapril in patients with severe chronic heart failure. N Engl J Med 1986; 315: 847–853
54 Osterziel WJ, Dietz R, Mikulaschek K et al. Comparison of captopril with enalapril in the treatment of heart failure: influence on haemodynamics and renal function. Z Kardiol 1988; 77: 378–384
55 Packer M, Lee WH, Medina N, Yushak M. Influence of renal function on the hemodynamic and clinical responses to long term captopril therapy in severe chronic heart failure. Ann Int Med 1986; 104: 147–154
56 Deedwania PC. Angiotensin-converting enzyme inhibitors in congestive heart failure. Arch Intern Med 1990; 150: 1798–1805
57 Meissner MD, Wilson AR, Jessup M. Renal artery stenosis in heart failure. Am J Cardiol 1988; 62: 1307–1308
58 Cowley AJ, Rowley JM, Stainer K, Hampton JR. Effect of captopril on abnormalities of the peripheral circulation and respiratory function in patients with severe heart failure. Lancet 1984; ii: 1120–1124
59 Drexler H, Banhardt U, Meinertz T et al. Contrasting peripheral short-term and long-term effects of converting enzyme inhibition in patients with congestive heart failure: a double blind, placebo-controlled trial. Circulation 1989; 79: 491–502
60 Arnolda L, Conway M, Dolecki M et al. Skeletal muscle metabolism in heart failure: a ^{31}P nuclear magnetic resonance spectroscopy study of leg muscle. Clin Sci 1990; 79: 583–589
61 Mancini DM, Coyle E, Coggan A et al. Contribution of intrinsic skeletal muscle changes to ^{31}P NMR skeletal muscle metabolic abnormalities in patients with chronic heart failure. Circulation 1989; 80: 1338–1346
62 Sullivan MJ, Green Howard J, Cobb FR. Skeletal muscle biochemistry and histology in ambulatory patients with long-term heart failure. Circulation 1990; 81: 518–527
63 Morrison WL, Gibson TNA, Rennie MJ. Skeletal muscle and whole body protein turnover in cardiac cachexia: influence of branch chain amino acid administration. Eur J Clin Invest 1988; 18: 648–654
64 McMurray J, Abdullah I, Shaprio D, Dargie HJ. Tumour necrosis factor may contribute to development of 'cardiac cachexia'. Br Heart J 1991; 66: 77
65 Hammond MD, Bauer KA, Sharp JT, Rocha RD. Respiratory muscle strength in congestive heart failure. Chest 1990; 98: 1091–1094
66 Davies SW, Emery TM, Watling MIL et al. A critical threshold of exercise capacity in the ventilatory response to exercise in heart failure. Br Heart J 1991; 65: 179–183
67 Buller NP, Poole-Wilson PA. Mechanism of the increased ventilatory response to exercise in patients with chronic heart failure. Br Heart J 1990; 63: 281–283
68 Editorial. Cardiac asthma. Lancet 1990; i: 693–694
69 Richardson A, Bayliss J, Scriven AJ et al. Double blind comparison of captopril alone

against frusemide plus amiloride in mild heart failure. Lancet 1987; ii: 709–711

70 Anand IS, Karla GS, Ferrari R et al. Enalapril as initial and sole treatment in severe chronic heart failure with sodium retention. Int J Cardiol 1990; 28: 341–346

71 Ellison DH. The physiologic basis of diuretic synergism: its role in treating diuretic resistance. Ann Int Med 1991; 114: 886–894

72 Kiyingi A, Field MJ, Pansey CC et al. Metolazone in treatment of severe refractory congestive cardiac failure. Lancet 1990; i: 29–31

73 Ikram H, Webster MWI, Nicholls MG et al. Combined spironolactone and converting-enzyme inhibitor therapy for refractory heart failure. Aust NZ J Med 1986; 16: 61–63

74 Editorial. Digoxin: new answers, new questions. Lancet 1989; ii: 79–80

75 Ferguson DW, Berg WJ, Sanders JS et al. Sympathoinhibitory responses to digitalis glycosides in heart failure patients. Circulation 1989; 80: 65–77

76 DiBianco R, Shabetai R, Kostuk W et al. A comparison of oral milrinone, digoxin and their combination in the treatment of patients with chronic heart failure. N Engl J Med 1989; 320: 677–683

76a Packer M, Carver JR, Rodeheffer RJ et al for the PROMISE Study Research Group. Effect of oral milrinone on mortality in severe chronic heart failure. N Engl J Med 1991; 325: 1468–1475

77 Kromer EP, Elsner D, Riegger GAJ. Digoxin, converting enzyme inhibition and the combination in patients with congestive heart failure functional class II and sinus rhythm. J Cardiovasc Pharmacol 1990; 16: 9–14

77a Packer M, Gheorghiade M, Young JB et al. Randomised double blind placebo controlled withdrawal study of digoxin in patients with chronic heart failure treated with converting enzyme inhibitors. J Am Coll Cardiol 1992; 19 (Suppl): 260A

78 Mahdyoon H, Battilana G, Rosman H et al. The evolving pattern of digoxin intoxication: observations at a large urban hospital from 1980 to 1988. Am Heart J 1990; 120: 1189–1194

79 Editorial. Xamoterol: stabilising the cardiac beta receptor? Lancet 1988; ii: 1401–1402

80 Editorial. New evidence on xamoterol. Lancet 1990; ii: 24

81 Firth BG. The multifacetted role of angiotensin converting enzyme inhibitors in congestive heart failure. Am J Med Sci 1988; 296: 275–288

81a Stevenson RN, Keywood C, Amadi AA et al. Angiotensin converting enzyme inhibitors and magnesium conservation in patients with congestive cardiac failure. Br Heart J 1991; 66: 19–21

82 Nishimura H, Kubo S, Ueyama M et al. Peripheral hemodynamic effects of captopril in patients with congestive heart failure. Am Heart J 1989; 117: 100–105

83 Cohen-Solal A. Improving exercise tolerance in patients with chronic heart failure: should we treat the heart or the periphery? Eur Heart J 1989; 10: 866–871

84 Riegger GAJ. Effects of quinapril on exercise tolerance in patients with mild to moderate heart failure. Eur Heart J 1991; 12: 705–711

85 Newman TJ, Maskin CS, Dennick LG et al. Effects of captopril on survival in patients with heart failure. Am J Med 1988; 84 (Suppl 3A): 140–144

86 Fonarow G, Chelimsky-Fallick C, Stevenson LW et al. Impact of vasodilator regimen on sudden death in advanced heart failure: a randomized trial of angiotensin-converting enzyme inhibition and direct vasodilatation. J Am Coll Cardiol 1991; 17 (Suppl): 92A

87 Baur LHB, Schipperheyn JJ, Baan J et al. Influence of angiotensin converting enzyme inhibition on pump function and cardiac contractility in patients with congestive heart failure. Br Heart J 1991; 65: 137–142

88 Metcalfe M, Ford I, Dargie HJ. Contribution of perindopril in the treatment of congestive heart failure. JAMA (SEA) 1990; 6 (12): 23–28

89 Kleber FX, Niemoller L, Fischer M, Doering W. Influence of severity of heart failure on the efficacy of angiotensin-converting enzyme inhibition. Am J Cardiol 1991; 88 (Suppl D): 121D–126D

90 Schofield PM, Brooks NH, Lawrence GP et al. Which vasodilator drug in patients with chronic heart failure? A randomised comparison of captopril and hydralazine. Br J Clin Pharmacol 1991; 31: 25–32

91 Scriven AJI, Lipkin DP, Anand IS et al. Double-blind, randomised cross-over comparison of oral captopril and enoximone added to diuretic treatment in patients with severe heart failure. J Cardiovasc Pharmacol 1988; 11: 45–50

92 Cowley AJ. Efficacy of flosequinan in heart failure. Am Heart J 1991; 121: 983–988

93 Cohn JN, Johnson G, Ziesche S et al. A comparison of enalapril with hydralazine–isosorbide dinitrate in the treatment of chronic congestive heart failure. N Engl J Med 1991; 325: 303–310

94 Cowley AJ, Stainer K, Fullwood L et al. Effects of enoximone in patients with heart failure uncontrolled by captopril and diuretics. Int J Cardiol 1990; 28 (Suppl 1): S45–54

95 Cleland JGF, Henderson E, McLenachan J et al. Effect of captopril, an angiotensin-converting enzyme inhibitor, in patients with angina pectoris and heart failure. J Am Coll Cardiol 1991; 17: 733–739

96 Kirlin PC, Dansby C, Laird CK, Willis PW. Discrepancy between first-dose converting enzyme inhibition at rest and subsequent inhibition during exercise in chronic heart failure. Clin Pharmacol Ther 1988; 43: 616–622

97 Giles TD, Katz R, Sullivan JM et al. Short and long acting angiotensin converting enzyme inhibitors: a randomized trial of lisinopril versus captopril in the treatment of congestive heart failure. J Am Coll Cardiol 1989; 13: 1240–1247

98 Pouleur H, Rousseau MF, Ryden L. Angiotensin converting enzyme inhibition and mortality in heart failure: is enalapril better than captopril? Circulation 1990; 82 (Suppl III): III-675

99 McMurray J, Chopra M. Influence of ACE inhibitors on free radicals and reperfusion injury: pharmacological curiosity or therapeutic hope. Br J Clin Pharmacol 1991; 31: 373–379

100 Hasford J, Bussmann W-D, Delius W et al. First dose hypotension with enalapril and prazosin in congestive heart failure. Int J Cardiol 1991; 31: 287–294

100a Cohn JN. Nitrates are effective in the treatment of chronic congestive heart failure: the protagonists' view. Am J Cardiol 1990; 66: 444–446

101 Cohn JN. Statistical significance of veterans administration vasodilator heart failure trial results. Am J Cardiol 1990; 66: 1507–1509

102 Weber KT, Kinasewitz GT, West JS et al. Long term vasodilator therapy with trimazosin in chronic cardiac failure. N Engl J Med 1980; 303: 242–250

103 DiBianco R, Parker JO, Chakko S et al. Doxazosin for the treatment of chronic congestive heart failure: results of a randomised double-blind and placebo controlled study. Am Heart J 1991; 121: 372–380

104 Anderson JL. Should complex ventricular arrhythmias in patients with congestive heart failure be treated? A protagonist's viewpoint. Am J Cardiol 1990; 66: 447–450

105 Echt DS, Liebson PR, Mitchell LB et al. Mortality and morbidity in patients receiving encainide, flecainide or placebo. N Engl J Med 1991; 324: 781–788

106 Podrid PJ, Wilson JS. Should asymptomatic ventricular arrhythmia in patients with congestive heart failure be treated? An antagonist's viewpoint. Am J Cardiol 1990; 66: 451–456

107 Burkart F, Pfisterer M, Kiowski W et al. Effect of antiarrhythmic therapy on mortality in survivors of myocardial infarction with asymptomatic complex ventricular arrhythmias: Basel antiarrhythmic study of infarct survival (BASIS). J Am Coll Cardiol 1990; 16: 1711–1718

108 Hamer AWF, Arkles LB, Johns JA. Beneficial effects of low dose amiodarone in patients with congestive cardiac failure: a placebo controlled trial. J Am Coll Cardiol 1989; 14: 1768–1774

109 Dargie HJ, Cleland JG. Arrhythmias in heart failure: the role of amiodarone. Clin Cardiol 1988; 11 (Suppl): 1126–1130

109a Pelissier C, Legendre M, Delorme G et al. Antianginal effects of amiodarone: a randomised double blind comparison with long acting propranolol. Arch Mal Coeur 1990; 83: 1467–1473

110 Uretsky BF, Jessup M, Konstain MA et al. Multicenter trial of oral enoximone in patients with moderate to moderately severe congestive heart failure: lack of benefit compared with placebo. Circulation 1990; 82: 774–780

111 Narahara KA. Oral enoximone therapy in chronic heart failure: a placebo controlled randomized trial. Am Heart J 1991; 121: 1471–1479

112 Cowley AJ, Wynne RD, Stainer K et al. Flosequinan in heart failure: acute haemodynamic and longer term symptomatic effects. Br Med J 1988; 297: 169–173

113 Elborn JS, Stanford CF, Nicholls DP. Effect of flosequinan on exercise capacity and symptoms in severe heart failure. Br Heart J 1989; 61: 331–335

114 Neuberg GW, Kukin ML, Penn et al. Hemodynamic effects of renin inhibition by enalkiren in chronic congestive heart failure. Am J Cardiol 1991; 67: 63–66

115 Neubert GW, Kukin ML, Penn J et al. Renin inhibition (but not plasma renin activity) predicts the response to converting enzyme inhibitors in chronic heart failure. J Am Coll Cardiol 1990; 15: 172A

116 Hunn D, Pedersen WR, Beaker R et al. Benefits of attending a heart failure clinic. Circulation 1990; 82 (Suppl III): 111-609

116a Falk RH. A plea for a clinical trial of anticoagulation in dilated cardiomyopathy. Am J Cardiol 1990; 65: 914–915

117 Sullivan MJ, Higginbotham MB, Cobb FR. Exercise training in patients with severe left ventricular dysfunction, haemodynamic and metabolic effects. Circulation 1988; 78: 506–515

118 Coats AJS, Adamopoulos S, Meyer TE et al. Effects of physical training in chronic heart failure. Lancet 1990; i: 63–66

119 Nicolozakes AW, Binkley PF, Leier CV. Hemodynamic effects of smoking in congestive heart failure. Am J Med Sci 1988; 296: 377–380

120 Levine AB, Levine TB. Patient evaluation for cardiac transplantation. Prog Cardiovasc Dis 1991; 33: 219–228

121 Stevenson LW. Selection of therapy for patients with advanced heart failure: tailored afterload reduction or cardiac transplantation. In: Lewis BS, Kinchi A, eds. Heart failure: mechanisms and management. Berlin: Springer-Verlag, 1991, pp 448–461

122 Graham TR, Lewis CT. Artificial hearts: ventricular assist systems are the best option. Br Med J 1989; 298: 843–844

123 Editorial. Cardiac myoplasty with the latissimus dorsi muscle. Lancet 1991; i: 1383–1384

5

Electrocardiographic diagnosis of tachycardias

J. E. Creamer   D. J. Rowlands

INTRODUCTION

Although there had been many previous isolated clinical descriptions of tachycardias,[1] and some attempts at their interpretation by the use of arterial and venous pulsation traces,[2] accurate diagnostic descriptions have depended on their registration by electrocardiography. Virtually all of the clinically important arrhythmias were recorded by Einthoven using his string galvanometer and reported in his two papers on clinical electro-cardiography.[3, 4] Major contributions to the identification and explanation of atrial fibrillation and flutter from the electrocardiogram (ECG) and polygraph were made by Lewis[5] and further advances in the understanding of tachycardias followed after description of the conducting system of the heart.[6]

The advent of 12 lead electrocardiography allowed further refinements in the analysis of almost all tachycardias. The major limitation of static electrocardiography is that it depends critically upon the presence of the pathological tachycardia at the time of recording. Most tachycardias are intermittent and transient and it is not always possible to obtain a recording during an event. This has led to the development of prolonged and ambulatory monitoring of the electrocardiogram, event recorders and ECG telemetry. In certain cases it is also possible to provoke clinical tachycardias if they have a clearly defined relationship to specific manoeuvres, for example exercise.

Clinical intracardiac electrophysiological techniques have been perfected over the last two decades and have enabled the mechanisms of tachycardias to be studied in detail.[7, 8] This allows the most accurate diagnosis of tachycardias to be made with respect to both site of origin and mechanism, and is especially useful where there is doubt about the diagnosis from surface electrocardiographic records. Another benefit from these techniques is the ability to provoke tachycardias in order to study them at the investigator's convienience rather than having to wait for a spontaneous event to occur.

THE 12 LEAD ECG IN THE DIAGNOSIS OF TACHYCARDIA: BASIC PRINCIPLES

This review considers the role of the 12 lead ECG in the diagnosis of tachycardias. It is important to keep a number of basic principles in mind with respect to the conducting system of the heart and the influence of tachycardias on its behaviour.

1.   Myocardial tissue conducts cardiac impulses at a constant velocity irrespective of the coupling interval between successive beats, whereas the atrioventricular node exhibits decremental conduction. This means that as the coupling interval between successive beats is shortened so the conduction velocity of the impulses is reduced, and conduction time prolonged, progressively. At a certain limit (the 'Wenckebach point') beats are dropped. This has the effect of preventing atrioventricular conduction at excessively rapid rates. This phenomenon is not seen with impulses conducted via most atrioventricular accessory pathways, which behave like other myocardial structures.

2.   Impulses occurring almost simultaneously in different sites within the heart may interact with each other and produce 'fusion' complexes on the surface ECG.

3.   Impulses originating from outside the specialized conducting tissue may penetrate areas of pacemaker activity and reset the timing of spontaneous pacemaker depolarization. However, occasionally areas of spontaneously depolarizing cells are insulated against such penetration.

The P waves are the electrocardiographic manifestation of atrial myocardial depolarization. They provide information about the approximate site of origin of that depolarization (thus, for example, in lead II of the 12 lead ECG, which is effectively 'viewing' the heart from the left inferiorly, maximally positive P waves imply depolarization transmitted from upper right to lower left as in sinus node or adjacent atrially initiated beats, whereas negative P waves in II, III and AVF suggest atrial depolarization initiated inferiorly and travelling superiorly as in atrial rhythms originating from near the AV node. The QRS complexes are the electrocardiographic manifestation of ventricular myocardial depolarization. They give information about the site of initiation of that depolarization (e.g. narrow ($ \leqslant 0.10 $ s) QRS complexes indicate that the depolarization arises above the bifurcation of the His bundle, beats of ventricular origin with a right bundle branch block configuration usually arise within the left ventricle and those with a left bundle branch block configuration usually arise within the right ventricle (though it should be noted that this is not always so)). The morphology of the P waves and QRS complexes is most useful in providing information about the origin of atrial and ventricular activity respectively but it also provides information about the pattern of conduction within the relevant part of the myocardium (this is particularly true in relation to the QRS complexes). The rhythm of the heart may be defined as the ordered sequence of depolarization of the myocardium and of the pacemaker conducting tissue and, in so far as it can be determined from the 12 lead ECG, it is dependent upon the rate, regularity and morphology of the P waves and of the QRS complexes and of the time relations between the two. Repolarization (indicated in the ECG by the Ta wave, the S-T segment and the T wave) is irrelevant to rhythm analysis.[9]

TECHNIQUES OTHER THAN THE 12 LEAD ECG IN TACHYCARDIA DIAGNOSIS

Single lead ECGs

Tachyarrhythmias are most commonly noted and documented by single lead recordings taken in an intensive care area. While accurate rhythm diagnosis from a 12 lead recording can be difficult, from a single lead recording it is often impossible. Whenever the precise nature of an arrhythmia is less than crystal clear from a single channel recording (and in every case where a broad QRS complex tachycardia is being analysed) a 12 lead record of high quality should be taken. Neglect of this important principle will lead to a greater risk of mis-diagnosis. The only exception to this rule is in the presence of cardiac arrest, where a single lead monitor recording is often sufficient. Availability of a 12 lead ECG during tachycardia and a previous 12 lead recording during sinus rhythm greatly increases the chance of a successful rhythm diagnosis.

Physiological manoeuvres

Physiological manoeuvres combined with surface electrocardiographic monitoring may give further help.[10] For example, carotid sinus pressure may increase the degree of atrioventricular block and reveal an underlying atrial tachycardia whereas the same manoeuvre is likely to terminate a junctional tachycardia, which includes the atrioventricular node in the tachycardia circuit, and have no effect on a tachycardia arising from the ventricles. Valsalva manoeuvres may also affect tachycardias but the responses are more difficult to characterize in practice. Exercise testing is a useful method for inducing tachycardias for study and assessment of therapy in some cases (Fig. 5.1).[11] Response to antiarrhythmic drugs, especially adenosine, may also give information of diagnostic significance in conjunction with electrocardiographic recordings.

Ambulatory monitoring

Changes in P wave and QRS morphology and their relationship during tachycardia give the most information about the site of origin and mechan-

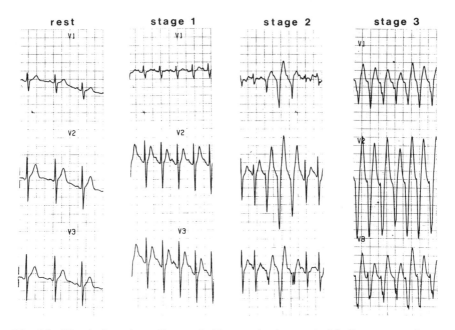

Fig. 5.1   Ventricular tachycardia provoked by exercise, in stage 3 of the Bruce protocol.

ism of tachycardias. However, temporal changes in rate of tachycardias, the mode of onset and cessation, and stability of rate may give additional information. These principles have been applied to the automatic tachycardia detection algorithms used in modern, sophisticated tachycardia termination devices.[12] Similarly, some evidence can be gained to distinguish so-called 'automatic' from re-entry type tachycardias.

Clinical electrophysiology

Currently this technique is the gold standard of rhythm diagnosis and is employed when surface electrocardiography fails to provide a conclusive diagnosis. Clinical electrophysiology employs multiple electrodes introduced percutaneously and positioned within the cavities of the heart and associated venous structures.[13] Using these electrodes electrocardiographic recordings can be made adjacent to the specialized conducting tissues and myocardium to plot accurately the patterns of excitation of the heart both in sinus rhythm and during tachycardias. The technique allows accurate visualization of atrial activity and its conduction pattern which is not always possible using the surface ECG during tachycardias. Patterns of activation and conduction can be explored and dynamic testing of physiological behaviour of various areas of interest within the heart can be performed using programmed electrical stimulation. Tachycardias can be induced and terminated by pacing methods which further helps in establishing the diagnosis as well as opening up therapeutic possibilities.

ELECTROCARDIOGRAPHIC FEATURES OF SPECIFIC TACHYCARDIAS

Tachycardias may originate from four broad areas of the heart: the sinus node, the atria, the junctional region or the ventricles (Table 5.1). Tachycardia circuits in the junctional tachycardias may be confined to the atrioventricular node or may include different combinations of atrioventricular bypass tracts and the bundle of His in various directions. These latter types also include segments of atrial and ventricular myocardium in the circuits.

Atrial tachyarrhythmias

Sinus tachycardia

There is usually no difficulty in recognizing sinus tachycardia, particularly if a 12 lead ECG is available. The rate is between 100 and 180 per minute (though for a resting patient the rate rarely exceeds 140), the P waves and QRS complexes have the morphology usual for that patient (e.g. if the patient has atrial hypertrophy or bundle branch block the P waves or QRS complexes show the appropriate abnormality consistently). The onset and cessation are usually gradual, occurring over several beats, and there may be slight variation in the rate with changes in body position, respiration or with time.

Table 5.1   Tachycardias: an anatomical classification

Sinus node tachycardias
    Sinus tachycardia (ST)
    SA nodal re-entrant tachycardia (SANRT)

Atrial tachyarrhythmias
    Atrial tachycardia (At.T)
    Atrial flutter   (At.Fl)
    Atrial fibrillation (At.Fib)

Junctional tachycardias
    Atrioventricular nodal re-entrant tachycardia (AVNRT)
    Atrioventricular re-entrant tachycardia (using bypass tracts) (AVRT)
    Coumel type of incessant tachycardia
    His bundle tachycardia
    Junctional tachycardias associated with nodoventricular pathways

Ventricular tachycardias (VT)
    Monomorphic ventricular tachycardia
    Multiple monomorphic tachycardia
    Polymorphic ventricular tachycardia
    Ventricular flutter

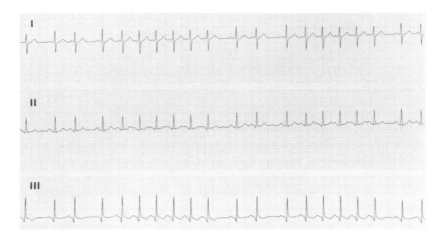

Fig. 5.2 Sinoatrial re-entrant tachycardia. Sinus beats are followed by either premature atrial beats or short bursts of tachycardia. The P wave morphology of these beats is identical to the sinus beats.

Sinoatrial nodal re-entrant tachycardia (SANRT)

In this rhythm the atrial impulses originate from the region of the sinus node.[14] The atrial activation pattern is normal and on a 12 lead ECG it may be impossible to distinguish from sinus tachycardia. In this case prolonged electrocardiographic monitoring may be helpful, showing a sudden onset with a premature beat or a sudden cessation (Fig. 5.2). If these features are not seen then the rate of tachycardia may be helpful since it hardly varies with time in the re-entrant tachycardia whereas there is usually a continual though gradual variation in rate in sinus tachycardia.

Atrial tachycardia

Atrial tachycardias arise from the atrial myocardium and may have a re-entrant basis[15] or may be due to abnormal automaticity.[16] The surface electrocardiographic features are that all QRS complexes are preceded by P waves and the P wave rate is faster than 100 beats per minute (usually 150 to 250 beats/min). The morphology of the P waves varies with the site of origin of the tachycardia but unless the site is very close to the sinoatrial node, the atrial activation pattern and, therefore, the P wave morphology is abnormal (Figs 5.3, 5.4).

Atrial tachycardia due to abnormal automaticity may be paroxysmal or incessant and may be difficult to distinguish from re-entrant tachycardia on the surface ECG. The P wave morphology is usually abnormal and may vary between beats.

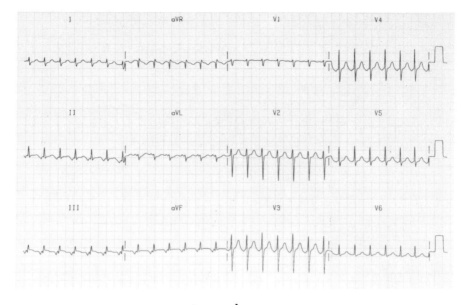

A

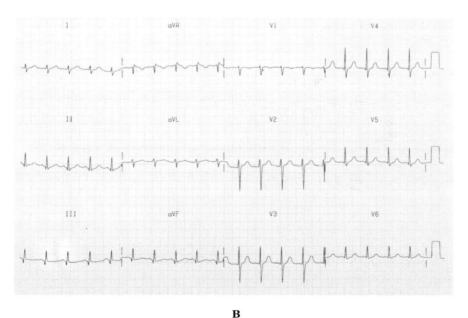

B

Fig. 5.3 **A** Atrial tachycardia. Note the abnormal P waves preceding each QRS complex with a short PR interval. **B** After flecainide, there is sinus tachycardia. Note the normal P wave morphology and normal PR interval.

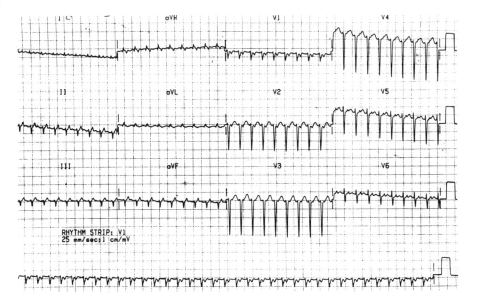

Fig. 5.4 Atrial tachycardia. In this example the PR interval is prolonged (though within normal limits) and the rate of the tachycardia is such that the abnormal P wave occurs close to the preceding QRS complex. It is difficult to distinguish from atrioventricular re-entrant tachycardia using a bypass tract. However, the P waves are positive in leads I, II, III, aVF and V6 but negative in aVR, aVL and V1, suggesting they originate at a site distant from the atrioventricular junction.

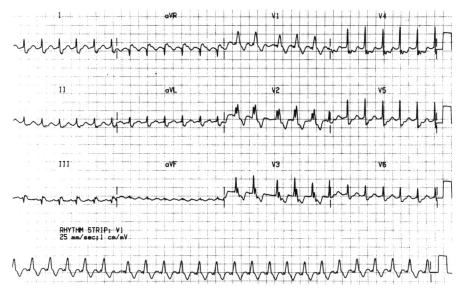

Fig. 5.5 Atrial flutter with 2:1 atrioventricular block and right bundle branch block. The diagnosis is confirmed by transient 3:1 block seen after the second QRS complex in leads V1, V2 and V3.

Atrial flutter

Atrial flutter should not be mistaken for atrial fibrillation in spite of the apparent similarity of their surface ECGs. Atrial flutter has been shown to be due to a macro re-entrant circuit in the atrium[17, 18, 19] whereas atrial fibrillation is probably due to multiple and changing micro re-entry circuits and results in completely disorganized atrial activity on intracardiac recording. The former, on the other hand shows regular atrial activity usually seen as flutter ('F') waves on at least one lead of the surface ECG. The atrial rate of atrial flutter is characteristically close to 300 beats/min, and, as few atrioventricular nodes are capable of conducting impulses at this rate at rest, is usually conducted with at least 2:1 atrioventricular block giving the characteristic ventricular rate of 150 beats/min (Figs 5.5, 5.6). Occasionally, the degree of atrioventricular block varies; usually in a fixed ratio but occasionally it may be so variable as to mimic atrial fibrillation. Atrial flutter may co-exist with, and degenerate into, atrial fibrillation. In patients with ventricular pre-excitation the ventricular response may be 1:1 at a rate of 300 beats/min and may progress to, and be indistinguishable from, ventricular flutter.

Atrial fibrillation

The typical electrocardiographic appearance of atrial fibrillation is of an irregular baseline with no recognizable discrete P wave activity and a completely irregular ventricular response. Occasionally the fibrillation may

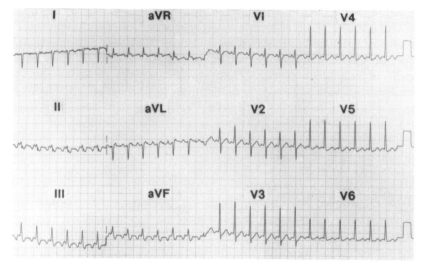

Fig. 5.6 Atrial flutter with 2:1 atrioventricular block. Note that it could easily be mistaken for sinus tachycardia if lead V1 alone was recorded. The flutter waves are more obvious in leads II, III and aVF.

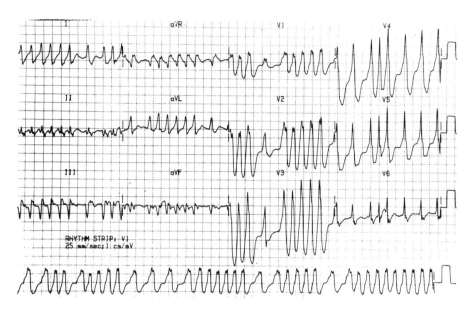

Fig. 5.7   Atrial fibrillation with pre-excitation in the Wolff–Parkinson–White syndrome. In any one lead the QRS complexes have the same basic shape, though with varying degrees of pre-excitation, but the *rate* is completely irregular.

be so fine as to lead to the appearance of absent atrial activity in all leads. In this case the second feature (a completely irregular ventricular rate) usually allows accurate diagnosis. This is so even when the complexes are abnormal, either due to bundle branch block or pre-excitation, though the rate will often be much faster in the latter case because the braking effect of the atrioventricular node is bypassed (Fig. 5.7). Usually, in atrial fibrillation, the QRS complexes are narrow ($\leqslant 0.10$ s) but if there is pre-existing bundle branch block or concurrent ventricular pre-excitation the QRS complexes may all be broad. It is common to find occasional QRS complexes which are broad ($\leqslant 0.14$ s) in a recording with otherwise normal QRS complexes. This is usually due to aberrant intraventricular conduction. It will probably occur at the end of a short R-R interval which has followed a long R-R interval.[20]

Junctional tachycardias

Junctional tachycardias are those which include junctional structures (atrioventricular node, His bundle, anomalous atrioventricular connections) as integral components of the tachycardia circuit. They are commonly mislabelled 'supraventricular' though, with the possible exception of some intra-atrioventricular nodal tachycardias, they also incorporate atrial and/or ventricular myocardium in the tachycardia circuit. The potential

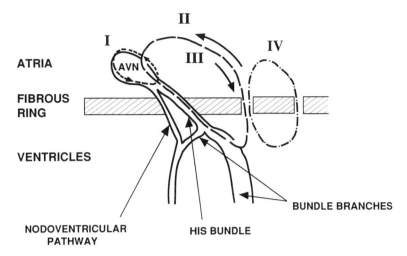

Fig. 5.8 Junctional tachycardia circuits. AVN = atrioventricular node; I = atrioventricular nodal re-entry circuit; II = orthodromic atrioventricular re-entry circuit via direct anomalous pathway and AVN/His bundle; III = antidromic circuit using the same pathways as II; IV = duodromic circuit using two direct anomalous atrioventricular connections. Note that the nodoventricular pathway may potentially be involved in these tachycardia circuits, or may act as a 'bystander' for atrioventricular conduction in circuit I.

tachycardia circuits are outlined in Figure 5.8. The QRS complex morphology may be normal and 'narrow', or may be 'wide', showing bundle branch block patterns or pre-excitation. In these latter cases the distinction from ventricular tachycardia is essential.

Atrioventricular nodal re-entrant tachycardia (AVNRT)

In these tachycardias the re-entrant circuit is located within the atrioventricular node (and also in the adjacent myocardium)[21, 22] (Circuit I, Fig. 5.8). Dual physiological conduction pathways can usually be demonstrated within the node. In the commonest type anterograde conduction through the node is via the slower pathway. Conduction of the impulse down the slow AV nodal pathway is followed by a ventricular depolarization via the His bundle (a fast pathway) and retrograde atrial depolarization via the fast AV nodal pathway so that atrial and ventricular depolarizations are virtually synchronous. As a result of this the P wave is usually buried within the QRS complex on the surface ECG. The P waves may occasionally be identified as negative deflections within the QRS complexes in leads II, III and aVF, especially when compared to the QRS morphology in these leads during sinus rhythm (Fig. 5.9). If the onset of the tachycardia is recorded it can be seen to be initiated usually by an atrial premature beat which conducts to the ventricles with a significantly prolonged PR interval, indicating conduction block in the fast pathway and conduction down the

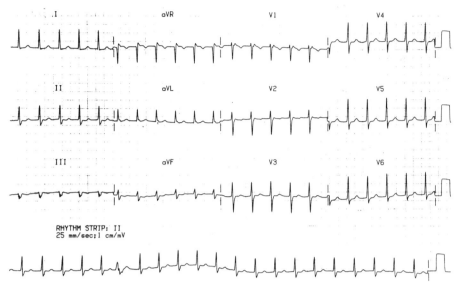

Fig. 5.9 Atrioventricular nodal re-entry tachycardia (AVNRT). Note the negative (retrograde) P waves located *within the QRS complexes* in leads II, III and aVF.

slow pathway. This interval is usually longer than the tachycardia cycle length either because of the decremental conduction properties of atrioventricular nodal tissue or the presence of multiple pathways. Cessation of the tachycardia is usually also abrupt, and may be caused by an atrial or ventricular premature beat or by transient changes in the electrophysiological properties of the components of the circuit.

A rare atypical form of this tachycardia uses the fast pathway in the anterograde direction and the slow pathway in the retrograde direction (the so-called 'fast slow' AV nodal re-entrant tachycardia). The surface ECG, electrophysiological features and repetitive and incessant behaviour mimics the long R-P' tachycardias using bypass tracts (see below).[23]

Atrioventricular re-entrant tachycardia (AVRT) using bypass tracts

The commonest form of tachycardia of this type involves a re-entrant circuit utilizing the AV node, an anomalous myocardial pathway connecting atrium and ventricle (which may either be overt, as in the Wolff–Parkinson–White syndrome,[24] or concealed[25]), and the intervening areas of atrial and ventricular myocardium.

In *orthodromic reciprocating tachycardia* (circuit II, Fig. 5.8) the re-entrant circuit involves antegrade conduction through the AV node (slowly conducting) and retrograde conduction via the accessory pathway (rapidly conducting). This gives rise to normal (narrow) QRS complexes (Fig. 5.10). Because the impulse has to travel via ventricular myocardium to gain

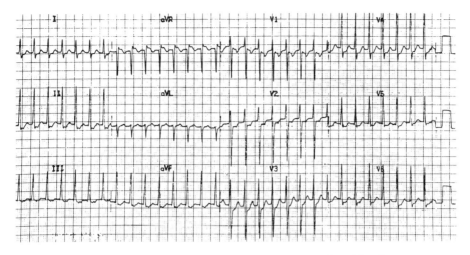

Fig. 5.10 Orthodromic atrioventricular re-entry tachycardia (AVRT). Here P waves are visible *within the ST segment*, best seen in leads II, III, and aVF.

access to the distal end of the accessory pathway before returning to the atria, the retrograde depolarization of the atria is delayed (despite rapid conduction through the accessory pathway) and the P waves occur well after the QRS complexes, usually during the early part of the ST-T segment. The morphology of the P waves during tachycardia varies with the location of the accessory pathway, being negative in those leads closest to the pathway (Fig. 5.11).

A less common form of AVRT is *antidromic reciprocating tachycardia* (circuit III, Fig. 5.8) in which retrograde conduction occurs via the atrio-ventricular node and antegrade conduction via the accessory pathway (Fig. 5.12). Because of the latter the QRS complexes are broad and abnormal (the ventricles are pre-excited). The difficult distinction in this case is from ventricular tachycardia. P waves may well be visible after the QRS complexes (and certainly one would expect atrial depolarization to occur well after the ventricular depolarization, partly because of the need for the re-entrant circuit to pass through the area of ventricular myocardium between the accessory pathway and the AV node and also because of slow retrograde conduction through the AV node) but this does not help in the diagnostic process since 1:1 ventriculoatrial conduction can infrequently occur in association with ventricular tachycardia. If a 12 lead ECG in sinus rhythm (taken before the onset of the tachycardia) is available and if this shows ventricular pre-excitation (i.e. if the pathway is revealed) then identical morphology of the QRS complexes during sinus rhythm with ventricular pre-excitation and during broad QRS complex tachycardia would strongly support the diagnosis of antidromic reciprocating atrioventricular tachy-cardia but would not, of course, prove it since there is no reason why

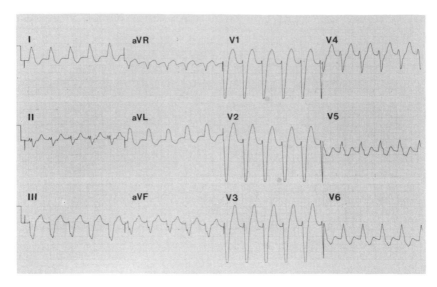

Fig. 5.11   Orthodromic atrioventricular re-entry tacycardia with left bundle branch block. Note that the P waves are negative in leads V5 and V6 and positive in leads III, aVR, V1 and V2 confirming that retrograde conduction is via a left lateral anomalous atrioventricular pathway. That this pathway is the site of retrograde conduction is also supported by the relatively slow rate of the tachycardia in the presence of left bundle branch block (compare with Fig. 5.10).

tachycardia of ventricular origin should not have very similar QRS morphological characteristics. The availability of a full 12 lead ECG recording during tachycardia and an identical recording during sinus rhythm would, however, be particularly important in the case of a diagnostic dilemma such as this.

Although the QRS complexes are usually normal in the cases of orthodromic reciprocating tachycardia there is, of course, no reason why there should not also be bundle branch block in such cases (Fig. 5.11) and this would, again, give rise to one of those situations of broad QRS complex tachycardia where the precise rhythm diagnosis might prove to be very difficult.

The morphology of the P wave during tachycardia may give some idea of the location of the bypass tract. The P waves are negative in those leads closest to the pathway. Further information about the location of the accessory pathway may occasionally be obtained when bundle branch block occurs fortuitously during tachycardia.[26, 27] If the ECG recording includes two or more beats of the tachycardia before the onset of bundle branch block and two or more beats of tachycardia after the onset of bundle branch block and if the cycle length prolongs with the onset of bundle branch block then one can conclude that the accessory pathway is on the same side as the bundle branch affected (Fig. 5.11). For example, if right bundle branch block occurs during tachycardia using a right-sided accessory pathway the

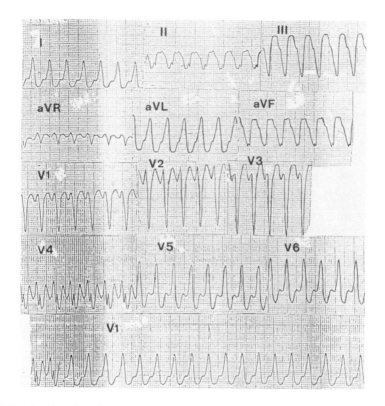

Fig. 5.12   Antidromic atrioventricular re-entrant tachycardia. The pre-excitation pattern, i.e. delta wave negative in II, III, aVF and V1, and positive in I, aVL, V5 and V6, suggests a right-sided accessory pathway. On the evidence of this one recording it is not possible, with certainty, to exclude ventricular tachycardia.

tachycardia cycle length would prolong slightly. The same would not occur in a tachycardia using a right-sided accessory pathway if left bundle branch block developed.

It is by no means always possible to determine the mechanism of a broad QRS complex tachycardia (see below) and invasive studies may be of benefit by allowing confident identification and mapping of the atrial activation pattern. The tachycardia may be further investigated by programmed electrical stimulation, whereby critically timed atrial and ventricular extra stimuli are used to reset and to terminate it.

More rarely these tachycardias may involve multiple pathways where many potential tachycardia circuits may occur. Tachycardias using bypass tracts for both the anterograde and retrograde limbs of the circuit are known as duodromic (circuit IV, Fig. 5.8) and are not easily diagnosed from the surface ECG.[28] Invasive studies are necessary to diagnose accurately their presence and the precise circuits involved.

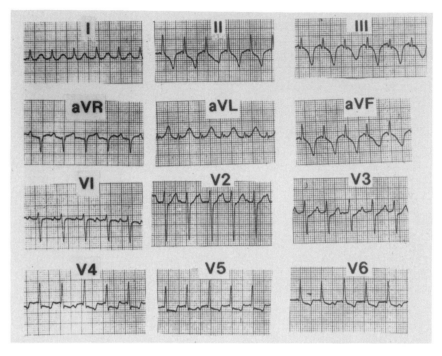

Fig. 5.13 Long R-P′ tachycardia. Note the pronounced retrograde P waves occurring just over halfway between successive QRS complexes. These tachycardias are often incessant.

The Coumel type of incessant tachycardia

Another rare form of atrioventricular re-entrant tachycardia using a bypass tract is the 'long R-P′ tachycardia of Coumel'.[23, 29] Here, as the name implies, retrograde conduction is via a slowly conducting pathway and the P waves therefore appear much later between successive QRS complexes, often at or around the mid point. The P waves are usually negative in the inferior leads. Because of the slow conduction in both limbs of the circuit these tachycardias have a wide initiation 'window' and are difficult to terminate. They therefore present as incessant tachycardia (Fig. 5.13).

Focal His bundle tachycardias

Also known as junctional ectopic tachycardia, this tachycardia occurs in children, and is thought to arise from an ectopic focus in the lower part of the atrioventricular node or His bundle.[30] The tachycardias are rapid and often incessant and resistant to drug treatment. QRS morphology is normal and there is often atrioventricular dissociation (giving rise to independent P waves and occasional capture beats).

Junctional tachycardias associated with nodoventricular pathways

Tachycardias may occur in patients with accessory pathways connecting the atrioventricular node with the ventricular myocardium,[31] usually the right ventricular septum, bypassing the bundle of His and producing a 'left bundle branch block' pattern of QRS complex morphology. It is not usually possible, from the surface ECG, to distinguish whether the pathway forms part of the tachycardia circuit or is acting as a 'bystander' in the presence of an atrioventricular nodal re-entry tachycardia.

Intracardiac studies may be necessary for the diagnosis of junctional tachycardias when P wave activity cannot readily be identified and empirical drug therapy has been unsuccessful, when they cannot otherwise be distinguished from ventricular tachycardia, or when the precise mechanism and anatomical localization of the tachycardia circuit is necessary for ablative therapy.

Ventricular tachycardias

The key feature in ventricular tachycardias is that the QRS complexes are abnormally wide and abnormally shaped. Almost any QRS configuration may occur but there are a number of characteristic patterns as indicated later.

The most common forms of ventricular tachycardia are those arising in the myocardium (usually in the subendocardial region) as a result of previous myocardial infarction. These have wider QRS complexes ($\geqslant 0.14$ s) with bizarre morphology as often seen with ventricular premature beats, because the impulses are conducted relatively slowly through the ventricular myocardium. Less common forms of ventricular tachycardia arise from the bundle branches and, as they occur in the specialized conducting tissue so that conduction is via the rapidly conducting pathways usually employed by sinus beats (albeit in a different direction), the QRS complexes are only marginally prolonged (i.e. 0.10 to 0.14 s) and often have a recognizable bundle branch block pattern. These tachycardias are also sensitive to calcium channel blockers, unlike the intramyocardial types.[32]

Atrial activation may occur in the retrograde direction via the His bundle and atrioventricular node or via accessory pathways when they happen to be present. The conduction may be 1:1 or may exhibit varying degrees of Wenckebach periodicity but most frequently there is complete ventriculoatrial dissociation. When this latter feature occurs the surface electrocardiogram shows P wave activity which is independent of the QRS complexes. Occasionally there may be 'capture beats' where a sinus beat occurs sufficiently early that the ventricular activation proceeds via the specialized conducting tissue but does not abolish the tachycardia circuit. This appears as a QRS complex of normal morphology occurring in the

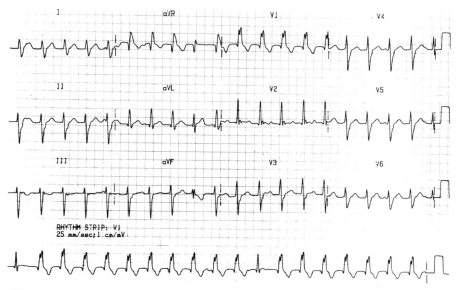

Fig. 5.14 Fascicular tachycardia, showing right bundle branch block morphology and left axis deviation (mean frontal QRS axis, −75°), with independent P wave activity and capture beats.

midst of the tachycardia (Fig. 5.14). If the sinus beat occurs a fraction of a second later the normally conducted beat and abnormal tachycardia beat occur simultaneously producing a fusion beat (Fig. 5.14) with morphology intermediate between normal sinus beats and tachycardia beats. The occurrence of the phenomena of capture beats and fusion beats is probably responsible for the slight variability of rate which is said to be characteristic of ventricular tachycardia.

The precise morphology of the tachycardia from the surface 12 lead ECG gives information about the localization of microscopic tachycardia circuits and the conduction pathway of macro re-entrant tachycardia circuits.[33] In the case of recurrent ventricular tachycardia this information is vital if ablative therapy is contemplated. Basic 12 lead ECGs are the templates for judging and localizing clinical tachycardias for this purpose, and should therefore be obtained in all cases before emergency reversion therapy is employed, except in the presence of cardiac arrest with loss of consciousness. If the patient is conscious an ECG should be recorded before giving anti-arrhythmic drugs or while arranging appropriate anaesthesia for DC cardioversion.

Monomorphic and multiple monomorphic tachycardia

These tachycardias usually have a fixed anatomical/physiological substrate and present with a monomorphic pattern (i.e. consecutive QRS complexes have the same shape). Occasionally, there may be recurrent episodes in

Table 5.2   Diagnostic features of ventricular
tachycardia

---

1. QRS duration > 140 ms
2. QRS axis − 30° to 180°
3. Specific QRS morphology
      R > R' in V1
      rS in V6
      Concordant patterns in precordial leads
4. Atrioventricular dissociation
      Independent P wave activity
      Fusion beats
      Capture beats

---

which, although a single pattern is present with each episode, separate
episodes may be associated with differing ventricular rates and QRS
morphologies (Fig. 5.15). These are the so-called multiple monomorphic
tachycardias and they represent different sites of origin or different tachycardia circuits. If these are suspected it is important to document all the
different types for the purposes of ensuring adequate treatment and monitoring of that treatment.

Numerous criteria have been presented for distinguishing monomorphic
ventricular tachycardia from other broad QRS complex tachycardias
(Table 5.2)[13] (i.e. for many of the atrial and junctional tachycardias listed in
Table 5.1 which occur in association with functional bundle branch block,
pre-exising bundle branch block or ventricular pre-excitation) and clinical
algorithms have been proposed for practical use.[34] If capture beats are seen
or if there are fusion beats or if the QRS rate is consistently greater than the
P wave rate then the rhythm is certainly ventricular tachycardia. If the QRS
duration is 0.14 s or more and it is known that a very recent record taken
during a supraventricular rhythm has a QRS duration of 0.10 s or less then
the rhythm is likely to be ventricular tachycardia although antidromic
tachycardia remains a possibility. If a previous record is available in which
the rhythm is clearly supraventricular but in which ventricular ectopic
beats are seen which have a QRS morphology identical in all 12 leads with
the QRS complexes seen during wide QRS complex tachycardia then the
rhythm is almost certainly ventricular tachycardia. If a previous record is
available in which the rhythm is unequivocally supraventricular and the
QRS complexes are identical in shape and dimensions to those seen in the
wide QRS complex tachycardia (in all 12 leads) then the rhythm is likely to
be supraventricular with a pre-existing intraventricular conduction abnormality. If the P waves can be recognized and there is evidence of atrioventricular dissociation then the rhythm is ventricular. Finally there are
various patterns of the QRS complexes in the precordial leads which
suggest the probability of (but do not prove the existence of) ventricular
tachycardia. These include Rs, Rr or QR in V1 and R, RS, QS and QR
configuration in V6.

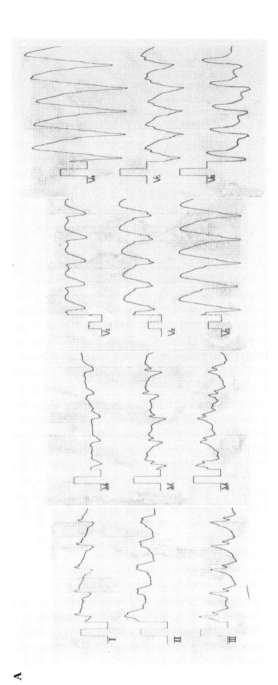

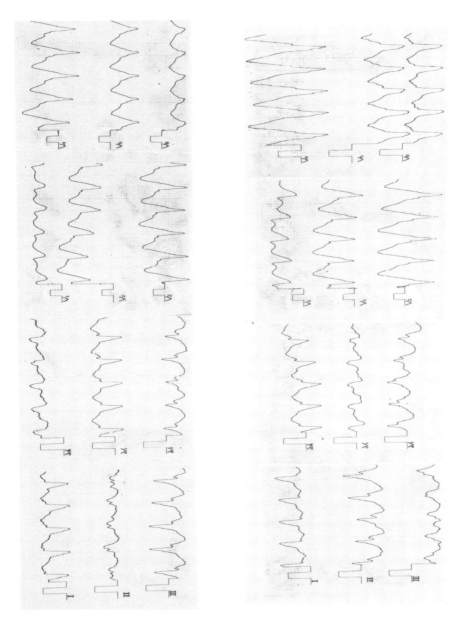

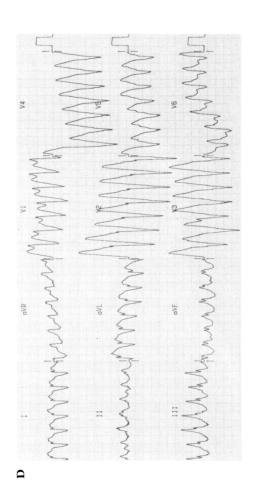

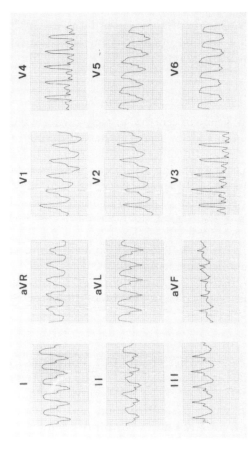

Fig. 5.15 Multiple monomorphic ventricular tachycardia. Five different episodes of ventricular tachycardia in one patient. **A, B** Left bundle branch block pattern, rates 178 and 165 respectively, mean frontal QRS $^+$105° and $^+$135°. **C, D** Concordant negative QRS complexes in precordial leads, rates 145 and 152, and mean frontal QRS axis $^+$105° and $^+$75° respectively. **E** Right bundle branch block pattern, rate 182, and mean frontal QRS axis $^+$150°. Each of these tachycardias was mapped during electrophysiologic study and found to originate from a different discrete area in the right or left ventricle.

The criteria for distinguishing monomorphic ventricular tachycardia from other broad QRS complex tachycardias have been evaluated recently.[35] Of the electrocardiographic criteria the most useful in practice, when present, are the various manifestations of atrioventricular dissociation. However, the single most highly correlated feature in the diagnosis of ventricular tachycardia is the history of a previous myocardial infarction!

Invasive studies are useful in ventricular tachycardia and should be considered in many cases, not only to confirm the ventricular origin but also to assess the inducibility of the arrhythmia in order to assess the effects of treatment and for precise location of the circuit (or its exit site into the myocardium) to guide ablative therapy.

Polymorphic ventricular tachycardia

This forms another major group of ventricular tachycardia in which successive QRS complexes within a given lead may have differing morphology. Often the morphology varies with subsequent beats in such a way that the QRS complexes appear to be rotating around the baseline, the so-called 'torsades des pointes' (Fig. 5.16). These tachycardias typically occur in the presence of marked prolongation of the QT interval caused either by profound electrolyte abnormalities, or the administration of drugs (anti-arrhythmic drugs, psychotrophic drugs, etc.), and in the inherited 'long QT syndromes' (Jervell–Lange–Neilsen and Romano–Ward syndromes). These tachycardias do not have an identifiable fixed anatomic substrate but may represent multiple changing re-entrant circuits. There is usually little doubt about their diagnosis even on a single lead of the ECG.

Ventricular flutter

This appears on the surface ECG as broad QRS complex tachycardia at a rate of approximately 300 beats/min (Fig. 5.17). It usually produces cardiovascular collapse and often degenerates into ventricular fibrillation. An analogy may be drawn with atrial fibrillation and flutter. The major differential diagnosis is from atrial flutter with pre-excitation. This is, in fact, academic at the time of presentation since the haemodynamic consequences (catastrophic if not immediately dealt with) and the management (immediate DC cardioversion) are identical. The distinction is usually made in retrospect (if at all!).

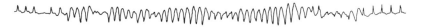

Fig. 5.16   Polymorphic ventricular tachycardia showing 'torsades des pointes' which can be easily diagnosed from a single lead. Note that unlike pre-excited atrial fibrillation (Fig. 5.7) the ventricular rate varies only slightly but the morphology varies significantly with successive beats.

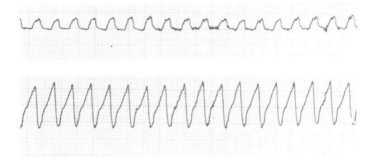

Fig. 5.17   Ventricular flutter. Usually a transient arrhythmia during the degeneration of ventricular tachycardia to ventricular fibrillation.

In clinical practice tachycardias have been loosely divided into narrow or broad QRS complex types. This has proved clinically useful in so far as the narrow QRS complex types are non-ventricular tachycardias and therefore their diagnosis and treatment have a different degree of urgency with a more favourable prognosis. However, this simplistic approach has probably also been responsible for the failure to seek an accurate diagnosis for individual tachycardias and for the frequent misdiagnosis of ventricular tachycardia.[36] The following section gives a practical approach to refining the diagnosis of tachycardias from this simple clinical starting point.

ELECTROCARDIOGRAPHIC ASSESSMENT OF NARROW QRS TACHYCARDIA

The following is a logical approach to the assessment of narrow QRS tachycardia.

1.   If the ventricular rate is grossly irregular (i.e. there is no correlation between the preceding and succeeding R-R intervals) the rhythm is likely to be atrial fibrillation. Look for an irregular pattern of atrial activity in parts of the record where the R-R interval is longer. The combination of an irregular or apparently absent atrial activity and an irregular ventricular rate confirm the diagnosis of atrial fibrillation.

2.   If there are variations in the ventricular rate consider whether these might represent Wenckebach periodicity (varying 2:1, 3:2, 4:3, 5:4, etc. conduction) or varying atrioventricular block (2:1, 3:1, 4:1, 5:1, etc.). These may occur in atrial tachycardia or atrial flutter and possibly rarely in atrioventricular nodal re-entrant tachycardia but their occurrence precludes the possibility of atrioventricular re-entrant tachycardia. If no spontaneous variation in ventricular rate occurs it is worthwhile considering carotid sinus massage to see if such variations can be induced. Variations induced in this way have the same significance as spontaneous

variations. It is particularly helpful to look for pauses (whether spontaneous or induced) within which the pattern of atrial activation is often revealed (Fig. 5.5). The 'saw-tooth' pattern is typical of atrial flutter (atrial rate 300 beats/min). In atrial tachycardia the atrial rate is slower (150–250 beats/ min) with the result that an isoelectric interval appears between consecutive atrial waves.

3.   If the rate is constant and is 150 beats/min the likely rhythm is atrial flutter. Look for the 'saw-tooth' pattern of atrial activity which may be best shown in lead II and V1. Variations in the degree of A-V block (2:1, 3:1, 4:1 and (rarely) possibly even 1:1 can occur). Instantaneous ventricular rates (i.e. the reciprocal of R-R intervals) are thus typically 150 (2:1 A-V block), 100 (3:1), 75 (4:1) or 300 (1:1). Tachycardias with these rates strongly suggest atrial flutter. Unless the conduction is 1:1 (very rare) or 2:1 the flutter waves are usually obvious.

4.   If the ventricular rate is regular consider sinus tachycardia or sinoatrial nodal re-entrant tachycardia. In each of these rhythms the P wave and QRS configuration are normal. In sinus rhythm the rate varies gently and cyclically and the initiation and termination are gradual. In SANRT the rate is constant and the onset and offset are abrupt. If the P waves are abnormal and precede the QRS complexes the rhythm is likely to be atrial tachycardia.

5.   When sinus tachycardia, SANRT, atrial tachycardia, atrial flutter and atrial fibrillation have been excluded the most important remaining possibilities are AVNRT, AVRT and His bundle tachycardia. If no P waves are visible and the rate is 150–250 beats/min the rhythm is likely to be AVNRT. If P waves are visible after the QRS (early in the S-T segment) the rhythm is likely to be AVRT. If P waves can be seen to be dissociated from the QRS complexes the rhythm is likely to be a His bundle tachycardia.

ELECTROCARDIOGRAPHIC ASSESSMENT OF BROAD QRS TACHYCARDIA

1.   If the ventricular rate is grossly irregular the rhythm is likely to be atrial fibrillation with ventricular pre-excitation or bundle branch block. If the rhythm is atrial fibrillation with bundle branch block the ventricular rate will be limited by the A-V node to less than 180 beats/min. In the case of atrial fibrillation with ventricular pre-excitation the ventricular rate may be in the region of 220–300 beats/min.

2.   Look for transient variations in the rhythm. These can be due to capture beats or fusion beats (both of which are diagnostic of VT) or to transient variations in the degree of A-V block which excludes VT and AVRT and suggests atrial flutter or tachycardia with bundle branch block or conduction down a bystander (not participating in the re-entrant circuit) accessory pathway.

3.   If P waves can be seen it is often possible to diagnose a rhythm. If the P wave rate is less than the QRS rate the rhythm is ventricular. If the P wave rate is greater than the QRS rate the rhythm could be ventricular (with coincidental atrial arrhythmia) or supraventricular. If the P wave rate is equal to the ventricular rate the rhythm could be atrial (with 1:1 A-V conduction), junctional or ventricular (with 1:1 V-A conduction). If the P waves are independent of the QRS complexes the rhythm is ventricular.

4.   The remaining criteria are 'soft'.

(a)   If a previous record is available in which the rhythm is clearly supraventricular and ventricular ectopic beats are seen which have a QRS morphology identical in all 12 leads to the QRS complexes during the wide QRS complex tachycardia then the rhythm is likely to be ventricular tachycardia.

(b)   If a previous record is available in which the rhythm is unequivocally supraventricular and the QRS complexes are identical in shape and dimensions to those shown in the wide QRS complex tachycardia then the rhythm is supraventricular with a pre-existing intraventricular conduction abnormality.

(c)   If the QRS duration is 0.14 s or more and it is known that a very recent record taken during a supraventricular rhythm has a normal (equal to or less than 0.10 s) duration then the rhythm is probably ventricular tachycardia.

(d)   If the frontal plane QRS axis during a tachycardia lies within the range $-30°$ to $-120°$ (travelling anticlockwise, i.e. it is a superior axis) then the rhythm is likely to be ventricular tachycardia.

(e)   If the QRS configuration in V1 is rS, Rr or QS or if the QRS configuration in V6 is R, RS, QS, or QR then the rhythm is likely to be ventricular. If the QRS complexes of all the chest leads are similar (i.e. concordant) the tachycardia is likely to be ventricular. Ultimately, however, it has to be stressed that there is no certainty that a broad QRS complex tachycardia can definitively be diagnosed from a 12 lead ECG. The commonest and most important residual area of doubt (when all reasonable assessments of the record have been made) concerns the distinction between ventricular tachycardia and antidromic antrioventricular re-entrant tachycardia. It should be obvious, but it bears re-stating, that the haemodynamic state of the patient makes no significant contribution to the distinction between ventricular and non-ventricular tachycardias. The haemodynamic state of the patient is likely to depend upon the underlying condition of the myocardium, the heart valves and the ventricular rate.

SUMMARY

Most tachycardias can be diagnosed with reasonable confidence from a good quality 12 lead ECG and every effort should be made to obtain such a recording during an attack, the only exception being in the case of a true cardiac arrest when treatment must take precedence.

The major problem in the electrocardiographic diagnosis of tachycardias is in recording what are usually transient events and thus prolonged recording and provocation testing may be of benefit in many cases.

Occasionally invasive studies are needed to clarify the diagnosis where non-invasive methods have proved inadequate, to guide the treatment of malignant ventricular tachycardias and other tachycardias resistant to drug therapy, and to provide further accurate localization of the tachycardia substrate to guide ablative therapy.

REFERENCES

1 Major RH. Classic descriptions of disease. 3rd ed. Springfield, Il: CC Thomas, 1978
2 Mackenzie J. Diseases of the heart. 3rd ed. Springfield, Il: CC Thomas, 1918
3 Einthoven W. Le telecardiogramme. Arch Int Physiol 1906; 4: 132–164
4 Einthoven W. Weiteres Uber das elektrocardiogramm. Nach gemeinschaftlich mit Dr Vaandrager angestellten versuchen mitgeteilt. Pflugers Archiv ges Physiol 1908; 122: 517–584
5 Lewis T. Observations upon flutter and fibrillation part IX. The nature of fibrillation as it occurs in patients. Heart 1921; 8: 193
6 Tawara S. Das Reizleitungssysem des saugetierherzens. Ein anatomisch-histologische studie uber das atrioventricularbundel und die Purkinjeschen faden. Gustav Fisher, Jena, Poland 1906
7 Wellens HJJ. Electrical stimulation of the heart in the study and treatment of tachycardias. University Park Press: Baltimore. 1971
8 Fisher JD. Role of electrophysiologic testing in the diagnosis and treatment of patients with known and suspected bradycardias and tachycardias. Prog Cardiovasc Dis 1981; 24: 25
9 Rowlands DJ. Clinical electrocardiograph. Gower Medical Publishing, 1991
10 Waxman MB, Wald RW, Sharma AD, Huerta F, Cameron DA. Vagal techniques for termination of paroxysmal supraventricular tachycardia. Am J Cardiol 1980; 46: 655
11 Podrid PJ, Venditti FJ, Levine PA, Klein M. The role of exercise testing in evaluation of arrhythmias. Am J Cardiol 1988; 62: 24–33H
12 Creamer JE, Davies DW, Nathan AW. Clinical experience with the Intertach pacemaker. PACE 1987; 10: 996 (abstract)
13 Ward DE, Camm AJ. Clinical electrophysiology of the heart. London: Arnold, 1987
14 Curry PVL, Evans TR, Krikler DM. Paroxysmal reciprocating sinus tachycardia. Eur J Cardiol 1977; 6: 199
15 Coumel P, Flammang D, Attuel P, Leclercq JF. Sustained intra atrial reentrant tachycardia; electrophysiologic study of 20 cases. Clin Cardiol 1979; 2: 167
16 Gillette PC, Garson A. Electrophysiologic and pharmacologic characteristics of automatic atrial ectopic tachycardia. Circulation 1977; 56: 571
17 Lewis T. Theory of circus movement and its application to atrial flutter. In: The mechanism and graphic registration of the heart beat. London: Shaw, 1925
18 Boineau JP. Atrial flutter: a synthesis of concepts. Circulation 1985; 72: 249
19 Waldo AL, MacLean WAH, Karp RB, Kouchoukos NT, James TN, Entrainment and interruption of atrial flutter with atrial pacing. Studies in man following open heart surgery. Circulation 1977; 56: 737
20 Gouaux JL, Ashman R. Auricular fibrillation with aberration simulating ventricular paroxysmal tachycardia. Am Heart J 1947; 34: 366
21 Scheinman MM. Atrioventricular nodal or atriojunctional reentrant tachycardia? J Am Coll Cardiol 1985; 6: 1393
22 Ross DL, Johnson DC, Denniss AR, Cooper MJ, Richards DA, Uther JB. Curative

surgery for atrioventricular junctional ('AV nodal') reentrant tachycardia. J Am Coll Cardiol 1985; 6: 1383

23 Coumel P, Cabrol C, Fabiato A, Gourgon R, Slama R. Tachycardie permanente par rhythme reciproque. I. Preuves du diagnostic par stimulation auriculaire et ventriculaire. Arch Mal Coeur 1967; 60: 1830

24 Wolff L, Parkinson J, White PD. Bundle branch block with short PR interval in healthy young people prone to paroxysmal tachycardia. Am Heart J 1930; 5: 685

25 Spurrell RAJ, Krikler DM, Sowton E. Concealed bypass of the atrioventricular node in patients with paroxysmal supraventricular tachycardia revealed by intracardiac electrical stimulation and verapamil. Am J Cardiol 1974; 33: 590

26 Coumel P, Attuel P. Reciprocating tachycardia in overt and latent preexcitation. Influence of functional bundle branch block on the rate of the tachycardia. Eur J Cardiol 1974; 1: 423

27 Wellens HJJ, Ross DL, Farre J, Brugada P. Functional bundle branch block during supraventricular tachycardia in man: observations on mechanisms and their incidence. In: Zipes D, Jalife J (eds). Cardiac electrophysiology and arrhythmias. 1985: Orlando: Grune & Stratton, p 435

28 Ward DE, Camm AJ, Spurrell RAJ. Reentrant tachycardia using two bypass tracts and excluding AV node in short PR interval, normal QRS syndrome. Br Heart J 1978; 40: 1127

29 Gallagher JJ, Sealy WC. The permanent form of junctional reciprocating tachycardia; further elucidation of the underlying mechanism. Eur J Cardiol 1978; 8: 413

30 Coumel P, Fidelle JE, Attuel P, Brechenmacher C et al. Tachycardies focales hissienes congeniales. Arch Mal Coeur 1975; 69: 899

31 Ward DE, Camm AJ, Spurrell RAJ. Ventricular preexcitation due to anomalous nodoventricular pathways: report of 3 cases. Eur J Cardiol 1979; 9: 111

32 Ward DE, Nathan AW, Camm AJ. Fascicular tachycardia sensitive to calcium antagonists. Eur Heart J 1984; 5: 896

33 Josephson ME, Horowitz LN, Waxman HL, Cain ME et al. Sustained ventricular tachycardia: role of the 12 lead electrocardiogram in localizing site of origin. Circulation 1981; 64: 257

34 Dancy M, Ward DE. Diagnosis of ventricular tachycardia: a clinical algorithm. B M J 1985; 291: 1036

35 Griffith M, de Belder MA, Linker NJ, Ward DE, Camm AJ. Multivariate analysis to simplify the differential diagnosis of broad complex tachycardia. Br Heart J 1991; 66: 166–174

36 Dancy M, Camm AJ, Ward DE. Misdiagnosis of ventricular tachycardia. Lancet 1985; 2: 320

6

Proarrhythmic effects of antiarrhythmic drugs

F. D. Murgatroyd   A. J. Camm

The notion that drugs prescribed to normalize the heart rhythm may sometimes have the opposite effect can be traced back two centuries, to Withering's descriptions of drug-induced tachycardia in digitalis intoxication.[1] For decades, quinidine therapy for atrial arrhythmias has been associated with a risk of ventricular fibrillation,[2,3] and the mechanism of this effect has been the focus of much research. In the last ten years, several studies have implicated antiarrhythmic agents as a possible cause of excess mortality in a variety of patient groups;[4-8] this has generated considerable interest, and speculation as to how prescribing habits should be modified.

The term 'proarrhythmia' has been coined to denote the creation or worsening of an arrhythmia, usually by an antiarrhythmic drug.[9] This chapter aims to give an overview of current knowledge in the field, starting with an outline of the various types of proarrhythmic response. The possible mechanisms by which drugs may give rise to cardiac arrhythmias will then be described, along with the evidence for each model. Finally, the methodological difficulties encountered in clinical research into proarrhythmia will be discussed, in the context of the more important recent studies in this field, and their implications for clinical practice.

TYPES OF PROARRHYTHMIC RESPONSE

Bradycardia

Although the term 'proarrhythmia' is most often used to refer to tachycardias, taken in its broadest sense the concept must also include drug-induced bradycardia, which is without doubt more common. This is hardly surprising, given that virtually all antiarrhythmic drugs reduce the excitability of cardiac tissue and depress conduction to some degree.[10] Thus, excessive doses of beta-blocking drugs, digitalis and most class I drugs cause sinus bradycardia, and can also do so in therapeutic dosage in the presence of sinus node disease.[11] These agents can similarly (again, even in therapeutic concentrations) aggravate atrioventricular (AV) conduction disease (as can calcium channel blockers), and ventricular (escape) bradyarrhythmias can result (Table 6.1).

Table 6.1 Classification of drug-induced arrhythmias, according to site of origin (After Bigger and Sahar)[12]

Drug-induced bradyarrhythmias

Aggravation or provocation of sinus bradyarrhythmias
1. Sinus automaticity (sinus bradycardia, sinus arrest)
2. Sino-atrial block

Aggravation or provocation of AV block
1. AV node
2. His–Purkinje system
3. Intraventricular block

Drug-induced tachyarrhythmias

Supraventricular
1. Atrial tachycardia with block
2. Non-paroxysmal AV junctional tachycardia

Ventricular
1. Prolonged QT with torsade de pointes multiform VT
2. New spontaneous sustained, uniform VT
   a. Episodic or sporadic
   b. Incessant
   c. Accelerated idioventricular rhythm
3. New spontaneous sustained multiform VT (QT not prolonged)
   a. Torsade de pointes VT
   b. Bidirectional VT (digitalis)
4. Increased frequency of spontaneous sustained uniform VT
   a. Similar morphology
   b. Different morphology
5. Increased spontaneous VPD morphology
   a. Fourfold increase in VPD frequency
   b. Tenfold increase in repetitive VPD
6. Response to programmed ventricular stimulation
   a. Conversion of unsustained to sustained VT
   b. Ruskin sequence
   c. VT rate faster during drug therapy
   d. VT easier to induce

In general, drug-induced bradycardias are associated either with very high plasma levels of antiarrhythmic agents, or with pre-existing sinus node dysfunction or conducting tissue disease. The risk of a drug-induced bradycardia is therefore theoretically predictable, and severe occurrences should be rare. However, inter-individual pharmacokinetic variation, drug interactions and electrolyte abnormalities are often overlooked. Furthermore, a predisposition to bradycardia may be difficult to detect without invasive electrophysiological studies (of, for example, sinus node recovery time and AV conduction intervals). Such investigations are not always readily available, but a period of Holter recording or inpatient monitoring prior to the initiation of therapy will detect the majority of high-risk patients. Close observation and a high index of suspicion for drug-induced bradycardia are necessary to detect the remaining sporadic cases sufficiently early to avoid serious adverse consequences.

Tachycardia

Proarrhythmic actions of drugs have given rise to a wide variety of tachyarrhythmias in various contexts. These have been classified by Bigger and Sahar according to their site of origin, clinical occurrence and morphology (Table 6.1).[12]

Certain tachycardias are so characteristic that their causal association with the drug seldom clinically gives rise to doubt. Amongst the arrhythmias of supraventricular origin, two tachycardias are characteristic of digitalis toxicity: atrial tachycardia with block (Fig. 6.1a) and nonparoxysmal AV junctional tachycardia.[89] Acquired torsade de pointes ventricular tachycardia in association with prolongation of the QT interval is usually caused by drugs, especially Vaughan Williams class Ia antiarrhythmic agents. It is classically associated with quinidine in toxic levels, or in association with bradycardia or serum electrolyte depletion.[60,62] Digitalis toxicity gives rise to two other 'characteristic' ventricular arrhythmias: bidirectional ventricular tachycardia (Fig. 6.1b), and accelerated idioventricular rhythm with AV block. The latter is faster than the ventricular escape rhythm usually seen with complete heart block, but slower than 120 beats/min.

In other cases the tachyarrhythmia itself is not characteristic, but the clinical situation leaves little doubt that it is drug induced. It is well established that, in a patient with the Wolff–Parkinson–White syndrome, digoxin or verapamil given during atrial fibrillation may favour conduction down the accessory pathway, and the resulting rapid ventricular response may degenerate into ventricular fibrillation (Fig. 6.1c). New incessant ventricular tachycardia (the term 'incessant' refers to a tachycardia that restarts immediately after terminating, and does not imply that the arrhythmia does not stop at all) in a patient on class Ia or Ic agents is almost always caused by the drug, and high concentrations of class Ia agents can cause these arrhythmias even in patients with normal hearts. Incessant ventricular tachycardia associated with class Ic drugs is typically of sinusoidal appearance (Fig. 6.1d), with marked broadening of the QRS complex and a relatively slow rate, in comparison to spontaneous ventricular tachycardia in the drug-free patient.

Finally, there is a large group of cases in which antiarrhythmic drugs are identified as a proarrhythmic factor in the absence of a distinctive electrocardiographic or clinical pattern. These include instances in which a drug causes a new arrhythmia (but one that is not uniquely identified with that drug), instances in which a drug causes an increase in the frequency and/or severity of an arrhythmia, and instances in which a drug 'worsens' the response of a patient to programmed ventricular stimulation. These groups

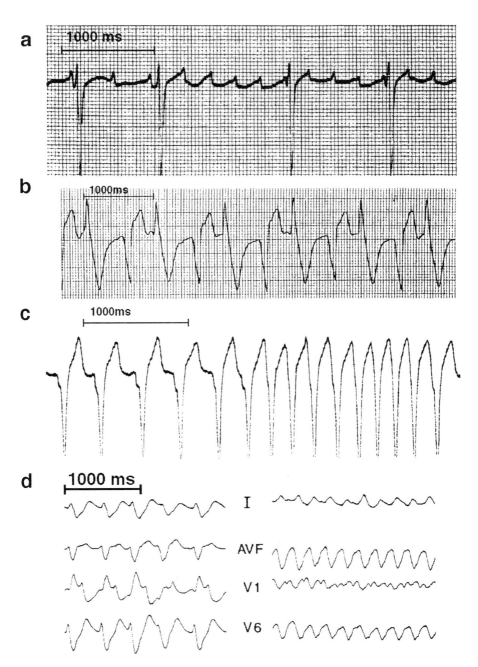

Fig. 6.1 Tachyarrhythmias characteristically associated with antiarrhythmic drugs. **a** Atrial tachycardia with AV block in a case of digitalis intoxication. **b** 'Bidirectional' ventricular tachycardia in digitalis intoxication. **c** Pre-excited atrial fibrillation in a patient with the Wolff–Parkinson–White syndrome. A dramatic increase in ventricular rate follows the administration of intravenous verapamil. **d** Ventricular tachycardia before (left) and after (right) flecainide. The rate is unusually high for a 'sinusoidal' tachycardia. (**a, b** and **d** are adapted, with permission, from Julian DG, Camm AJ, Fox KM, Hall RJC and Poole-Wilson PA (eds): *Diseases of the heart*, London: Bailliere Tindall, 1989; **c** is by courtesy of Dr C Garratt)

probably represent the majority of cases of proarrhythmic responses and certainly the majority of difficulties in their identification, management and avoidance. They will be discussed in more detail later in this chapter.

MECHANISMS FOR PROARRHYTHMIA

The mechanisms by which tachycardias may arise can be divided into those of abnormal impulse initiation and those of abnormal impulse conduction: these will be reviewed first in general terms, then with respect to their importance in drug-induced arrhythmias.

Abnormalities of impulse initiation

Enhanced automaticity (Fig. 6.2)

Certain cardiac cells in the sino-atrial and atrioventricular nodes, and in the conducting system of the heart, exhibit a slow inward current in the resting state (phase 4 of the action potential), which causes a gradual loss of polarization. If these cells are not first depolarized by an action potential arriving from another part of the heart, this slow depolarization continues until a threshold is reached, when an action potential is initiated by the opening of fast sodium channels (phase 0). Thus these groups of cells possess the inherent property of 'automaticity', and can all act as cardiac pacemakers. The automaticity is affected by alterations in the phase 4 current of these cells, or in their threshold potentials. Physiologically, this mechanism governs sinus node automaticity (and hence heart rate) in response to vagal and sympathetic influences;[16,17] it may also be the mechanism by which ectopic foci arise, causing some atrial tachycardias. Enhanced automaticity is probably the mechanism responsible for certain drug-induced arrhythmias, particularly those caused by sympathomimetic inotropes and phosphodiesterase inhibitors.[18] This is unlikely to be an important mechanism, however, for arrhythmias caused by antiarrhythmic agents, as their effects on automaticity tend to be depressive. An important exception to this rule is digitalis. In addition to its vagotonic action, which slows AV conduction, in toxic levels digoxin also has a centrally mediated sympathomimetic effect,[19] and this combination may be responsible for two tachycardias classically seen in digitalis toxicity: paroxysmal atrial tachycardia with AV block, and non-paroxysmal junctional tachycardia.[13]

Triggered activity

In certain circumstances, abnormal oscillations are seen during the plateau and repolarization phases of the cardiac action potential (phases 2 and 3), or during phase 4. These are, respectively, termed early and delayed after-depolarizations (EADs and DADs). Such oscillations can trigger abnormal

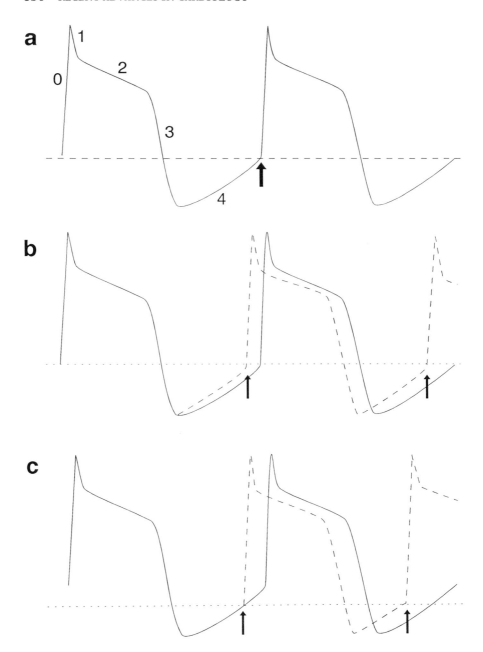

Fig. 6.2   Mechanisms of enhanced automaticity. The cardiac action potential in normal 'pacemaker' tissue is represented in **a**: the phases of the action potential are labelled. During diastole, a slow inward current causes gradual loss of the negative intracellular potential (phase 4); when this reaches the threshold potential (broken line), 'fast' sodium channels open (phase 0), initiating another action potential. If the threshold potential becomes more negative (**b**), or the slope of the phase 4 depolarization is increased (**c**), the threshold is reached earlier, and the automatic rate is increased.

action potentials. The term 'triggered activity' refers to the initiation of an abnormal action potential by a preceding impulse; this dependent relationship differentiates this mechanism from that of enhanced automaticity. However, the two are often grouped together as sources of tachycardia arising from a single focus, as opposed to a re-entrant circuit.

Early afterdepolarizations have been studied most extensively using microelectrode techniques in isolated canine Purkinje fibre preparations, in which they can be produced by agents such as caesium and barium,[20,21] but importantly also by quinidine, even (though with difficulty) in concentrations similar to those found in therapeutic use.[15] These EADs also give rise to triggered activity.[22] The cellular mechanism accounting for EADs is unclear, but probably relates to alterations in the balance between inward sodium and outward potassium transmembrane currents during phases 2 and 3 of the action potential.[23] Techniques using monophasic action potential recordings in intact animal hearts have demonstrated that EADs with very similar appearances can be produced, that give rise to polymorphic ventricular arrhythmias, in a variety of experimental circumstances, including caesium administration and reperfusion following ischaemia.[24,25] In general, EADs are seen in conditions favouring delayed repolarization and, in particular, the combinations of a slow heart rate, hypokalaemia and certain chemical stimuli predispose to their generation, whereas they can be inhibited by increasing the heart rate and administering magnesium.[26–30]

The importance of these experimentally produced EADs and triggered activity lies in their remarkable similarities with the clinical syndromes of torsade de pointes associated with prolonged repolarization, seen in some congenital conditions and frequently in quinidine toxicity. The experimental and clinical tachycardias are morphologically indistinguishable: both are aggravated by bradycardia and hypokalaemia, and both can be suppressed by magnesium and rapid pacing.[31,32] Typically, torsade de pointes does not commence with an 'R-on-T' ectopic beat (as does re-entrant ventricular tachycardia – see later), but following the beat succeeding a pause induced by a premature complex. This 'short–long–short' initiation pattern closely resembles the pacing sequences which experimentally produce EADs and triggered activity.[32] Furthermore, monophasic action potentials recorded from the right ventricle of patients with familial and drug-induced long QT syndromes demonstrate 'EADs', followed sometimes by triggered activity and torsade de pointes (Fig. 6.3).[31,33] However, these findings have not yet been widely reproduced, and intact-heart animal models of quinidine-induced torsade require an extra factor, such as ischaemia or the administration of aconitine.[34,35] Studies using microelectrode mapping techniques have demonstrated that the electrocardiographic appearance of torsade probably arises from competition between two or more ventricular activation sequences,[34] though there remains controversy as to whether these originate in EADs and triggered activity or

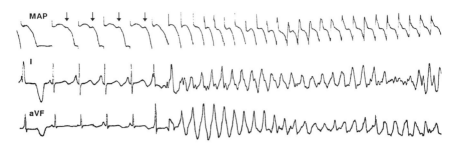

Fig. 6.3 Early afterdepolarizations (EADs) and torsade de pointes in a human subject with a hereditary long QT syndrome. This recording was made at electrophysiological study. The top trace was recorded from the right ventricle with a monophasic action potential electrode (MAP); the other two traces are surface electrocardiogram leads. The MAP trace shows 'humps' at the end of the plateau phase (arrowed), which resemble experimental recordings of EADs. The first beat of torsade is not, however, demonstrably initiated by an EAD at the site of the electrode; nor does it follow the typical short–long–short sequence of RR intervals. Whether such recordings represent the same mechanism as experimental EADs and torsade remains a source of controversy. (By courtesy of Dr NJ Linker)

re-entrant circuits occurring within a substrate of non-uniform repolarization within the myocardium.[36,37]

Delayed afterdepolarizations and triggered activity have been produced experimentally by a variety of means, including ischaemia associated with infarction,[38,39] sympathetic activation by stimulation of the stellate ganglion,[40] specific beta-adrenergic stimulation[41,42] and exposure to digitalis.[43,44] Thus these factors (singly or in combination), as well as enhancing the physiological automaticity of cardiac myocytes as described earlier, may also generate abnormal impulses by a separate mechanism. DADs are associated with intracellular calcium overload, possibly giving rise to an inward sodium current during phase 4 of the action potential.[45] The extent to which digitalis causes DADs by directly increasing intracellular calcium, as opposed to via the sympathetic nervous system, is unknown. In contrast to EADs, DADs are more likely to give rise to triggered activity and arrhythmias at high heart rates.[46] The evidence appears quite strong that triggered activity arising from DADs is the mechanism for certain digitalis-induced arrhythmias, particularly non-paroxysmal AV junctional tachycardia.[47] However, this link remains to be demonstrated in the clinical setting.

Abnormalities of impulse conduction

Re-entrant circuits

Most clinical tachycardias are thought to arise from re-entrant circuits. This view of tachycardias arose from animal experiments around the turn of the century, and the classical model was refined when basic electrophysiological techniques became available.[48] In this model, circus move-

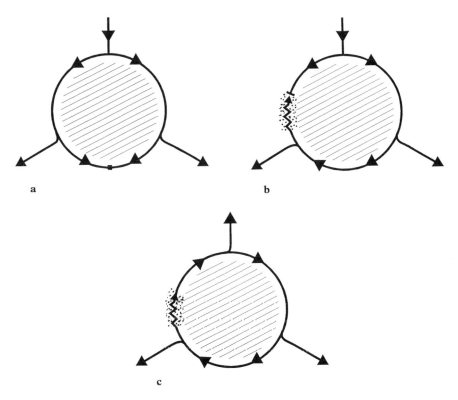

Fig. 6.4   The classical model of re-entry. The hatched area represents a fixed anatomical obstacle to conduction. In sinus rhythm, the cardiac impulse passes around the obstacle in both directions (**a**). An area of partial block (dotted) may halt the early forward conduction of an impulse while allowing the slow conduction of the impulse arriving later from the other side of the obstacle (**b**). If conduction is slowed sufficiently in this area, the impulse that emerges encounters tissue which has regained excitability, and a re-entrant circuit is established (**c**).

ment of the electrical impulse takes place around a fixed anatomical obstacle (Fig. 6.4). For this to occur, certain conditions must be satisfied. First, there must be an area of undirectional block to the initiating impulse in one of the two paths around the obstacle (this often arises temporarily when the initiating impulse is premature). Second, conduction of the impulse in the other direction must be sufficiently slow to allow previously excited tissue to recover from refractoriness. Continued conduction around the circuit depends on the propagating wavefront continuing to arrive at tissue which has recovered excitability: the cycle length of the tachycardia must exceed the refractory period of all parts of the circuit.

This model is critically dependent on delay and inhomogeneity in the conduction of the cardiac impulse. In the case of the AV re-entrant tachycardia of the Wolff–Parkinson–White syndrome, the anatomical basis for this model has been demonstrated: the fixed obstacle is the insulating

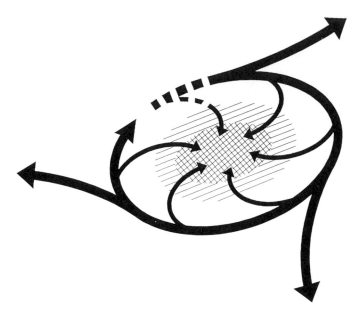

Fig. 6.5   The 'leading circle' model of re-entry. This model dispenses with the need for a fixed anatomical obstacle, by proposing that re-entry can occur around an area of tissue (hatched) which is maintained functionally refractory by inward wavefronts from the re-entrant circuit itself.

AV septum; the second pathway around it is provided by the accessory bundle, and the area of slowed conduction is within the (normal) AV node. A more recent model, based on a rabbit atrial preparation, proposes that re-entrant circuits may exist without a fixed anatomical centre: the continuous centripetal wavefront arising from the circuit itself maintains the refractoriness of the central zone (Fig. 6.5).[49] The 'eye of the storm' is functional, rather than anatomical, and is therefore not necessarily fixed: multiple migrating circulating wavefronts of this nature have long been suggested as the mechanism of fibrillation. [50,51]

The structural and functional changes caused by myocardial infarction can provide the conditions, enumerated earlier, of anatomical or functional obstacles, delayed and blocked conduction, necessary for re-entry to occur. Studies mapping the activation sequence during ventricular tachycardia associated with infarction in animal models[52-54] and humans[55,56] support the re-entrant model of tachycardia for these arrhythmias. A further degree of sophistication to the model comes from canine subendocardial infarction experiments, in which mapping demonstrates the commonest pattern of excitation to arise from one critical fixed slowly conducting pathway, and two (or more) return limbs, forming a pair of re-entrant circuits, in a 'figure-of-eight'.[57]

In addition to these mapping studies, evidence from the behaviour of tachycardias in response to programmed electrical stimulation supports the view that most arise from re-entrant mechanisms.[58] In the classical circus model described above, one would expect a correctly timed extrastimulus to initiate tachycardia in the same manner as a spontaneous premature beat, typically of the 'R-on-T' variety. Furthermore, the re-entrant circuit would be predicted to have an 'excitable gap' of tissue between the repolarization of one wavefront and the depolarization of the next. Correctly timed extrastimuli delivered during this excitable gap might be expected to either terminate tachycardia by rendering the gap refractory, or 'reset' the tachycardia by starting a new depolarizing wavefront ahead of the old. Similarly, pacing at or above the tachycardia rate might be expected to 'entrain' the tachycardia to the pacing sequence, producing a rate-dependent degree of fusion in the surface ECG between the pure tachycardia pattern and a pure paced pattern.[59] Mapping of clinical tachycardias is currently only available during open-heart surgery, and these pacing techniques are therefore largely relied on to investigate the mechanisms of tachycardia in humans. Most regular clinical tachycardias have been demonstrated by these methods to be initiated and terminated by programmed extrastimuli, and to show properties consistent with the presence of an excitable gap.

Antiarrhythmic agents and re-entrant mechanisms

The conditions necessary for re-entrant circuits to be initiated, and become sustained, depend critically on the relationships between the speed of impulse conduction and the refractoriness of the tissues forming the circuit. It is simple to speculate, from experimental knowledge of the properties of antiarrhythmic agents, in what ways they might interfere with the re-entrant mechanism.

Drugs which prolong the myocardial action potential will delay the recovery of excitability of tissue in a circuit, and if this delay is insufficient the re-entering wavefront will be extinguished when it arrives at refractory tissue (Fig. 6.6). Classes Ia and III antiarrhythmic drugs have this property, and this is thought to be the mechanism of their therapeutic action in re-entrant arrhythmias. On the other hand, drugs which slow conduction in a circuit may have two effects, depending on the properties of the circuit. If they turn an area of unidirectional block into one of bidirectional block, or change an area of slowed conduction into one of blocked conduction, the circuit will be broken and the tachycardia extinguished. Conversely, by creating an area of unidirectional block or causing an area of critically slowed conduction, the drug may actually create the substrate for re-entry where there was none. All class I drugs affect the conduction velocity of the cardiac impulse by their action on the sodium channel responsible for phase 0 depolarization, and could therefore cause re-entrant arrhythmias by this mechanism. In the re-entry model, the relative effects of a drug on conduction velocity and repolarization will determine whether the sub-

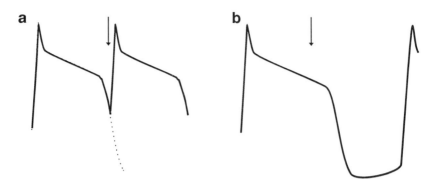

Fig. 6.6   Extinction of re-entry by prolongation of the action potential duration. The maintenance of tachycardia depends on the time of arrival of the re-entering wavefront (arrow) in relation to the action potential of the tissue. In **a**, the tissue is no longer refractory, and a second action potential is triggered. If the action is sufficiently prolonged by an antiarrhythmic drug, the tissue is still refractory and the circuit is extinguished (**b**).

strate for tachycardia is abolished or created: this has been represented graphically by Campbell (Fig. 6.7).[60]

Class I drugs also differ in the characteristics of their binding to the sodium channel, and this may affect their antiarrhythmic and pro-arrhythmic properties. The binding of disopyramide, for example, is increased at fast heart rates: this property is not shared by lignocaine, but the latter has a specific effect on conduction in ischaemic tissue; these individualities, as well as the differing effects on repolarization may partly explain the differences in response between the class I drugs.[61]

Our knowledge of the interactions between antiarrhythmic agents and re-entrant circuits is less advanced than that regarding afterdepolarizations and triggered activity; in fact, there is no direct evidence for the mechanisms just described. However, if drugs do cause re-entrant arrhythmias by their effect on conduction, certain predictions regarding this behaviour can be made, and these are indeed borne out by clinical observations.[62] First, the tachycardia associated with early afterdepolarizations and triggered activity in animal models resembles the torsade de pointes classically associated with proarrhythmic responses to drugs which prolong the action potential. By the same token, one would expect the morphology of tachycardias caused by drugs that slow ventricular conduction to resemble those produced by known re-entrant circuits, and to have broad QRS complexes due to the slow propagation of the tachycardia. Drugs producing the greatest sodium channel blockade and hence the greatest slowing of propagation should have the greatest propensity to produce this form of tachycardia. This is seen clinically; the sustained, monomorphic, broad-QRS 'sinusoidal' ventricular tachycardia is most frequently associated with class Ic agents, which are the most powerful sodium channel blockers.[63–65] In contrast, the least commonly implicated class I agents are the class Ib

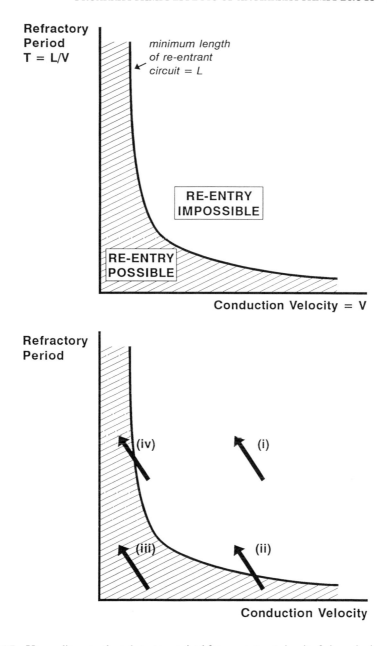

Fig. 6.7   Upper diagram: the substrate required for a re-entrant circuit of given size is determined by the conduction velocity and the refractory period of the tissue. Only if conduction is slow enough for the impulse to continually encounter tissue which has regained excitability can re-entry continue. Lower diagram: the arrows represent the four possible actions of an antiarrhythmic drug which slows conduction and prolongs the refractory period of cardiac tissue. (i) *No arrhythmia*: the substrate cannot support re-entry. (ii) *Antiarrhythmic effect*: the substrate is altered and re-entry becomes impossible. (iii) *Ineffective therapy*: re-entry remains possible. (iv) *Proarrhythmia*: the drug creates the substrate for re-entry.

subgroup, and these have the least effect on impulse propagation.[7] Second, the model depends on the drug's effects on conduction creating the substrate for re-entry, and structurally abnormal hearts will have many potential re-entrant circuits. One would therefore expect to see sustained, wide-complex, monomorphic tachycardia as a complication of anti-arrhythmic therapy far more frequently in structural heart disease than in normal hearts, and this is indeed the case.[66] Finally, as interventions to terminate tachycardia, such as pacing and cardioversion, do not alter the substrate for re-entry itself, one would expect drug-induced re-entrant tachycardias to recur immediately, as they usually do, until the agent responsible has been eliminated.

Mechanisms for proarrhythmia: Summary

Two models for the mechanisms of drug-induced tachycardia dominate. Triggered activity induced by early afterdepolarizations may account for the polymorphic ventricular tachycardia associated with antiarrhythmic drugs which prolong repolarization (Vaughan Williams classes Ia and III), and triggered activity arising from late afterdepolarizations may account for some of the arrhythmias seen in digitalis intoxication. These mechanisms can occur with equal ease in structurally normal and abnormal hearts. Drugs which delay conduction of the cardiac impulse are associated with

Table 6.2   Clinical features of drug-induced arrhythmias (After Horowitz et al)[9]

I.   Primary or secondary
   1. Primary: unrelated to any identifiable arrhythmogenic factor other than underlying arrhythmia or heart disease
   2. Secondary: requiring adjunctive factor, such as high plasma concentrations, concomitant medications, electrolyte disturbances, ischaemia

II. Type
   1. Bradyarrhythmias
     a. Sinus node dysfunction
     b. Atrioventricular block
   2. Tachyarrhythmias
     a. Supraventricular tachyarrhythmias
     b. Ventricular tachyarrhythmias

III. Level of certainty that response is drug-induced
   1. Confirmed (definite): reproducible
   2. Probable (without rechallenge): new onset of serious arrhythmias or statistically significant change in frequency of existing arrhythmia, arrhythmia in close temporal relationship to initiation of drug, change in dose or development of contributing factors such as hypokalaemia
   3. Possible: other than the two aforementioned levels

IV. Clinical relevance
   1. Significant: spontaneous occurrence of life-threatening or significantly symptomatic arrhythmia
   2. Unknown: increased frequency of asymptomatic arrhythmia or response to programmed electrical stimulation

sustained or incessant monomorphic, broad-complex ventricular tachy-cardias, and may exert these proarrhythmic effects by causing re-entrant circuits. As would be expected, this is more commonly found with more potent sodium-channel blockers, and in structurally abnormal hearts. Direct evidence in humans for these mechanisms of proarrhythmia is largely anecdotal and based on responses to programmed electrical stimu-lation, but the comparisons between drug-induced tachycardias and both animal models and spontaneous clinical tachycardias are compelling.

CLINICAL STUDIES OF PROARRHYTHMIA

Attention will now be turned to clinical studies of the proarrhythmic effects of antiarrhythmic drugs. A great deal has been written about these studies in recent years, based on remarkably little primary clinical data. This partly reflects the fact that general recognition of the importance of proarrhythmia has been relatively recent, but also that death from proarrhythmia seems to be a rare enough occurrence that its systematic evaluation would require very large studies. The problems in defining proarrhythmia will be discussed first. A description of the more important clinical studies will follow, with discussions of the other methodological difficulties which they illustrate.

The definition of proarrhythmia

Perhaps the greatest difficulties hitherto in the clinical study of proarrhyth-mia have been in the lack of uniformity in both the definitions of pro-arrhythmic responses, and the description of the various types. Consensus is emerging, however, in both of these areas.

Types of proarrhythmic response

A full description of a proarrhythmic response requires the detailing of several clinical parameters in addition to the electrocardiographic features: the cause of the arrhythmia, its clinical importance, and the level of certainty with which the drug is implicated (Table 6.2)[9]

Non-invasive criteria for proarrhythmia

When a new arrhythmia, especially one of the 'characteristic' types de-scribed at the beginning of this chapter, occurs in association with the initiation of antiarrhythmic therapy, the causal link is easily made. How-ever, where the proarrhythmic response consists of an increase in the frequency or severity of an existing arrhythmia, there has been great variation as to what criteria should be used. In particular, there has been divergence of opinion as to what constitutes a significant rise in the frequency of ventricular premature complexes (VPCs). An improved understanding of the spontaneous variability in the frequency of VPCs has led to proposals for strict criteria which can be applied uniformly;[67,68] less stringent criteria were applied to some important early studies, which should be interpreted in this light. An increase in the heart rate sufficient to cause haemodynamic effects where none existed before is generally considered to constitute a proarrhythmic response to a drug, and this has been observed with atrial arrhythmias as well as ventricular tachycardia. In the former case, a possible mechanism is a reduction in the rate of the atrial arrhythmia sufficient to allow the AV node to conduct 1:1, and hence cause a rise in ventricular rate.[69,70] On the other hand, changes in the morphology alone of a tachycardia are no longer considered a manifestation of proarrhythmia. A further difficulty arises with the marked increase in QRS duration often seen with class Ic drugs: it can be difficult to distinguish ventricular tachycardia from supraventricular arrhythmias with aberrant conduction. It can be argued that this distinction is unimportant, and that

Table 6.3 Non-invasive criteria for proarrhythmia (After Morganroth and Pratt)[72]

- Proarrhythmic death

- Serious proarrhythmic events
  Spontaneous new onset of polymorphic VT, VFL or VF
  Spontaneous new onset of haemodynamically significant non-sustained VT or, if no haemodynamic significance, ≥ 100 VT events per day

- Non-serious proarrhythmic events
  Asymptomatic change in the frequency of previously documented VPCs or non-sustained VT, including:
  – Increase in the frequency of VPCs required for proarrhythmia (except when due predominantly to sustained VT):

Mean VPCs per hour	
Baseline	Fold increase
10–50	30
51–100	15
101–300	5
301–500	4
501–1000	3
> 1000	2

– Increase in frequency of VT events required for proarrhythmia:

VT events per day	
Baseline	Fold increase
1	≥ 100
2–5	50
6–50	20
> 50	10

- Or a change from no symptoms or palpitations or presyncope to syncope, cardiac arrest or death

Table 6.4   Criteria for proarrhythmia at electrophysiological testing (After Horowitz et al)[77]

Initiation of sustained VT or VF in a patient in whom only non-sustained VT was provoked by the complete stimulation protocol during baseline testing

Conversion while on drug therapy of induced sustained VT that, during the baseline study, could be terminated by programmed stimulation, to sustained VT or VF requiring cardioversion for termination during the drug evaluation

Initiation of sustained VT or VF during drug evaluation by an induction mode less aggressive than that required to initiate the arrhythmia during baseline testing

Development of spontaneous sustained VT during drug evaluation in a patient who required programmed stimulation to initiate the arrhythmia during baseline testing

the ventricular rate is the determinant of risk. On the other hand, the ventricular activation sequence differs between the two arrhythmias, and this may affect both the coordination of contraction and the likelihood of degeneration into ventricular fibrillation.

Based on these considerations, certain definitions have been proposed, and are in current use for the evaluation of new agents (Table 6.3);[71,72] it is hoped that greater uniformity and comparability between studies will result.

Criteria for proarrhythmic responses at electrophysiological testing

The empirical prescription of long-term antiarrhythmic therapy following myocardial infarction and out-of hospital cardiac arrest has not been found to improve mortality and may actually increase the incidence of sudden cardiac death.[73,74] Programmed ventricular stimulation has been used to establish a suspected causal relationship between antiarrhythmic drugs and out-of-hospital cardiac arrest.[4,75] Serial electrophysiological studies, in combination with non-invasive techniques, are now routinely used in the selection of antiarrhythmic drugs for dangerous arrhythmias, although there is a degree of spontaneous variability in a patient's response.[76-79] Again, consensus is emerging as to what constitutes a proarrhythmic response (Table 6.4).[77] The value of electrophysiological testing in predicting proarrhythmic responses will be discussed later in this chapter.

Early studies of class Ic agents: Risk factors for proarrhythmia

Increased awareness of the danger of ventricular proarrhythmia led in the early 1980s to close monitoring of two new class Ic drugs currently being introduced at that time: flecainide and encainide. Reports from early studies of these agents represented the first systematic attempts to collate findings into a database from which information regarding proarrhythmic effects could be extracted. Unfortunately, the studies differed not only in the types of patients included, but more importantly in the definitions used to determine proarrhythmic responses. For this reason, it is difficult to derive evaluations of absolute overall safety from these studies, or to compare the proarrhythmic risk of each drug, other than within the context of the patient group and methods used for each individual study. Earlier data are even more lacking in homogeneity of methods, although the technique of meta-analysis has been used to yield some results (see below).

These studies can, however, tell us a great deal about clinical factors which predispose to proarrhythmic responses. Information from the flecainide and encainide databases identifies the following risk factors: (1) the presence of structural heart disease; (2) sustained ventricular tachycardia (VT) as the presenting arrhythmia (as opposed to non-sustained VT or frequent ventricular premature complexes (VPCs)); (3) inpatient initiation of therapy (presumably a marker of illness severity); and (4) rapid dose escalation, as opposed to careful prescribing following pharmacokinetic principles.[66,80] Non-invasive inpatient evaluation of a wide variety of antiarrhythmic agents (see below) gives broadly the same findings: Podrid et al found that a history of ventricular tachycardia or fibrillation, and poor left ventricular function, are the major risk factors for proarrhythmic responses, whereas age, sex and type of heart disease are not.[81] Drug-induced changes in the surface electrocardiogram, although often associated with drug-induced tachycardias, have not been found to be good predictors of proarrhythmic response (assessed either non-invasively or by electrophysiological testing).[77,82,83]

Comparative inpatient studies of antiarrhythmic drugs

Two large series have been reported which compare the frequency of proarrhythmic events observed with a large number of different antiarrhythmic agents tested acutely.[7,8] Velebit et al, in 1982, presented the results of a retrospective analysis of patients referred with ventricular arrhythmias who underwent a protocol of short-term serial drug testing. After a control period of 48 hours off antiarrhythmic therapy (digitalis was allowed), a single substantial oral dose of a drug was administered, and if it was deemed effective the drug was given for 48 hours. Evaluation was by Holter monitoring and maximal exercise stress testing. In total, 722 drug tests (including single doses) were given to 155 patients. Proarrhythmia was noted in 53 (34.2%) of the patients, and 80 (11.1%) of the tests. Tocainide, quinidine, and the beta-blocking drugs pindolol and propranol were the agents most frequently implicated.

Stanton et al reported a larger series, of 506 patients undergoing 1268 drug trials, in 1989. Again, patients were observed on admission during a two-day washout period, and this was used as a reference. In this case, only spontaneously occurring arrhythmias were entered into analysis. The findings were markedly different in many respects from those of the earlier study. Proarrhythmic responses were recorded in only 35 (6.9%) of the patients and 43 (3.4%) of the drug trials. The incidence of arrhythmogenic effects was highest for newer, largely class Ic drugs not included in the first study, but quinidine accounted for only one proarrhythmic response and tocainide and beta-blockers none at all.

There are many possible reasons for the large discrepancies between these studies. First, although the populations studied were very similar in terms of age, sex and accompanying cardiac diagnoses, the presenting arrhythmias were different. The proportions of patients in the study of Stanton et al with ventricular fibrillation and ventricular tachycardia (sustained and non-sustained) were, respectively, 25.7% and 74.3%, whereas in the group reported by Velebit et al they were 41.9% and 35.5% – the remaining 22.6% had symptomatic single ventricular premature complexes as their presenting arrhythmia. Second, each study employed a different definition of proarrhythmia. Velebit et al included significant increases in VPCs and repetitive forms, and the first occurrence of sustained VT if not present in the control period; Stanton et al required the presence of a new spontaneous symptomatic ventricular tachyarrhythmia associated temporally with commencing the drug, and disappearing with discontinuation of the drug. As mentioned earlier, exercise provocation was not used. Finally, and most importantly, both studies were retrospective and neither was randomized: the choice of drugs in each will probably have reflected current clinical practice (which will have been better informed in the second study, published seven years later). Indeed, Stanton et al state specifically that drugs were chosen on the basis of each patient's clinical and therapeutic history, and agents known to be negatively inotropic were avoided in patients with overt heart failure: this factor probably accounts for the discrepancy between the two studies regarding beta-blockers and disopyramide.

The hypothesis that the choice of antiarrhythmic drug may have been better suited to the individual patient in the later study is supported by updated results from the series of Velebit et al, published in 1987.[81] The series, now of 1287 drug tests performed according to the same protocol as before, used the same criteria for proarrhythmia, but included a range of class Ic agents not in the first study. It is interesting to note that the proportionate incidence of proarrhythmic response to the apparently 'worse' drugs in the first series had fallen: in the case of tocainide, from 12/76 to 14/180, and in the case of quinidine, from 20/130 to 20/180 (results for beta-blockers were not given in the second series). These figures strongly suggest that drug selection was much improved in the interval between the two reports.

Quinidine for the prevention of atrial fibrillation (AF)

A meta-analysis of randomized controlled trials of quinidine therapy in the maintenance of sinus rhythm after cardioversion has recently been published.[6] The authors selected six trials from 52 publications relating to the subject, on the basis of methodology alone: other trials were rejected largely because they were not randomized, not controlled, or controlled against other drugs. The results of the meta-analysis suggest that quinidine is an

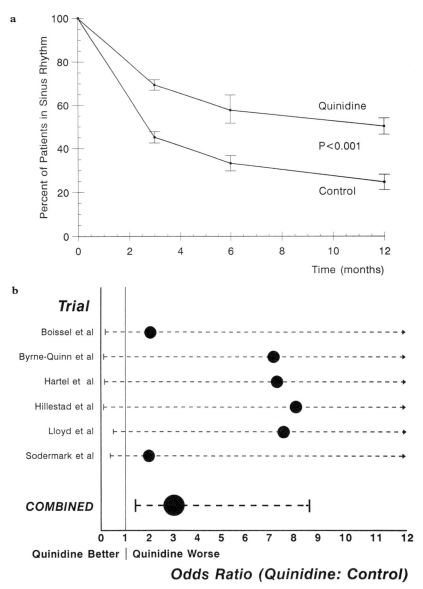

Fig. 6.8 **a** Effectiveness of quinidine in the prevention of recurrence of atrial fibrillation following cardioversion: results of a meta-analysis of randomized controlled trials. **b** Total mortality in patients receiving quinidine during the randomized controlled trials, expressed as an odds ratio (quinidine versus control) with 95% confidence intervals for each trial, and for the pooled data (bottom). (Adapted from Coplen et al)[6]

effective treatment, but that it is associated with an increase in overall mortality (Fig. 6.8).

The techniques of meta-analysis offer the possibility of pooling data from multiple trials, the findings of which individually fail to achieve statistical significance because of insufficient size. However, caution must be exercised in drawing firm conclusions from such studies. First, care must be taken to avoid bias in the selection of the data to be incorporated in the meta-analysis. In this case, the authors undertook a computer-based literature search; from the results of this, they selected suitable studies while blinded to their provenance and results. While this method is clearly the best in choosing amongst published reports, it cannot correct for publication bias in favour of positive findings, and although the authors give good reason why they feel that this is not an important effect, it cannot be excluded. Second, meta-analysis usually combines results from studies undertaken over a long period of time (during which clinical practice may have changed) and with a variety of methods. This can be regarded both as a strength and a potential weakness. For example, four of the six studies were undertaken before the importance of the quinidine–digoxin interaction was fully recognized, and it is not clear whether any of the deaths were in patients taking digoxin. Furthermore, the mortality figures are quite small: 12 out of 413 patients on quinidine died, and 3 out of 387 controls. Sudden cardiac death was established in only 3 of the 12 deaths on quinidine (the mode of death was not known in a further 7 cases and in one of the 3 controls who died). While the *all-cause* mortality for patients on long-term treatment with quinidine is higher (odds ratio for death on treatment = 3.1), this does not quite reach conventional statistical significance, and all-cause mortality is not a satisfactory marker of proarrhythmic risk. A very high level of statistical significance would have to be achieved in order for mortality from causes with no clear pathophysiological relationship to a drug to be attributed to that drug.

Meta-analysis is a powerful statistical tool: it has been particularly useful in providing pilot data for the design of large-scale clinical trials. However, it is the latter that provide more definitive answers to questions of efficacy and safety. The quinidine meta-analysis can be regarded as a useful indicator of the potential risks of antiarrhythmic therapy and of the need for further investigation in the field, but its direct relation to clinical practice in the 1990s and beyond can be debated.

Flecainide, encainide and the CAST study

Patients who survive acute myocardial infarction (AMI) remain at an increased risk of death compared with comparable controls: even beyond one year, the relative risk is four to eightfold.[84] More than a third of deaths occurring late after AMI are sudden, and the majority of these are presumed to be due to ventricular arrhythmias.[85] The recognition of this risk, and the advent of powerful new agents in the 1970s and early 1980s, may partly explain the substantial increase in antiarrhythmic drug prescribing in this period.[86] There was (and remains) great interest in identifying patients at high risk of sudden death following AMI, and finding treatments that might reduce that risk.

The presence of VPCs is a predictor of mortality after AMI independent of left ventricular function.[87] In the mid-1980s, the Cardiac Arrhythmia Pilot Study (CAPS) examined the efficacy of flecainide, encainide, imipramine (a tricyclic antidepressant with antiarrhythmic properties) and moricizine in the suppression of VPCs following AMI, using a randomized, placebo-controlled design.[88] It found that flecainide and encainide were very effective, and moricizine and imipramine less so, but still greater than placebo. Imipramine had a high incidence of intolerable side effects. Flecainide and encainide were often found to be effective in patients unresponsive to moricizine. CAPS was not designed to detect any effects on mortality.

Based on these findings, the Cardiac Arrhythmia Suppression Trial (CAST) set out to test the hypothesis that suppression of ventricular arrhythmias following AMI will reduce sudden cardiac death. In order to have sufficient power to detect effects on mortality, the study was large (4400 patients were initially to be recruited) and included only patients with impaired left ventricular function, who are known to have a higher mortality. An initial period of inpatient open-label titration identified patients responding to flecainide, encainide or moricizine, and these patients were then randomized to receive the drug to which they responded, or placebo. The primary endpoint of the study was death due to arrhythmia (or resuscitation requiring defibrillation).

The preliminary findings of the CAST investigators were published in August 1989, following the recommendation of the Data and Safety Monitoring Board that flecainide and encainide be discontinued.[89] The Board had analysed interim results of the study to date, and found that, overall, patients receiving active therapy had a statistically higher mortality than those assigned to placebo; this difference was entirely attributable to encainide and flecainide (Fig. 6.9). The relative risks of death from arrhythmia or cardiac arrest for these drugs, were 3.4 and 4.4, respectively, and the results for all-cause mortality were virtually identical. A statistically significant increase in mortality was not seen with moricizine, although later on a trend in this direction was seen of sufficient magnitude to predict that CAST would not be able to detect a benefit from this drug. The trial was therefore discontinued altogether in August 1991.

These findings have without doubt brought the issue of proarrhythmia into the limelight more than any other study. Very soon after their publication, the manufacturers of flecainide restricted their recommendations for the use of the drug to life-threatening arrhythmias. This decision was felt by many to be premature,[90] as there is no good reason to extrapolate the

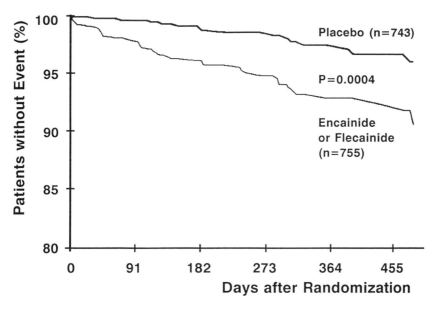

Fig. 6.9 Actuarial survival curves for death or cardiac arrest due to arrhythmia in patients receiving flecainide, encainide or placebo in the CAST study. (Adapted from Echt et al)[94]

data from a study of ventricular arrhythmias in post-AMI patients to all other patient groups, on which considerable safety data already existed.[63,65,66,91] Nonetheless, the preliminary findings of CAST have probably done more to alter cardiac drug prescribing than any other single recent trial, with the exception of those regarding thrombolysis.

Two features emerge from the CAST study which may throw some light on its striking findings. First, the mortality in the patient group randomized to placebo treatment was under 4% – a much lower finding than in most post-infarction studies. This is probably explained by the selection procedure: only patients who responded to treatment in the initial open-label dose-titration phase were randomized. When this effect is corrected for, the 'natural' overall mortality rate for patients initially enrolled is between 6.3% and 8.4%.[92] The non-responders in the open-label phase had more extensive coronary disease and a higher mortality rate than those randomized to placebo.[93] The finding of low placebo mortality of the patients randomized is important, as the trial may not have had sufficient power to detect any beneficial effect of the agents tested, which may have been present in addition to the detrimental effect.

Second, it is interesting to speculate on the causes of excess death in the treatment group. Surprisingly, this group did not exhibit a higher incidence of non-lethal arrhythmic events, such as proarrhythmia, VT, syncope or need for permanent pacing. The mortality in the treatment group was higher, not only from arrhythmic deaths, but also from other causes, largely acute myocardial ischaemia and cardiogenic shock. The total number of deaths and non-fatal ischaemic events in the treatment and placebo groups were virtually identical. These findings strongly suggest that active treatment increased the likelihood of ischaemic events becoming fatal: this could either have been due to the facilitation of fatal arrhythmias, or the adverse result of the negatively inotropic effects of flecainide and encainide in the acutely ischaemic heart.[94]

Although some would argue that features of its design make it difficult to generalize from its results, the CAST study has important implications for the future use of antiarrhythmic therapy, and draws attention to the need for further large-scale placebo-controlled trials.[95-97] In particular, it is clear from CAST and other studies that proarrhythmic responses to drugs may occur late in patients who initially appear to respond to treatment without adverse effects. However, Kennedy has pointed out that it is not clear whether this is a manifestation of a delayed primary proarrhythmic response, or secondary to an interaction with some form of change in the patient's underlying condition.[98,99]

Proarrhythmic effects of other drugs

This chapter has concentrated largely on proarrhythmic responses to Vaughan Williams class I drugs, as these have been the most frequently reported and the closest studied. No class of antiarrhythmics is without risk, however. Beta-adrenergic antagonists and calcium-channel blockers, as discussed earlier, can give rise to both bradyarrhythmias and consequent escape rhythms, and occasionally exacerbate tachycardias. The class III drugs amiodarone and sotalol are generally thought to be 'safer' than class Ic agents from the point of view of proarrhythmia, and their use is probably limited more by their other side effects. However, both drugs have been associated with torsade de pointes, which is hardly surprising as their principal electrophysiological effect is to prolong repolarization. In a review of 1288 patients entered into early trials of sotalol for supraventricular and ventricular arrhythmias, 4.3% of cases developed a proarrhythmic response. This was usually torsade de pointes associated with QT prolongation, but neither the QT interval, hypokalaemia nor bradycardia were predictive of proarrhythmia.[100] Amiodarone predictably increases the QT interval, and has been implicated in the genesis of torsade de pointes, especially in high doses,[101] although it is also an effective therapy for torsade.[102]

Mention should briefly be made of arrhythmias caused by drugs other than antiarrhythmic agents. The risks of tachycardias induced by beta-adrenergic agonists and phosphodiesterase inhibitors probably relate to enhanced automaticity, as mentioned earlier. Where these arrhythmias occur in critically ill cardiac patients, they are easily recognized, but the causal relation is not always clear. On the other hand, the induction of tachycardia is the main factor limiting the doses of salbutamol and theophylline that can be used in acute asthma. Overdosage of many drugs, especially tricyclic antidepressants, has long been known to cause fatal arrhythmias. Recently, a variety of drugs, only some of which are used in cardiac arrhythmias, have been sporadically linked with QT interval prolongation and torsade de pointes. These include the calcium-channel antagonists prenylamine, lidoflazine and bepridil, and terodiline, an anticholinergic agent used as a bladder relaxant. [103-110] Recent experimental evidence suggests that these agents may share a common mechanism of prolonged ventricular repolarization related to their actions on the slow inward calcium current.[111,112] Although these occurrences are rare, the drug can easily be identified as the likely cause if there is no prior history of arrhythmia.

Can the risk of proarrhythmia be predicted for an individual?

If a patient on antiarrhythmic therapy suffers a serious arrhythmia, it is often not clear whether the occurrence is due to inadequate treatment or a proarrhythmic effect. In a study of six patients suffering out-of-hospital cardiac arrest while on antiarrhythmic therapy, Ruskin et al found that programmed ventricular stimulation (PVS) provoked VT in four cases, and high-grade AV block developed in a fifth, at therapeutic levels of the drugs concerned. In no case could VT be provoked when antiarrhythmic therapy was withheld, and all but one patient (who died in chronic heart failure) remained well.[4] PVS can thus be used to establish a causal relationship between a spontaneous arrhythmia occurring in a patient on drug therapy, and the drug concerned. It has been suggested that adverse responses might be predicted, at the time therapy is initiated, by similar techniques.

As mentioned earlier, in the management of VT and ventricular fibrillation (VF), specialist centres use PVS, in addition to continuous (real-time or Holter) monitoring and exercise electrocardiography, to evaluate patients' responses to antiarrhythmic agents.[113] The choice of long-term therapy can be guided by serially testing a variety of drugs and their combinations in this manner. The effectiveness of the non-invasive techniques in evaluating treatment response is limited by their insensitivity: the frequency of VT, and particularly VF, is usually too low for a significant change to be detectable: indirect measures, such as VPC frequency, have to be used instead. On the other hand, PVS attempts to provoke arrhythmia in artificial circumstances, and the significance of a positive response, are unclear. In up to 80% of cases, VT or VF remain inducible despite antiarrhythmic therapy, yet a clinical recurrence (VT or sudden death) occurs in less than half of these.[114] In the series of Velebit and Podrid, proarrhythmic response to PVS occurred in 12.9% of single-drug tests, and this proportion is comparable to that seen with non-invasive testing.[82] However, it is not known whether PVS can predict a spontaneously occurring proarrhythmic response, as in most published series drug therapy has been discontinued when an arrhythmia is induced. Thus, non-invasive methods can be regarded as insensitive but specific measures of drug efficacy, while the converse may hold for PVS.

Brugada et al, recognizing these difficulties, have instituted a 'parallel' study, in which, uniquely, response to therapy will be tested by monitoring, exercise electrocardiography and PVS, but therapy is only altered if *spontaneous* recurrence of the clinical tachycardia occurs.[115] Early results from this study suggest that proarrhythmic effects observed during PVS (22% of 65 tests) may not have any prognostic significance, and should not preclude continuation of a potentially beneficial drug.[114] It is to be hoped that much may be learned from this study about the predictability of beneficial and adverse responses to antiarrhythmic agents. However, the CAST study, the meta-analysis of quinidine trials and the observations of Kennedy suggest that late proarrhythmia (whether primary, or related to a change in the electrophysiological substrate) may continue to be difficult to predict.

SUMMARY: CLINICAL IMPLICATIONS

All antiarrhythmic drugs carry the risk of causing or aggravating arrhythmia. Torsade de pointes, associated with prolonged repolarization, is particularly associated with class Ia agents. While this can occur in patients with normal hearts and no apparent predisposing factors, clinicians can minimize the risk of torsade by avoiding high drug doses and hypokalaemia, and being aware of the added risk conferred by bradycardia and concomitant antiarrhythmic therapy. When this proarrhythmic response does occur, potassium replacement and magnesium supplementation are of value, and overdrive pacing can be used to suppress the arrhythmia while the causative agent is withdrawn.

Incessant broad-complex ventricular tachycardia, typically associated with class Ic agents, can be much harder to treat. The risk of this occurrence is greatest in those with structural heart disease, impaired ventricular function, and the more serious arrhythmias. In general, their use should be avoided in such patients, who should be referred to specialized centres. When such patients respond well to acute therapy in hospital, the clinician should remember the risk of late proarrhythmia, and continue close monitoring in the long term, with regular non-invasive testing and review of the need for antiarrhythmic therapy. The indication for treating asymptomatic or mildly symptomatic 'minor' arrhythmias, such as ventricular premature complexes, must be questioned. Dosing of all antiarrhythmic drugs should be tailored to the individual, and the danger of drug interactions and electrolyte abnormalities should not be overlooked.[116,117]

SUMMARY: FUTURE PROSPECTS

Good models exist for the mechanisms of proarrhythmic response to drugs, but their validity has not yet been fully established. If these models hold, then it is the very properties that make these drugs effective that can also create or worsen arrhythmias, and the potential for proarrhythmia will remain an inevitable accompaniment of all antiarrhythmic drugs. Indeed, as a general rule, the more potent antiarrhythmic agents have the greatest propensity to adverse responses. It will not be possible to reliably predict the occurrence of proarrhythmia in an individual case until the substrate for arrhythmia in that individual can be characterized with great precision. With the possible exception of the Wolff–Parkinson–White syndrome (because of its anatomical simplicity), this goal remains distant. However, awareness of the risk of proarrhythmia has greatly increased in recent years, and it is hoped that standardization of research methods and large-scale studies with long-term follow-up will enable future selection of anti-arrhythmic therapy to be safer and more effective. Serial drug testing with a combination of non-invasive techniques and programmed ventricular stimulation remains the strategy of choice for the patient with a life-threatening ventricular arrhythmia,[113] and if no satisfactory drug is found patients can now be considered for an automatic implantable cardioverter–defibrillator. The use of these devices is likely to increase greatly in the near future, and early use may even become cheaper than serial drug testing.[118]

REFERENCES

1 Withering W. An account of the foxglove and some of its medical uses with practical remarks on dropsy and other diseases. Birmingham, UK: Sweeney, 1785
2 Kerr WJ, Bender WL. Paroxysmal ventricular fibrillation with cardiac recovery in a case of auricular fibrillation and complete heart-block while under quinidine sulphate therapy. Heart 1922; 9: 269–281
3 Selzer A, Wray HW. Quinidine syncope: paroxysmal ventricular fibrillation occurring during treatment of chronic atrial arrhythmias. Circulation 1964; 30: 17–26
4 Ruskin JN, McGovern B, Garan H, DiMarco JP, Kelly E. Antiarrhythmic drugs: a possible cause of out-of-hospital cardiac arrest. N Engl J Med 1983; 309: 1302–1305
5 Preliminary report: effect of encainide and flecainide on mortality in a randomized trial of arrhythmia suppression after myocardial infarction. The Cardiac Arrhythmia Suppression Trial (CAST) Investigators. N Engl J Med 1989; 321: 406–412
6 Coplen SE, Antman EM, Berlin JA, Hewitt P, Chalmers TC. Efficacy and safety of quinidine therapy for maintenance of sinus rhythm after cardioversion: a meta-analysis of randomized control trials. Circulation 1990; 82: 1106–1116
7 Velebit V, Podrid P, Lown B, Cohen BH, Graboys TB. Aggravation and provocation of ventricular arrhythmias by antiarrhythmic drugs. Circulation 1982; 65: 886–894
8 Stanton MS, Prystowsky EN, Fineberg NS, Miles WM, Zipes DP, Heger JJ. Arrhythmogenic effects of antiarrhythmic drugs: a study of 506 patients treated for ventricular tachycardia or fibrillation. J Am Coll Cardiol 1989; 14: 209–215
9 Horowitz LN, Zipes DP, Bigger JT Jr et al. Proarrhythmia, arrhythmogenesis or aggravation of arrhythmia: a status report, 1987. Am J Cardiol 1987; 59: 54E–56E
10 Singh BN, Opie LH, Harrison DC, Marcus FI. Antiarrhythmic agents. In: Opie LH, ed. Drugs for the heart. Orlando FL: Grune and Stratton, 1987; pp 54–90
11 Ferrer MI. The sick sinus syndrome. In: Katz AM, Selwyn A, eds. The cardiac arrhythmias. Sunderland: Sinauer, 1983, pp 47–57
12 Bigger JT Jr, Sahar DI. Clinical types of proarrhythmic response to antiarrhythmic drugs. Am J Cardiol 1987; 59: 2E–9E
13 Bigger JT Jr. Digitalis toxicity. J Clin Pharmacol 1985; 25: 514–521

14 Bauman JL, Bauernfeind JL, Hoff JV, Strasberg B, Swiryn S, Rosen KM. Torsade de pointes due to quinidine: observations in 31 patients. Am Heart J 1984; 107: 425–430

15 Roden DM, Hoffman BF. Action potential prolongation and induction of abnormal automaticity by low quinidine concentrations in canine Purkinje fibers: relationship to potassium and cycle length. Circ Res 1985; 56: 857–867

16 Jalife J, Moe GK. Phasic effects of vagal stimulation on pacemaker activity of the isolated sinus node of the young cat. Circ Res 1979; 45: 595–608

17 Hutter OF, Trautwein W. Vagal and sympathetic effects on the pacemaker fibers in the sinus venosus of the heart. J Gen Physiol 1956; 39: 715–733

18 Naccarelli GV, Goldstein RA. Electrophysiology of phosphodiesterase inhibitors. Am J Cardiol 1989; 63: 35A–40A

19 Somberg JC, Smith TW. Localization of the neurally mediated arrhythmogenic properties of digitalis. Science 1979; 204: 321–323

20 Takanaka C, Singh BN. Barium-induced nondriven action potentials as a model of triggered potentials from early afterdepolarizations: significance of slow channel activity and differing effects of quinidine and amiodarone. J Am Coll Cardiol 1990; 15: 213–221

21 Dangman KH. Effects of procainamide on automatic and triggered impulse initiation in isolated preparations of canine cardiac Purkinje fibers. J Cardiovasc Pharmacol 1988; 12: 78–87

22 Cranefield PF. Action potentials, afterpotentials, and arrhythmias. Circ Res 1977; 41: 415–423

23 Rosen MR. Mechanisms for arrhythmias. Am J Cardiol 1988; 61: 2A–8A

24 Patterson E, Szabo B, Scherlag BJ, Lazzara R. Early and delayed afterdepolarizations associated with cesium chloride-induced arrhythmias in the dog. J Cardiovasc Pharmacol 1990; 15: 323–331

25 Priori SG, Mantica M, Napolitano C, Schwartz PJ. Early afterdepolarizations induced in vivo by reperfusion of ischemic myocardium: a possible mechanism for reperfusion arrhythmias. Circulation 1990; 81: 1911–1920

26 Kaseda S, Gilmour RFJ, Zipes DP. Depressant effect of magnesium on early afterdepolarizations and triggered activity induced by cesium, quinidine, and 4-aminopyridine in canine cardiac Purkinje fibers. Am Heart J 1989; 118: 458–466

27 Davidenko JM, Cohen L, Goodrow R, Antzelevitch C. Quinidine-induced action potential prolongation, early afterdepolarizations, and triggered activity in canine Purkinje fibers: effects of stimulation rate, potassium, and magnesium. Circulation 1989; 79: 674–686

28 el Sherif N, Zeiler RH, Craelius W, Gough WB, Henkin R. QTU prolongation and polymorphic ventricular tachyarrhythmias due to bradycardia-dependent early afterdepolarizations: afterdepolarizations and ventricular arrhythmias. Circ Res 1988; 63: 286–305

29 Nayebpour M, Nattel S. Pharmacologic response of cesium-induced ventricular tachyarrhythmias in anesthetized dogs. J Cardiovasc Pharmacol 1990; 15: 552–561

30 Bailie DS, Inoue H, Kaseda S, Ben David J, Zipes DP. Magnesium suppression of early afterdepolarizations and ventricular tachyarrhythmias induced by cesium in dogs. Circulation 1988; 77: 1395–1402

31 el Sherif N, Bekheit SS, Henkin R. Quinidine-induced long QTU interval torsade de pointes: role of bradycardia-dependent early afterdepolarlizations. J Am Coll Cardiol 1989; 14: 252–257

32 Cranefield PF, Aronson RS. Torsade de pointes and other pause-induced ventricular tachycardias: the short–long–short sequence and early afterdepolarizations. PACE 1988; 11: 670–678

33 Bonatti V, Rolli A, Botti G. Recording of monophasic action potentials of the right ventricle in long QT syndromes complicated by severe ventricular arrhythmias. Eur Heart J 1983; 4: 168–179

34 Bardy GH, Ungerleider RM, Smith WM, Ideker RE. A mechanism of torsade de pointes in a canine model. Circulation 1983; 67: 52–59

35 Leichter D, Danilo PJ, Boyden P, Rosen TS, Rosen MR. A canine model of torsades de pointes. PACE 1988; 11: 2235–2245

36 Habbab MA, el Sherif N. Drug-induced torsades de pointes: role of early afterdepolarizations and dispersion of repolarization. Am J Med 1990; 89: 241–246

37 Surawicz B. Electrophysiologic substrate of torsade de pointes: dispersion of
    repolarization or early afterdepolarizations? J Am Coll Cardiol 1989; 14: 172–184
38 Gough WB, el Sherif N. Dependence of delayed afterdepolarizations on diastolic
    potentials in ischemic Purkinje fibers. Am J Physiol 1989; 257: H770–H777
39 Dangman KH, Dresdner KPJ, Zaim S. Automatic and triggered impulse initiation in
    canine subepicardial ventricular muscle cells from border zones of 24-hour transmural
    infarcts: new mechanisms for malignant cardiac arrhythmias? Circulation 1988; 78:
    1020–1030
40 Priori SG, Mantica M, Schwartz PJ. Delayed afterdepolarizations elicited in vivo by left
    stellate ganglion stimulation. Circulation 1988; 78: 178–185
41 Priori SG, Yamada KA, Corr PB. Influence of hypoxia on adrenergic modulation of
    triggered activity in isolated adult canine myocytes. Circulation 1991; 83: 248–259
42 Gilat E, Aronson RS, Nordin C. Triggered activity induced by K(+)-free, Na(+)-
    deficient solution in guinea pig ventricular muscle: the effects of ouabain, lidocaine, and
    Ca^{2+} channel blockers. J Cardiovasc Pharmacol 1990; 16: 267–275
43 Rosen MR, Merker C, Gelband H, Hoffman BF. Effects of ouabain on phase 4 of
    Purkinje fiber transmembrane potentials. Circulation 1983; 47: 681–689
44 Gorgels AP, de Wit B, Beekman HD, Dassen WR, Wellens HJ. Triggered activity
    induced by pacing during digitalis intoxication: observations during programmed
    electrical stimulation in the conscious dog with chronic complete atrioventricular block.
    PACE 1987; 10: 1309–1321
45 Tseng GN, Wit AL. Effects of reducing $[Na^+]_o$ on catecholamine-induced delayed
    afterdepolarizations in atrial cells. Am J Physiol 1987; 253: H115–H125
46 Damiano B, Rosen MR. The effects of pacing on early afterdepolarizations and triggered
    activity. Circulation 1984; 69: 1013–1025
47 Rosen MR, Fisch C, Hoffman BF, Danilo PJ, Lovelace DE, Knockel SB. Can
    accelerated atrioventricular junctional escape rhythm be explained by delayed
    afterdepolarizations? Am J Cardiol 1980; 45: 1272–1284
48 Schmitt FO, Erlanger J. Directional differences in the conduction of the impulse
    through heart muscle and their possible relation to extrasystolic and fibrillary
    contractions. Am J Physiol 1928; 87: 326–347
49 Allessie MA, Bonke FIM. Circus movement in rabbit atrial muscle as a mechanism of
    tachycardia. III. The 'leading circle' concept: a new model of circus movement in
    cardiac tissue without the involvement of an anatomical obstacle. Circ Res 1977; 41: 9–18
50 Mines GR. On the dynamic equilibrium in the heart. J Physiol 1913; 46: 349–383
51 Mines GR. On circulating excitations in heart muscles and their possible relation to
    tachycardia and fibrillation. Trans R Soc Can 1914; 8: 43–52
52 Wit AL, Allessie MA, Bonke FIM. Electrophysiologic mapping to determine the
    mechanism of experimental ventricular tachycardia in initiated by premature impulses.
    Am J Cardiol 1982; 49: 166–185
53 el Sherif N, Mehra R, Gough WB. Ventricular activation pattern of spontaneous and
    induced ventricular rhythms in canine one-day-old myocardial infarction: evidence for
    focal and reentrant mechanisms. Circ Res 1982; 51: 152–166
54 el Sherif N, Mehra R, Gough WB, Zeiler RH. Reentrant ventricular arrhythmias in the
    late myocardial infarction period. Circulation 1983; 68: 644–656
55 Josephson M, Buxton A, Marchlinski F. Sustained ventricular tachycardia in coronary
    artery disease: evidence for reentrant mechanism. In: Zipes DP, Jalife J, eds. Cardiac
    electrophysiology and arrhythmias. New York: Grune and Stratton, 1985, pp 409–418
56 Harris L, Downar E, Mickleborough L et al. Activation sequence of ventricular
    tachycardia: endocardial and epicardial mapping studies in the human ventricle. J Am
    Coll Cardiol 1987; 10: 1040–1047
57 Mehra R, Zeiler RH, Gough WB, el Sherif N. Reentrant ventricular arrhythmias in the
    late myocardial infarction period: electrophysiologic–anatomic correlation of reentrant
    circuits. Circulation 1983; 67: 11–23
58 Ward DE, Camm AJ. Mechanisms of tachycardia. In: Clinical electrophysiology of the
    heart. London: Edward Arnold, 1987, pp 127–149
59 Waldo AL, Maclean WAH, Karp RB, Kouchoukos NT, James TN. Entrainment and
    interruption of atrial flutter with atrial pacing: studies in man following open heart
    surgery. Circulation 1977; 56: 737

60 Campbell TJ. Proarrhythmic actions of antiarrhythmic drugs: a review. Aust NZ J Med 1990; 20: 275–282
61 Rosen MR, Wit AL. Arrhythmogenic actions of antiarrhythmic drugs. Am J Cardiol 1987; 59: 10E–18E
62 Levine JH, Morganroth J, Kadish AH. Mechanisms and risk factors for proarrhythmia with type Ia compared with Ic antiarrhythmic drug therapy. Circulation 1989; 80: 1063–1069
63 Nathan AW, Hellestrand KJ, Bexton RS, Banim SO, Spurrell RAJ, Camm AJ. Proarrhythmic effects of the new antiarrhythmic agent flecainide acetate. Am Heart J 1984; 107: 222–228
64 Winkle RA, Mason JW, Griffin JC, Ross DL. Malignant ventricular tachyarrhythmias associated with the use of encainide. Am Heart J 1981; 102: 857–864
65 Morganroth J, Horowitz LN. Flecainide: its proarrhythmic effect and expected changes on the surface electrocardiogram. Am J Cardiol 1984; 53: 89B–94B
66 Morganroth J, Anderson JL, Gentzkow GD. Classification by type of ventricular arrhythmia predicts frequency of adverse cardiac events from flecainide. J Am Coll Cardiol 1986; 8: 607–615
67 Morganroth J, Borland M, Chao G. Application of a frequency definition of ventricular proarrhythmia. Am J Cardiol 1987; 59: 97–99
68 Pratt CM, Hallstrom A, Theroux P, Romhilt D, Coromilas J, Myles J. Avoiding interpretive pitfalls when assessing arrhythmia suppression after myocardial infarction: insights from the long-term observations of the placebo-treated patients in the Cardiac Arrhythmia Pilot Study (CAPS). J Am Coll Cardiol 1991; 17: 1–8
69 Feld GK, Chen P-S, Nicod P, Fleck P, Meyer D. Possible atrial proarrhythmic effects of class 1c antiarrhythmic drugs. Am J Cardiol 1990; 66: 378–383
70 Marcus FI. The hazards of using type 1c antiarrhythmic drugs for the treatment of paroxysmal atrial fibrillation. Am J Cardiol 1990; 66: 366–367
71 Pratt CM. Proarrhythmic potential of moricizine: strengths and limitations of a data base analysis. Am J Cardiol 1990; 65: 51D–55D
72 Morganroth J, Pratt CM. Prevalence and characteristics of proarrhythmia from moricizine (Ethmozine). Am J Cardiol 1989; 63: 172–176
73 Moosvi AR, Goldstein S, VanderBrug Medendorp S et al. Effect of empiric antiarrhythmic therapy in resuscitated out-of-hospital cardiac arrest victims with coronary artery disease. Am J Cardiol 1990; 65: 1192–1197
74 Hine LK, Laird NM, Hewitt P, Chalmers TC. Meta-analysis of empirical long-term antiarrhythmic therapy after myocardial infarction. JAMA 1989; 262: 3037–3040
75 Ruskin JN, DiMarco JP, Garan H. Out of hospital cardiac arrest. Electrophysiologic observations and selection of long term antiarrhythmic therapy. N Engl J Med 1980; 303: 607–613
76 Rae AP, Kay HR, Horowitz LN, Spielman SR, Greenspan AM. Proarrhythmic effects of antiarrhythmic drugs in patients with malignant ventricular arrhythmias evaluated by electrophysiologic testing. J Am Coll Cardiol 1988; 12: 131–139
77 Horowitz LN, Greenspan AM, Rae AP, Kay HR, Spielman SR. Proarrhythmic responses during electrophysiologic testing. Am J Cardiol 1987; 59: 45E–48E
78 Josephson ME, Horowitz LN, Spielman SR, Greenspan AM. Electrophysiologic and hemodynamic studies in patients resuscitated from cardiac arrest. Am J Cardiol 1980; 46: 948–955
79 McPherson CA, Rosenfeld LE, Batsford WP. Day-to-day reproducibility of responses to right ventricular programmed stimulation: implications for serial drug testing. Am J Cardiol 1985; 55: 689–695
80 Morganroth J. Risk factors for the development of proarrhythmic events. Am J Cardiol 1987; 59: 32E–37E
81 Podrid P, Lampert S, Graboys TB, Blatt CM, Lown B. Aggravation of arrhythmia by antiarrhythmic drugs: incidence and predictors. Am J Cardiol 1987; 59: 38E–44E
82 Poser RF, Podrid PJ, Lombardi F, Lown B. Aggravation of arrhythmia induced with antiarrhythmic drugs during electrophysiologic testing. Am Heart J 1985; 110: 9–16
83 Stavens CS, McGovern B, Garan H, Ruskin JN. Aggravation of electrically provoked ventricular tachycardia during treatment with propafenone. Am Heart J 1985; 110: 24–29
84 May GS, Eberlein KA, Furberg CD, Passamani ER, DeMets DL. Secondary

prevention after myocardial infarction: a review of long-term trials. Prog Cardiovasc Dis 1982; 24: 331–332

85 The Multicenter Postinfarction Research Group. Risk stratification and survival after myocardial infarction. N Engl J Med 1983; 309: 331–336.

86 Hine LK, Gross TP, Kennedy DL. Outpatient antiarrhythmic drug use from 1970 through 1986. Arch Intern Med 1989; 149: 1524–1527

87 Bigger JT Jr, Fleiss JL, Kleiger R, Miller JP, Rolnitzky LM, Multicenter Post-Infarction Research Group. The relationships among ventricular arrhythmias, left ventricular dysfunction and mortality in the 2 years after myocardial infarction. Circulation 1984; 69: 250–258

88 The Cardiac Arrhythmia Pilot Study (CAPS) Investigators. Effects of encainide, flecainide, imipramine, and moricizine on ventricular arrhythmias during the year after acute myocardial infarction: the CAPS. Am J Cardiol 1988; 61: 501–509

89 The Cardiac Arrhythmia Suppression Trial (CAST) Investigators. Preliminary report: effect of encainide and flecainide on mortality in a randomized trial of arrhythmia suppression after myocardial infarction. N Engl J Med 1989; 321: 406–412

90 Anonymous. Editorial. Flecainide and CAST. Lancet 1989; ii: 481–482

91 Anderson JL, Jolivette DM, Fredell PA. Summary of efficacy and safety of flecainide for supraventricular arrhythmias. Am J Cardiol 1988; 62: 62D–66D

92 Epstein AE, Bigger JT Jr, Wyse DG, Romhilt DW, Reynolds-Haertle RA, Hallstrom AP. Events in the Cardiac Arrhythmia Suppression Trial (CAST): mortality in the entire population enrolled. J Am Coll Cardiol 1991; 18: 14–19

93 Wyse DG, Hallstrom A, McBride R, Cohen JD, Steinberg JS, Mahmarian J. The Cardiac Arrhythmia Suppression Trial (CAST) Investigators: events in the cardiac arrhythmia suppression trial (CAST): mortality in patients surviving open label titration but not randomized to double-blind therapy. J Am Coll Cardiol 1991; 18: 20–28

94 Echt DS, Liebson PR, Mitchell B et al. The Cardiac Arrhythmia Suppression Trial (CAST) Investigators: mortality and morbidity in patients receiving encainide, flecainide, or placebo. N Engl J Med 1991; 12: 781–788

95 Pratt CM, Moye LA. The Cardiac Arrhythmia Suppression Trial: background, interim results and implications. Am J Cardiol 1990; 65: 20B–29B

96 Anderson JL. Reassessment of benefit–risk ratio and treatment algorithms for antiarrhythmic drug therapy after the cardiac arrhythmia suppression trial. J Clin Pharmacol 1990; 30: 981–989

97 Bigger JT Jr. Implications of the cardiac arrhythmia suppression trial for antiarrhythmic drug treatment. Am J Cardiol 1990; 65: 3D–10D

98 Kennedy HL. Late proarrhythmia and understanding the time of occurrence of proarrhythmia. Am J Cardiol 1990; 66: 1139–1143

99 Kennedy HL, Sprague MK, Homan SM et al. Natural history of potentially lethal ventricular arrhythmias in patient treated with long-term antiarrhythmic drug therapy. Am J Cardiol 1989; 64: 1289–1297

100 Soyka LF, Wirtz C, Spangenberg RB. Clinical safety profile of sotalol in patients with arrhythmias. Am J Cardiol 1990; 65: 74A–81A

101 Lazzara R. Amiodarone and torsade de pointes. Ann Intern Med 1989; 111: 549–551

102 Mattioni TA, Zheutlin TA, Sarmiento JJ, Parker M, Lesch M, Kehoe RF. Amiodarone in patients with previous drug-mediated torsade de pointes: long-term safety and efficacy. Ann Intern Med 1989; 111: 574–580

103 Abinader EG, Shahar J. Possible female preponderance in prenylamine-induced 'torsade de pointes' tachycardia. Short communication. Cardiology 1983; 70: 37–40

104 Fraser AG, Ikram S. Torsade de pointes with prenylamine: do we still need the drug? Lancet 1986; ii: 572

105 Kaden F, Kubler W. [Recurrent, atypical tachycardia 'torsade des pointes' following administration of lidoflazine]. Med Welt 1978; 29: 1047–1048

106 Fazekas T, Kiss Z. Torsade de pointes ventricular tachycardia associated with lidoflazine therapy. Eur Heart J 1984; 5: 343

107 Manouvrier J, Sagot M, Caron C et al. Nine cases of torsade de pointes with bepridil administration. Am Heart J 1986; 111: 1005–1007

108 Sagot M, Ducloux G, Pauchant M, Thery C. [Torsade de pointes under bepridil (apropos of 5 cases)]. LARC Med 1983; 3: 369–371

109 Connoly MJ, Astridge PS, White EG, Morley CA, Campbell Cowan J. Torsades de pointes ventricular tachycardia and terodiline. Lancet 1991; 338: 344–345
110 Committee on Safety of Medicines. Terodiline (Micturin) and adverse cardiac reactions. London: CSM 1991
111 Campbell RM, Woosley RL, Iansmith DH, Roden DM. Lack of triggered automaticity repolarization abnormalities due to bepridil and lidoflazine. PACE 1990; 13: 30–36
112 Zipes DP. Personal communication, 1991
113 Wellens HJ, Brugada P, Stevenson WG. Programmed electrical stimulation: its role in the management of ventricular arrhythmias in coronary heart disease. Prog Cardiovasc Dis 1986; 29: 165–180
114 Brugada P, Lemery R, Talajic M, Della Bella P, Wellens HJ. Treatment of patients with ventricular tachycardia or ventricular fibrillation: first lessons from the 'parallel study'. In: Brugada P, Wellens HJJ, eds. Cardiac arrhythmias: where to go from here? Mount Kisco, NY: Futura, 1987, pp 457–470
115 Brugada P, Wellens HJJ. Need and design of a prospective study to assess the value of different strategic approaches of management of ventricular tachycardia or fibrillation. Am J Cardiol 1986; 57: 1180–1184
116 Woosley RL. Pharmacokinetics and pharmacodynamics of antiarrhythmic agents in patients with congestive heart failure. Am Heart J 1987; 114: 1280–1291
117 Woosley RL, Roden DM. Pharmacologic causes of arrhythmogenic actions of antiarrhythmic drugs. Am J Cardiol 1987; 57: 19E–25E
118 O'Donoghue S, Platia EV, Brooks-Robinson S, Mispireta L. Automatic implantable cardioverter–defibrillator: is early implantation cost-effective? J Am Coll Cardiol 1990; 16: 1258–1263

7

Medical and surgical management of patients with Wolff–Parkinson–White syndrome

H-T. Shih   W. M. Miles   L. S. Klein   D. P. Zipes

Wolff–Parkinson–White (WPW) syndrome is characterized by the presence of atrioventricular accessory pathways that are responsible for the pre-excitation of the ventricles, i.e. the delta wave and short PR interval in the surface electrocardiogram, and for the associated tachycardias. Depending on the rate and frequency of tachycardias and the corresponding haemodynamic status, patients may be completely asymptomatic or experience symptoms such as palpitations, chest discomfort, dyspnea, dizziness, presyncope, syncope and, uncommonly, sudden cardiac death. In patients with accessory pathways that cause incessant tachycardias such as the permanent form of junctional reciprocating tachycardia (PJRT), dilated cardiomyopathy and heart failure may result.[1] Ventricular fibrillation and death have been reported in patients who developed atrial fibrillation and very rapid ventricular response due to fast anterograde conduction and short refractoriness of the accessory pathway.[2, 3] Drugs, antitachycardia pacemakers, surgical ablation procedures and, most recently, catheter ablation techniques have been used to suppress or eliminate the arrhythmias. This review will concentrate on the management of the arrhythmias involving overt and concealed accessory pathways, PJRT, and tachycardias caused by pathways with 'Mahaim fibre' properties (Fig. 7.1). For simplicity, the term 'WPW patients' is used in the test to include all patients with an accessory pathway.

DRUG THERAPY

The principle of drug therapy is to prolong conduction time and/or increase the refractoriness of a portion of the pathway(s) used by the tachycardia, acutely to terminate the tachycardia and chronically to prevent a recurrence. The arrhythmias in patients with accessory pathways are of two kinds: those that incorporate the accessory pathway in the re-entrant circuit as the retrograde limb (orthodromic atrioventricular (AV) reciprocating tachycardia) or the anterograde limb (antidromic atrioventricular reciprocating tachycardias); and those in which the accessory pathway does not

RECIPROCATING TACHYCARDIAS

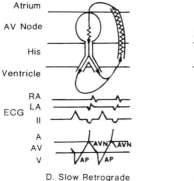
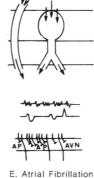
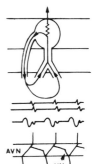

Fig. 7.1   Schematic diagram of tachycardias associated with accessory pathways. The top portion of each example shows the presumed anatomical pathways and the bottom half depicts the electrocardiographic presentation and the explanatory ladder diagram. **A** Orthodromic tachycardia with anterograde conduction over the AV node–His bundle system and retrograde conduction over the accessory pathway (left-sided for this example as depicted by left atrial activation preceding right atrial activation). **B** Orthodromic tachycardia and ipsilateral functional bundle branch block. **C** Antidromic tachycardia with anterograde conduction over the accessory pathway and retrograde conduction over the AV node–His bundle. **D** Orthodromic tachycardia with a slowly conducting accessory pathway as in the permanent form of junctional reciprocating tachycardia (PJRT). **E** Atrial fibrillation with the accessory pathway as a bystander. **F** Anterograde conduction over a portion of the AV node and a nodoventricular pathway ('Mahaim fibre') and retrograde conduction over the AV node. (Adapted from Zipes DP, Specific arrhythmias: diagnosis and treatment. In: Braunwald E (ed): Heart disease: a textbook of cardiovascular medicine, 3rd edn. Philadelphia: Saunders, 1988, p. 690)

take part in sustaining the tachycardia but conducts anterogradely to produce a rapid ventricular response (such as in atrial fibrillation) (Fig. 7.1). In the first situation, block in either the anterograde limb or the retrograde limb of the re-entrant loop, i.e. either the AV node–His system or the accessory pathway, interrupts the re-entry and stops the tachycardia.

Table 7.1   Site of primary antiarrhythmic effect

AV node	Accessory pathway	AV node and accessory pathway
Digitalis	Procainamide	Flecainide
Beta-blockers	Quinidine	Encainide
Calcium entry blockers	Disopyramide	Propafenone
Adenosine, ATP	Ajmaline	Amiodarone
		Sotalol

In the second case, however, blocking conduction in the AV node may enhance the anterograde conduction over the accessory pathway and increase the ventricular rate or even induce ventricular fibrillation.[4–7] To determine the correct antiarrhythmic agent to use, accurate interpretation of the arrhythmias, usually with an electrophysiology study, is necessary. Agents used to treat WPW syndrome are listed in Table 7.1 according to their preferential action on either the AV node or the accessory pathways.

Digitalis preparations

Digitalis is one of the most frequently used agents to treat supraventricular tachycardias. Intravenous ouabain (0.75–1.5 mg or 0.01–0.015 mg/kg) injection rendered AV reciprocating tachycardia non-inducible or more difficult to induce by electrical stimulation in 10–100% of patients with inducible tachycardia at control state, due to its direct and indirect effects in prolonging conduction time and refractoriness in the AV node.[8–10] However, in patients with atrial fibrillation associated with pre-excited ventricular complexes, i.e. QRS complexes with a delta wave due to conduction over the accessory pathway, digitalis has been shown to increase the pre-excited ventricular rate and may even precipitate ventricular fibrillation.[4] It is therefore important to differentiate carefully among various wide QRS tachycardias and avoid giving digitalis to patients with atrial fibrillation and anterograde conduction over the accessory pathway. Because patients with AV reciprocating tachycardia can develop atrial fibrillation, digitalis should probably not be used as a single drug in patients with WPW syndrome and tachyarrhythmias.

Beta-adrenoceptor blockers

Although predominantly affecting the AV node, when sympathetic tone is enhanced or the initiation of tachycardia is related to exercise, beta-blockers may affect both the AV node and the accessory pathway and terminate or prevent recurrences of AV reciprocating tachycardia. Several beta-blockers, including propranolol,[11, 12] metoprolol[13] and nadolol,[14] have been shown acutely to terminate AV reciprocating tachycardias in up to 30% of patients and chronically to suppress the occurrence of the tachycardia in approximately 40% of the WPW patients. However, a single bolus of intravenous esmolol injection (as much as 280 mg) was not found effective in terminating AV reciprocating tachycardias.[15] In addition, in patients with atrial fibrillation and ventricular pre-excitation, intravenous propranolol[16] and flestolol[17] increased the proportion of pre-excited ventricular complexes, although the overall ventricular rate was decreased in some patients. Neither drug affected conduction or refractoriness of the accessory pathway. Thus, beta-blockers as single agents are not very effective in acutely terminating or chronically preventing recurrences of accessory pathway-related tachycardias.

Calcium entry blockers

Verapamil[7, 18] and diltiazem[19, 20] both prolong conduction time and refractoriness in the AV node but do not directly affect the accessory pathway. Bepridil[21] has an additional property of increasing the anterograde and retrograde refractoriness in the accessory pathway. Calcium entry blockers have been found effective in terminating and preventing recurrences of orthodromic AV reciprocating tachycardia.[7, 19−24] Similar to digitalis, intravenous verapamil and diltiazem can shorten the pre-excited RR interval and increase the ventricular rate during atrial fibrillation[5−7, 19] and precipitate ventricular fibrillation.[5−7] Because of this, intravenous calcium entry blockers are contraindicated in patients with atrial fibrillation and anterograde conduction over an accessory pathway. As a general rule, these drugs intravenously are contraindicated in any patients who have a wide QRS complex tachycardia. Oral verapamil and diltiazem exert different effects compared with intravenous administration, and can be used.

Adenosine and adenosine triphosphate

Adenosine and adenosine triphosphate (ATP) prolong conduction time or block conduction in the AV node.[25] Adenosine given as an intravenous bolus (6–10 mg) terminates more than 90% of episodes of 'supraventricular tachycardia', including AV and AV nodal re-entrant tachycardias (see Fig. 7.2 for mechanisms).[26] Its efficacy compares favourably with that of verapamil but has an onset of action in seconds versus minutes.[27, 28] While adenosine and ATP shorten the action potential duration of the atrial myocardium and can have the propensity of inducing atrial flutter/fibrillation, they do not cause measurable haemodynamic deterioration in WPW patients with atrial fibrillation, even though the ventricular rate can increase transiently after ATP boluses.[29] Because of their rapid onset of action, ultra-short half-life (< 10 s), lack of negative inotropic effect, safety in patients with wide QRS tachycardia, and potential of being used for a diagnostic test to differentiate tachycardias, adenosine and ATP have become the initial drugs of choice for acute termination of supraventricular

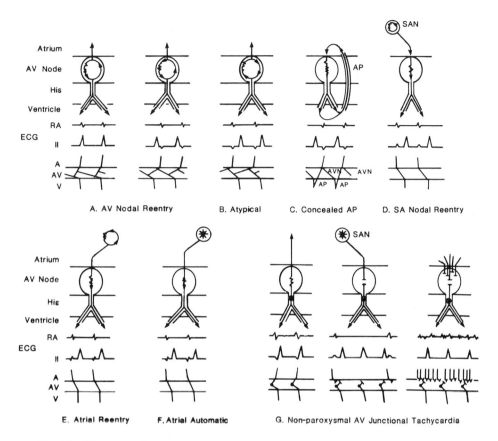

Fig. 7.2 Diagrammatic representation of various narrow QRS tachycardias. Format as in Figure 1A. **A** AV nodal re-entry. In the left-hand example, re-entrant excitation is drawn confined to the AV node, with retrograde atrial activity occurring simultaneously with ventricular activity owing to anterograde conduction over the slow AV nodal pathway and retrograde conduction over the fast AV nodal pathway. In the right-hand example, atrial activity occurs slightly later than ventricular activity, owing to retrograde conduction delay. **B** Atypical AV nodal re-entry due to anterograde conduction over a fast AV nodal pathway and retrograde conduction over a slow AV nodal pathway. **C** Concealed accessory pathway. Reciprocating tachycardia is due to anterograde conduction over the AV node and retrograde conduction over the accessory pathway. Retrograde P waves occur after the QRS complex. **D** Sinus nodal re-entry. The tachycardia is due to re-entry within the sinus node, which then conducts to the rest of the heart. **E** Atrial re-entry. Tachycardia is due to re-entry within the atrium, which then conducts to the rest of the heart. **F** Automatic atrial tachycardia. Tachycardia is due to automatic discharge in the atrium, which then conducts to the rest of the heart; it is difficult to distinguish from atrial re-entry. **G** Non-paroxysmal AV junctional tachycardia. Various presentations of this tachycardia are depicted with retrograde atrial capture, AV dissociation with the sinus node in control of the atria and AV dissociation with atrial fibrillation. (Adapted from Zipes DP, Specific arrhythmias: diagnosis and treatment. In: Braunwald E, ed. Heart disease: a textbook of cardiovascular medicine, 3rd edn. Philadelphia: Saunders, 1988, p 668)

tachycardia, including AV reciprocating tachycardia. It should be remembered that, due to the ultra-short half-life, adenosine and ATP should be administered rapidly as an intravenous bolus followed by flushing with intravenous fluid in order to maximize the effects.

Class I antiarrhythmic agents

The class Ia agents, procainamide, quinidine, and disopyramide, have been the mainstay of treatment for WPW syndrome in the last two decades. They primarily prolong conduction time or block conduction and prolong refractoriness in the accessory pathway. Intravenous ajmaline[30] and procainamide[31] have been used to identify patients who have accessory pathways with short anterograde effective refractory period (< 270 ms) and who might be at risk for developing rapid ventricular rates should they have atrial fibrillation. As stated earlier, a very rapid rate on occasion can precipitate sudden death. It should be noted, however, that intravenous ajmaline has been associated with the death of a patient.[32]

The class Ic antiarrhythmic drugs prolong conduction time and the refractory period of both the AV node and the accessory pathway.[33] In a summary of 80 reports on treatment of supraventricular arrhythmias with flecainide,[34] intravenous flecainide was found to terminate 88% of AV reciprocating tachycardias and 73% of supraventricular tachycardias related to the WPW syndrome. Oral flecainide was effective in chronic prevention of recurrences in 81% of patients with AV reciprocating tachycardias and 61% of patients with supraventricular tachycardias related to WPW syndrome. In the 695 patients with adverse effects reported, 6.9% reported cardiac side effects including worsened arrhythmia (28 patients), conduction disturbances (15 patients), and congestive heart failure (5 patients).

The effects of encainide are similar to flecainide.[33] Short-term oral encainide rendered AV reciprocating tachycardia non-inducible during electrophysiological study in 34–53% of the patients and prolonged the tachycardia cycle length in most of the patients in whom AV reciprocating tachycardia was still inducible.[35–37] Long-term follow-up for a mean of 18–38 months revealed that 71–93% of the patients taking oral encainide remained asymptomatic or had less frequent and severe symptoms without drug side effects.[36–38] In our series of 36 WPW patients with atrial fibrillation, 58% of the patients remained asymptomatic and another 29% experienced only rare, brief palpitations during chronic oral encainide therapy for a mean of 30.1 months.[35] Encainide is generally well tolerated but aggravation of tachycardia and new-onset ventricular tachycardia can occur in a small number of patients.[35] Isoproterenol can reverse the blocking of accessory pathway conduction and suppression of tachycardia induction by both flecainide[39] and encainide[40] and may be helpful in identifying the patients who may have a recurrence. Encainide is no longer available commercially.

Propafenone, a class Ic agent, also possesses beta-blocking properties. Its effects on the normal conduction system and the accessory pathway are similar to flecainide and encainide.[33] Intravenous propafenone at a dose of 1.5–2 mg/kg has been shown to convert 75–93% of episodes of reciprocating tachycardia to sinus rhythm[41, 42] and 30–46% of episodes of atrial fibrillation could be terminated.[42, 43] In a series of 43 patients receiving chronic oral propafenone therapy, 17 did not report any episode of symptomatic tachycardia, 18 had rare, slower, and self-terminating tachycardia, and 3 were without change.[44] The side effects have been mostly minor, such as nausea, dry mouth, dizziness, visual disturbance and constipation.[44]

Class III antiarrhythmic agents

Amiodarone and sotalol both prolong the conduction time and the refractory periods of the accessory pathway, the AV node, and the atrial and ventricular myocardium. Sotalol also possesses beta-blocking properties.[33] The response to intravenous amiodarone may predict the effects of oral amiodarone in preventing the occurrence of AV reciprocating tachycardia.[45] In 10 patients with atrial fibrillation (5 of whom previously also developed ventricular fibrillation), none had recurrence of atrial fibrillation or ventricular fibrillation within the 8–59 months of oral amiodarone therapy.[46] Because of the long loading period and serious side effects, amiodarone is usually reserved as second-line therapy and the adverse reactions should be closely monitored.

Intravenous sotalol at a dose of 0.6 mg/kg suppressed the electrical induction of reciprocating tachycardia in 5 of 9 patients, mainly due to AV nodal block.[47] Kunze et al[48] found that, after sotalol (1.5 mg/kg) was given intravenously to 15 patients, AV reciprocating tachycardia was no longer inducible in 1 patient and became non-sustained in another 10 patients. In 16 patients who received oral sotalol (240–320 mg per day) for a median of 36 months, 9 had no symptoms and 6 reported lessened symptoms though still experienced episodes of palpitations. In another 11 WPW patients, sotalol at a dose of 407 ± 149 mg per day suppressed induced orthodromic AV reciprocating tachycardia and prolonged the shortest RR interval during atrial fibrillation to 400 ms or greater in 4 patients; the same effects were achieved with a dose of 924 ± 337 mg per day in another 4 patients.[49] All 8 patients experienced no recurrence of sustained AV reciprocating tachycardia during a follow-up period of 15 ± 12 months.

Whereas the newer antiarrhythmic agents such as flecainide, encainide and propafenone are effective in acutely terminating and chronically preventing 70–90% of AV reciprocating tachycardia or suppressing the preexcited ventricular response during atrial fibrillation,[34–44] the increasing use of radiofrequency catheter ablation has replaced pharmacological therapy as the first-line treatment in centres with experienced electro-physiologists because of the safety and efficacy of radiofrequency ablation (see below). Of note is that encainide has been removed from the market in the United States, almost three years after the termination of phase I of the CAST trial.[50]

ANTITACHYCARDIA PACEMAKERS

Several types of antitachycardia pacemakers have been tested in small series of selected patients to terminate supraventricular tachycardias.[51-54] Fully automatic and externally activated systems have been used. The externally activated pacemakers rely on the patients to recognize the occurrence of tachycardia and activate the pacemakers to deliver either asynchronous or synchronous burst pacing. The antitachycardia pacemakers appear to be effective in terminating tachycardias and provide patient well-being.[51] The frequency of hospital admission is decreased. However, almost all patients still require antiarrhythmic therapy and the pacemakers can induce addi-tional tachycardias, especially atrial arrhythmias.[51-53] These devices have not been widely used and, because of catheter ablation, probably will never become a popular choice.

ABLATIVE PROCEDURES

Although pharmaceutical agents can prevent the recurrences of arrhyth-mias in up to 90% of patients with WPW syndrome, patients require long-term medication without complete assurance that the arrhythmias will not recur. It was not until 1968, when Sealy et al[55] successfully performed surgical ablation of the accessory pathway, that 'cure' could be offered to patients with WPW syndrome.

Surgical ablation

Until recently, surgical ablation has provided the only curative procedure for patients with WPW syndrome. However, the number of surgical operations performed for WPW patients has substantially decreased since the emergence of catheter ablation with radiofrequency current.

Endocardial approach[56]

The procedure initially described by Sealy et al was 'epicardial',[55] but it was the 'endocardial approach' that became the 'standard' procedure. After thoracotomy, epicardial electrophysiological mapping is performed with a probe electrode or multiple electrode band. Mapping determines the earliest activation point in the ventricles during either sinus rhythm or atrial pacing to locate the ventricular insertion of the accessory pathway(s), and the earliest activation point in the atria during orthodromic AV reciprocating tachycardia or ventricular pacing to locate its atrial insertion. Once the accessory pathway is located, the atriotomy is done under normothermic cardiopulmonary bypass and endocardial mapping is performed to confirm the location of the pathway. Incision at the pathway site is then made endocardially a few millimetres above the AV valve annulus. To separate the ventricular insertion of the accessory pathway from the ventricle, dissection through the fat pad is then made toward the ventricular side of the coronary sulcus until the epicardial reflection is reached (Fig. 7.3). Cryoablation has also been used for the same purpose.[57–59] With modifications in the dissection techniques, the success rate improved from 70% in the first 100 patients to nearly 100% in the more recent series.[56, 58–64] The recurrence rate ranged from 6.3% to 14%.[58, 64] The operative mortality rate in elective, uncomplicated cases has been 0–0.8%.[56, 59] The complications in recent larger series are infrequent and mostly are related to the nature of open heart surgery.[59, 60] Complete AV block may be of concern in the ablation of septal pathways.

Epicardial approach[65]

The epicardial approach was first advocated by Guiraudon et al.[66] In this approach, the primary dissection is carried out from the epicardial reflection off the atrium and extended to the ventricular side of the coronary sulcus in order to interrupt the atrial insertion of the accessory pathway (Fig. 7.3). The posteroseptal and right free wall pathways are usually ablated without cardiopulmonary bypass and atriotomy. The dissection of the left free wall, due to the spatial orientation of the heart in the chest, usually requires cardiopulmonary bypass to avoid haemodynamic compromise when the heart is lifted out of the chest. More recently, left free wall dissection without cardiopulmonary bypass has been done.[65–67, 68] Atriotomy and endocardial cryoablation are usually required in anteroseptal and the 'subendocardial' pathways, as epicardial dissection alone for the latter is insufficient to ablate the pathways. Other modifications include the use of ultrasonic aspirator for dissection of the fat pads.[67, 68] Because of the proximity of the right coronary artery to the anteroseptal space, cryoablation in this region may cause obstruction of the right coronary artery due to thrombus formation or injury to the arterial wall. Care should be exercised when applying the cryoprobe to the septal region to preserve AV conduction. The success rate, recurrence rate and complication rate are comparable to those found with the endocardial approach.[61, 65–70] Serious complications include inadvertent dissection of the coronary sinus or right coronary artery, and AV block. Compared with the endocardial technique, the epicardial approach has the advantage of not requiring cardiopulmonary bypass and atriotomy in most cases and the feasibility of dissecting the pathways associated with coronary sinus diverticulum. It

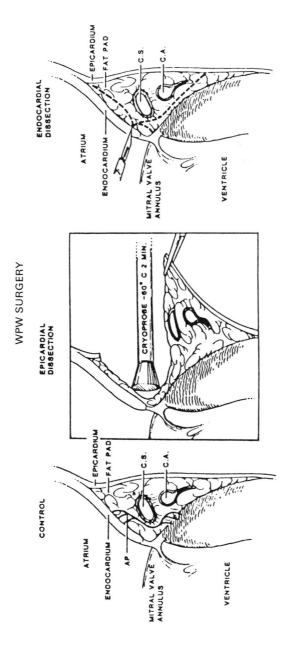

Fig. 7.3 The two different approaches for surgical ablation of the accessory pathway. The left-hand panel depicts the left AV groove and its vascular contents, the coronary sinus (C.S.), and circumflex coronary artery (C.A.). Multiple accessory pathways (AP) course through the fat pad. The middle panel shows the epicardial dissection approach while the right-hand panel exhibits the endocardial dissection. Both approaches clear out the fat to interrupt any accessory pathways. WPW = Wolff–Parkinson–White syndrome. (Reproduced with permission from Zipes DP, Cardiac electrophysiology: promises and contributions. J Am Coll Cardiol 1989; 13: 1329)

also appears to be easier in ablating posteroseptal pathways. Which approach used is generally decided by the experience of the surgeon.

The long-term costs of drug treatment and surgical ablation have been compared. [71] By projection, the two treatment modalities would incur the same amount of cost 12.5 years after the onset of treatment. However, patients receiving drug treatment remain at risk for a symptomatic recurrence. Thus, surgery appears to be a more resonable choice than drug treatment for symptomatic patients who otherwise require chronic drug therapy.

Catheter ablation

Direct current shock

It was reported in 1982 that delivering a high-energy direct current (DC) shock between a catheter placed close to the AV node and a reference electrode interrupted AV conduction in patients with refractory supraventricular tachyarrythmias.[72] The high-energy electrical discharge caused: (1) formation of an electric field; (2) pressure waves due to the formation and collapse of a vapour globe that is produced by water vaporization and hydrolysis of the water into hydrogen and oxygen gases; and (3) generation of heat. The tissue damage appears to be due to the intense electric field that causes cellular disruption. There is little evidence that the shock waves create significant barotrauma except in confined spaces such as the coronary sinus. In addition, it has been shown that lesions can be produced by applying DC shocks with very short durations that do not generate significant pressure waves. Although the electrical charges create a large amount of heat, the heat is quickly dissipated and little is transmitted to the tissue to cause significant damage.[73] The DC shock technique was soon applied to patients with WPW syndrome. Less commonly, patients received AV junction ablation to interrupt AV conduction that served as one limb of a re-entrant circuit because the His bundle was easier to identify and approach.[74, 75] This treatment was undesirable because of the high incidence of atrial arrhythmia and conduction over the accessory pathway, which required antiarrhythmic therapy, as well as pacemaker dependency (continuous conduction over the accessory pathway could not be relied upon). More frequently, DC shock was utilized to ablate the accessory pathway. Initially, the catheters were placed in the coronary sinus os for ablation of posteroseptal pathways. After rupture of the coronary sinus and cardiac tamponade were observed in the early series, the technique was modified. Instead of applying DC shock through the distal electrode, the pulse was delivered from the more proximal electrode (e.g. the third electrode in a quadripolar catheter) close to, but outside of, the coronary sinus os.[73–76] This modification substantially reduced the risk of rupture of the coronary sinus. The success rate of DC ablation of the posteroseptal pathways has been approximately 70%.[76, 77]

Recently, DC ablation of accessory pathways at all locations has been more satisfactory when mapping and ablation are done from within the cardiac chambers ('direct approach'). In 248 patients, Warin et al[78] successfully ablated 238 of 254 accessory pathways (94%) and impaired the function of another 8 pathways, using either two consecutive 160 J shocks or one 240 J shock per attempt. During a follow-up period of 3–64 months, 96% of the patients were free of arrhythmia recurrence. Their criteria for a desirable ablation site were: (1) recording the accessory pathway potential; (2) onset of local ventricular potential earlier than or equal to the onset of the delta wave during sinus rhythm or atrial pacing; (3) an accurate pace-map (QRS morphology during pacing from the mapping site) concordance with the major ventricular pre-excitation; (4) recording the shortest VA interval during orthodromic reciprocating tachycardia (mean = 80 ms); and (5) loss of the delta wave due to catheter pressure on the accessory pathway. Complications were infrequent but could be serious, such as cardiac perforation, cardiogenic shock, coronary artery spasm, AV block and late-onset ventricular fibrillation.[73, 76–79]

The disadvantage of high-energy DC ablation is that the energy release cannot be controlled, general anaesthesia is required to relieve patient discomfort, only woven Dacron electrode catheters have been tested for safe delivery of high amounts of DC energy, and the catheter has to be changed after each use because arcing may have occurred and damaged the catheter. Low-energy DC ablation (up to 30 J), successful in ablating 97% of the left free wall and 80% of the posteroseptal accessory pathways in a series of 45 patients, may be safe with the other types of catheters[80] and repeated use of the same catheter may be possible so that the mapping and ablation time may be shortened.

Radiofrequency energy[81]

The first successful ablation of an accessory pathway in humans with radiofrequency (RF) energy was reported in 1987.[82] With technical refinement, RF energy catheter ablation has become widely utilized and appears to be the best available curative procedure for WPW patients at the present time.

RF is an alternating electrical current with a frequency ranging from 30 kHz to 300 MHz. It was first reported to be effective in cutting living tissues in 1911. Because of its cutting and coagulating effects, RF current devices are widely utilized in the operating room by surgeons. Since unmodulated RF current produces coagulation necrosis, it has been applied to transcatheter ablation of the cardiac tissue involved in cardiac arrhythmias. The most important mechanism of action appears to be conversion of electrical energy into heat. A closed circuit is required for the flow of an electrical current. In the case of catheter ablation with RF current, the system has four components: the RF generator, the connecting wires, the electrodes, and the target tissue between the electrodes. The electrical current may be delivered between two 'active' electrodes in the same catheter (bipolar current delivery) or between the distal ('active') electrode of the catheter and a patch ('passive' electrode) on the body surface (unipolar delivery). As RF current flows through the tissue, ions in the tissue are accelerated and resistive heating occurs at the point where current density is high and electrical conductivity is relatively low. Thus temperature increases at the contact point of the 'active' electrode(s) and tissue surface, with maximal heat occurring at the electrode–tissue interface and decreasing as a function of current density.

To ablate successfully an accessory pathway with RF, in addition to the criteria for a desirable site noted for DC ablation,[78] several other factors are also important: large-tipped catheters (4 mm);[83, 84] good catheter contact with the tissue as demonstrated by simultaneously recording recognizable local atrial and ventricular potentials with low gain; a 1:1 ratio of the amplitude of the atrial and ventricular potentials; and delivery of RF current for more than 12 s per application if impedance has not increased and the catheter has not moved.[85] Figure 7.4 demonstrates the successful RF ablation of a left lateral pathway. The procedure does not require general anaesthesia and can be performed in a single session combined with diagnostic electrophysiological study.[86] The success rate for elimination of the accessory pathway conduction has been 83–99%, with 3–9% recurrence rate.[83, 86 – 90] However, most of the patients with recurrences have had successful results when the RF ablation was repeated. Because the longest

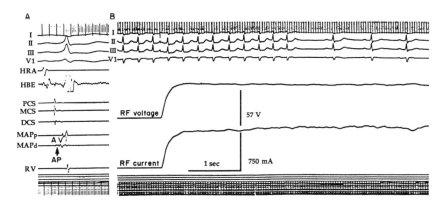

Fig. 7.4   Successful catheter ablation of the accessory pathway with RF current. **A** The accessory pathway potential (arrow) was recorded by the ablating catheter, which was inserted retrogradely across the aortic valve into the left ventricle and placed under the mitral valve at the left lateral position. **B** The tachycardia terminated with retrograde VA block 2.6 s after the onset of the RF pulse, indicating that the conduction of the accessory pathway had been interrupted by the RF energy. I, II, III, V1 were surface ECG leads; HRA = high right atrium; HBE = His bundle electrogram; PCS = proximal coronary sinus; MCS = middle coronary sinus; DCS = distal coronary sinus; MAPp = proximal mapping electrogram; MAPd = distal mapping electrogram: RV = right ventricle.

follow-up reported so far is 43 months, the long-term efficacy of RF ablation remains to be determined.

No deaths have been reported due to the catheterization, mapping or RF ablation. The complication rate has been low in the large series.[83, 86, 87] The complications related to actual mapping and RF ablation include pericardial effusion, complete AV block, thromboembolism (including intracardiac thrombi and pulmonary embolism), haemopericardium and cardiac tamponade (due to application of RF pulse in a small venous branch of the proximal coronary sinus), and myocardial infarction in a patient because of inadvertent delivery of RF current into the left coronary artery with occlusion of the left circumflex artery.[83, 86–89] None of the other patients have developed electrocardiographic evidence of myocardial infarction, though serum creatine kinase and the MB isozyme levels were elevated in a small portion of patients. The use of antiplatelet/anticoagulation therapy for thromboembolism varies in different centres. A multicentre trial may be necessary to determine whether such therapy is required and, if so, which regimen to choose. Another important issue is whether patients and physicians receive excessive radiation exposure. The average duration of radiation may vary from institution to institution because of the difference in the catheterization procedure, the diagnostic protocol, and the limitation in the access time to the fluoroscopic facility. In some uncomplicated cases, we have been able to complete a diagnostic study and successful ablation in one session with less than 20 minutes of fluoroscopic time. It remains to be determined whether long-term complications will occur due to several hours of fluoroscopic exposure and whether the radiation complications will be too serious to offset the symptomatic relief from RF ablation. Very likely further experience with the technique will reduce fluoroscopic exposure time considerably. Cost–benefit analysis has favoured catheter ablation over surgical ablation.[91, 92]

TREATMENT STRATEGY

The risk of sudden death in untreated asymptomatic patients with WPW syndrome is approximately 1 per 1000 patient-year.[93] However, patients with accessory pathways not uncommonly have symptoms that affect their lifestyles. Hence the rationale for treating patients with WPW syndrome would be: (1) to reduce the risk of sudden death; (2) to relieve symptoms associated with the tachycardias; (3) to prevent the occurrence of tachycardias; and (4) to eliminate the need for long-term drug therapy and the associated side effects, cost and discomfort.

Acutely, when a patient develops symptoms associated with tachycardia, a 12-lead electrocardiogram is almost always required to interpret the cardiac rhythm. The differential diagnosis of a narrow QRS tachycardia include AV nodal re-entrant tachycardia, orthodromic AV reciprocating tachycardia, PJRT, non-paroxysmal junctional tachycardia, and atrial flutter/fibrillation and atrial or sinus tachycardia without ventricular pre-excitation (Fig. 7.2). Vagal manoeuvres such as carotid sinus massage may terminate the re-entrant tachycardias, transiently interrupt but not terminate PJRT, or slow the ventricular response without changing the atrial rate in atrial tachycardia. Adenosine and ATP, because of their AV nodal blocking effect and very short half-life, have become the favourite drugs in terminating the re-entrant tachycardias and proving the diagnosis of narrow QRS tachycardia. Intravenous verapamil, digitalis, diltiazem, beta-blockers, procainamide and other antiarrhythmics have also been safely used. When the electrocardiogram reveals a wide QRS tachycardia, anti-dromic AV reciprocating tachycardia (often associated with multiple accessory pathways), orthodromic AV reciprocating tachycardia or AV nodal re-entrant tachycardia with functional right or left bundle branch block, atrial flutter/fibrillation with pre-excited ventricular complexes, and ventricular tachycardia have to be differentiated. In patients with haemodynamic instability, DC cardioversion appears to be the best approach in that most wide QRS tachycardias will be terminated. Intravenous procainamide or other class I agents may be helpful. It cannot be overemphasized that intravenous digitalis and calcium entry blockers must be avoided in patients with wide QRS tachycardias since acceleration of pre-excited ventricular rate[4–7, 19] and induction of ventricular fibrillation in WPW patients with atrial fibrillation can result following injection of these drugs.[4–7]

Chronic therapy should be guided by cardiac electrophysiological study.[94] Electrophysiological study provides valuable information such as: the location and characteristics of the accessory pathway(s); the nature of the tachycardia(s); the limb of the re-entrant circuit(s) in which conduction is most marginal at the tachycardia rate ('weak limb'); and the performance of the accessory pathway(s) during induced atrial fibrillation. Identification and localization of the accessory pathway(s) is the prerequisite for a successful ablation procedure. Determination of the 'weak limb' of the re-entrant circuit is helpful in deciding whether to use a drug that effects predominantly the AV node or the accessory pathway.[95] Survivors of ventricular fibrillation as a consequence of accessory pathway-related arrhythmias invariably are found to have an effective refractory period of the accessory pathway less than 270 ms and/or a shortest pre-excited RR interval less than 250 ms.[93] Chronic therapy should be aimed at completely blocking the conduction of the accessory pathway or at least prolonging the accessory pathway refractoriness and the shortest pre-excited RR interval during atrial fibrillation to decrease the risk of ventricular fibrillation in these patients. We would favour RF ablation in these patients.

Our present approach to symptomatic patients is to inform patients of the nature and risks of the diagnostic electrophysiological study and catheter ablation, offer RF energy catheter ablation as the first-line therapy, and perform the diagnostic study and catheter ablation in the same session with the consent from the patients. DC ablation serves as an alternative procedure to RF ablation. The presence of multiple pathways has not been a contraindication to catheter ablation. For patients with other cardiac structural abnormalities requiring surgical correction and highly symptomatic patients who failed attempts at catheter ablation, surgical ablation is recommended. In less symptomatic patients who failed catheter ablation, options of drug therapy or surgical ablation are presented and, if drug treatment is chosen, antiarrhythmic therapy is initiated with electrophysiological guidance. In institutions where ablation expertise is not available, best drug therapy should be chosen based on the electrophysiological findings. However, class Ic agents probably should be avoided in patients who belong to the same population as those enrolled in the CAST trial.[50] It is preferable to refer highly symptomatic patients for ablation of the accessory pathway(s).

The best management for asymptomatic patients with incidental finding of ventricular pre-excitation remains unclear. Non-invasive tests such as Holter recording and periodic electrocardiographic examinations, when identifying intermittent block in the accessory pathway, suggest that conduction over the pathway is marginal and predict that a slower pre-excited ventricular rate will result in the event of atrial fibrillation. The same inference can be derived when sudden loss of accessory pathway conduction occurs at a critical heart rate during exercise testing. Loss of pre-excitation after intravenous administration of a class I agent (e.g. procainamide and ajmaline) can identify patients with longer accessory pathway effective refractory period (> 270 ms)[30,31] but may depend on the dose of the antiarrhythmic used.[93] These measures are certainly no substitute for determination of the ventricular response to the actual induction of atrial fibrillation in the electrophysiological study. However, it is difficult to weigh the benefits against the risks of electrophysiological study in these patients, since 17% of the asymptomatic patients have a shortest pre-excited RR interval of less than 250 ms at electrophysiological study, but the sudden death rate is very low.[96] It is probably reasonable first to inform asymptomatic patients of the potential outcomes and reach a mutual agreement whether to proceed with an electrophysiological study on an individual basis. Patients who are found to have a shortest pre-excited RR interval of less than 250 ms, inducible reciprocating tachycardia, multiple pathways, or an average shortest RR interval of 360 ms or less probably should be considered for catheter ablation or drug prophylaxis, especially when even a small risk of serious arrhythmia will interfere with the patient's career or lifestyle.[93]

SUMMARY

Patients with accessory pathways frequently have symptoms caused by tachyarrhythmia, and a very small number of patients with excellent accessory pathway function are at risk of sudden death because of ventricular fibrillation induced by atrial fibrillation with rapid pre-excited ventricular response. Drug therapy has been the major choice for treatment of symptomatic patients, with antitachycardia pacemakers as an adjunct therapy, and surgical ablation indicated in highly symptomatic patients. Drug therapy should be guided by electrophysiological study, and agents that affect either limb of the re-entrant loop are effective in treating AV reciprocating tachycardia. Only drugs affecting the accessory pathway (preferably both the accessory pathway and the AV node) should be used in atrial fibrillation with pre-excited ventricular complexes, and intravenous digitalis and calcium entry blockers must be avoided. Surgical ablation consists of two different approaches—endocardial and epicardial—and both are equally effective. Catheter ablation with DC shock or RF energy has success rates comparable to that of surgical ablation but involves much shorter hospital stay and much less trauma and cost. RF ablation appears to be the most cost-effective treatment for symptomatic patients and has replaced both drug therapy and surgical ablation as the first-line therapy. Its long-term efficacy and complication rate remain to be determined. DC ablation may be a useful alternative to RF ablation when the latter has been unsuccessful. In asymptomatic patients, non-invasive tests may be useful but the electrophysiological study offers more definitive information and should be considered on an individual basis. Asymptomatic patients with risk factors of sudden cardiac death probably should not be treated because the risk of sudden death is very low.

ACKNOWLEDGEMENTS

This work was supported in part by the Herman C. Krannert Fund; by grants HL-42370 and HL-07182 from the National Heart, Lung and Blood Institute of the National Institutes of Health, US Public Health Service; and the American Heart Association, Inc., Indiana Affiliate.

REFERENCES

1 O'Neill BJ, Klein GJ, Guiraudon GM et al. Results of operative therapy in the permanent form of junctional reciprocating tachycardia. Am J Cardiol 1989; 63: 1074
2 Klein GJ, Bashore TM, Sellers TD et al. Ventricular fibrillation in the Wolff–Parkinson–White syndrome. N Engl J Med 1979; 30: 1080
3 Montoya PJ and the European Registry on Sudden Death in Wolff–Parkinson–White Syndrome. Ventricular fibrillation in the Wolff–Parkinson–White syndrome. Circulation 1988; 78(suppl II): II-88
4 Sellers TD Jr, Bashore TM, Gallagher JJ. Digitalis in the pre-excitation syndrome: analysis during atrial fibrillation. Circulation 1977; 56: 260
5 McGovern B, Garan H, Ruskin JN. Precipitation of cardiac arrest by verapamil in patients with Wolff–Parkinson–White syndrome. Ann Intern Med 1986; 104: 791
6 Garratt C, Antoniou A, Ward D, Camm AJ. Misuse of verapamil in pre-excited atrial fibrillation. Lancet 1989; i(8634): 367
7 Rinkenberger RL, Prystowsky EN, Heger JJ et al. Effects of intravenous and chronic oral

verapamil administration in patients with supraventricular tachycardias. Circulation 1980; 62: 996

8 Dhingra RC, Palileo EV, Strasberg B et al. Electrophysiologic effects of ouabain in patients with pre-excitation and circus movement tachycardia. Am J Cardiol 1981; 47: 139

9 Jedeikin R, Gillette PC, Garson A Jr et al. Effect of ouabain on the anterograde effective refractory period of accessory atrioventricular connections in children. J Am Coll Cardiol 1983; 1: 869

10 Wellens HJ, Durrer D. Effect of digitalis on atrioventricular connection and circus movement tachycardias in patients with Wolff–Parkinson–White syndrome. Circulation 1973; 47: 1229

11 Denes P, Cummings JM, Simpson R et al. Effects of propranolol on anomalous pathway refractoriness and circus movement tachycardias in patients with pre-excitation. Am J Cardiol 1978; 41: 1061

12 Barrett PA, Jordan JL, Mandel WJ et al. The electrophysiologic effects of intravenous propranolol in the Wolff–Parkinson–White syndrome. Am Heart J 1979; 98: 213

13 Gmeiner R, Ng CK. Metoprolol in the treatment and prophylaxis of paroxysmal reentrant supraventricular tachycardia. J Cardiovasc Pharmacol 1982; 4: 5

14 Chang MS, Sung RJ, Tai T-Y et al. Nadolol and supraventricular tachycardia: an electrophysiologic study. J Am Coll Cardiol 1983; 22: 894

15 Greer GS, Ramirez WM, Fananapazir L et al. Bolus esmolol in the treatment of supraventricular tachycardia. Circulation 1987; 76 (suppl IV): IV-67 (Abstract)

16 Morady F, DiCarlo LA Jr, Baerman JM, de Buitleir M. Effect of propranolol on ventricular rate during atrial fibrillation in the Wolff–Parkinson–White syndrome. PACE 1987; 10 (3 pt 1): 492

17 Swerdlow CD, Peterson J, Liem LB. Effect of flestolol on ventricular rate during atrial fibrillation in Wolff–Parkinson–White syndrome. Am J Cardiol 1988; 62: 78

18 Zipes DP, Fischer JC. Effects of agents which inhibit the slow channel on sinus node automaticity and atrioventricular conduction in the dog. Circ Res 1974; 34: 124

19 Shenasa M, Fromer M, Faugere G et al. Efficacy and safety of intravenous and oral diltiazem for Wolff–Parkinson–White syndrome. Am J Cardiol 1987; 59: 301

20 Rozanski JJ, Zaman L, Castellanos A. Electrophysiologic effects of diltiazem hydrochloride on supraventricular tachycardia. Am J Cardiol 1982; 49: 621

21 Touboul P, Atallah G, Kirkorian G et al. Electrophysiological action of bepridil on atrioventricular accessory pathways. Br Heart J 1987; 58: 333

22 Hamer A, Peter T, Platt M et al. Effects of verapamil on supraventricular tachycardia in patients with overt and concealed Wolff–Parkinson–White syndrome. Am Heart J 1981; 101: 600

23 Huycke EC, Sung RJ, Dias VC et al. Intravenous diltiazem for termination of reentrant supraventricular tachycardia: a placebo-controlled, randomized, doubleblind multicenter study. J Am Coll Cardiol 1989; 13: 538

24 Prystowsky EN. Electrophysiologic and antiarrhythmic properties of bepridil. Am J Cardiol 1985; 55: 59C

25 DiMarco JP, Sellers TD, Berne RM et al. Adenosine: electrophysiologic effects and therapeutic use for terminating paroxysmal supraventricular tachycardia. Circulation 1983; 68: 1254

26 Belardinelli L, Wu SN, Visentin S. Adenosine regulation of cardiac electrical activity. In: Zipes DP, Jalife J, eds. Cardiac electrophysiology: from cell to bedside. Philadelphia, Saunders, 1990, p 284

27 Sellers TD, Kirchoffer JB, Modesto TA. Adenosine: a clinical experience and comparison with verapamil for the termination of supraventricular tachycardias. Prog Clin Biol Res 1987; 230: 283

28 Belhassen B, Glick A, Laniads S. Comparative clinical and electrophysiologic effects of adenosine triphosphate and verapamil on paroxysmal reciprocating junctional tachycardia. Circulation 1988; 77: 795

29 Sharma AD, Klein GJ, Yee R. Intravenous adenosine triphosphate during wide QRS complex tachycardia: safety, therapeutic efficacy, and diagnostic utility. Am J Med 1990; 88: 337

30 Wellens HJJ, Bär FW, Gorgels AP, Vanagt EJ. Use of ajmaline in patients with the Wolff–Parkinson–White syndrome to disclose short refractory period of the accessory pathway. Am J Cardiol. 1980; 45: 13

31 Wellens HJJ, Braat S, Brugada P et al. Use of procainamide in patients with the Wolff–Parkinson–White syndrome to disclose a short refractory period of the accessory pathway. Am J Cardiol 1982; 50: 1087

32 Wellens HJJ, Bär FW, Vanagt EJ. Death after ajmaline administration. Am J Cardiol 1980; 45: 905

33 Packer DL, Prystowsky EN. Wolff–Parkinson–White syndrome: further progress in evaluation and treatment. Prog Cardiol 1988; 1/1: 147

34 Anderson JL, Jolivette DM, Fredell PA. Summary of efficacy and safety of flecainide for supraventricular arrhythmias. Am J Cardiol 1988; 62: 62D

35 Rinkenberger RL, Naccarelli GV, Miles WM et al. Encainide for atrial fibrillation associated with Wolff-Parkinson-White syndrome. Am J Cardiol 1988; 62: 26L

36 Miles WM, Zipes DP, Rinkenberger RL et al. Encainide for treatment of atrioventricular reciprocating tachycardia in the Wolff–Parkinson–White syndrome. Am J Cardiol 1988; 62: 20L

37 Prystowsky EN, Klein GJ, Rinkenberger RL et al. Clinical efficacy and electrophysiologic effects of encainide in patients with Wolff–Parkinson–White syndrome. Circulation 1984; 69: 278

38 Markel ML, Prystowsky EN, Heger JJ et al. Encainide for treatment of supraventricular tachycardias associated with the Wolff–Parkinson–White syndrome. Am J Cardiol 1986; 58: 41C

39 Brembilla-Perrot B, Admant P, Le Helloco A, Pernot C. Loss of efficacy of flecainide in the Wolff–Parkinson–White syndrome after isoproterenol administration. Eur Heart J 1985; 6: 1074

40 Akhtar M, Niazi I, Naccarelli GV et al. Role of adrenergic stimulation by isoproterenol in reversal of effects of encainide in supraventricular tachycardia. Am J Cardiol 1988; 62: 45L

41 Shen EN, Keung E, Huycke E et al. Intravenous propafenone for termination of reentrant supraventricular tachycardia: a placebo-controlled, randomized, doubleblind crossover study. Ann Intern Med 1986; 105: 655

42 Dubuc M, Kus T, Campa MA et al. Electrophysiologic effects of intravenous propafenone in Wolff–Parkinson–White syndrome. Am Heart J 1989; 117: 370

43 Boahene KA, Klein GJ, Yee R et al. Termination of acute atrial fibrillation in the Wolff–Parkinson–White syndrome by procainamide and propafenone: importance of atrial fibrillatory cycle length. J Am Coll Cardiol 1990; 16: 1408

44 Breithardt G, Borggrefe M, Wiebringhaus E, Seipel L. Effect of propafenone in the Wolff–Parkinson–White syndrome: electrophysiologic findings and long-term follow-up. Am J Cardiol 1984; 54: 29D

45 Wellens HJ, Brugada P, Abdollah H, Dassen WR. A comparison of the electrophysiologic effects of intravenous and oral amiodarone in the same patients. Circulation 1984: 69: 120

46 Feld GK, Nademanee K, Stevenson W et al. Clinical and electrophysiologic effects of amiodarone in patients with atrial fibrillation complicating the Wolff–Parkinson–White syndrome. Am Heart J 1988; 115 (pt 1): 102

47 Touboul P, Atallah G, Kirkorian G et al. Effects of intravenous sotalol in patients with atrioventricular accessory pathways. Am Heart J 1987; 114: 545

48 Kunze KP, Schlüter M, Kuck KH. Sotalol in patients with Wolff–Parkinson–White syndrome. Circulation 1987; 75: 1050

49 Mitchell LB, Wyse DG, Duff HJ. Electropharmacology of sotalol in patients with Wolff–Parkinson–White syndrome. Circulation 1987; 76: 810

50 Cardiac Arrhythmia Suppression Trial (CAST) Investigators. Preliminary report: effect of encainide and flecainide on mortality in a randomized trial of arrhythmia suppression after myocardial infarction. N Engl J Med 1989; 321: 406

51 den Dulk K, Brugada P, Smeets JLRM, Wellens HJJ. Pacing for supraventricular tachycardia. In: Zipes DP, Jalife J, eds. Cardiac electrophysiology: from cell to bedside. Philadelphia: Saunders, 1990, p 934

52 Fromer M, Gloor H, Kus T, Shenasa M. Clinical experience with a new software based antitachycardia pacemaker for recurrent supraventricular and ventricular tachycardias. PACE 1990; 13: 890

53 Holt P, Crick JC, Sowton E. Antitachycardia pacing: a comparison of burst overdrive, self-searching, and adaptive table scanning programs. PACE 1986; 9: 490

54 Portillo B, Medina-Ravell V, Portillo-Leon N et al. Treatment of drug resistant A-V

reciprocating tachycardia with multiprogrammable dual demand A-V sequential (DVI, MN) pacemakers. PACE 1982; 5: 814
55 Sealy WC, Hattler BG Jr, Blumenschein SD, Cobb FR. Surgical treatment of Wolff–Parkinson–White syndrome. Ann Thorac Surg 1969; 8: 1
56 Ferguson TB Jr, Cox JL. Surgical treatment for the Wolff–Parkinson–White syndrome: the endocardial approach. In: Zipes DP, Jalife J, eds. Cardiac electrophysiology: from cell to bedside. Philadelphia, Saunders, 1990, p 897
57 Gallagher JJ, Sealy WC, Anderson RW et al. Cryosurgical ablation of accessory atrioventricular connections: a method for correction of the pre-excitation syndrome. Circulation 1977; 55: 471
58 Selle JG, Sealy WC, Gallagher JJ et al. The complex posterior septal space in the Wolff–Parkinson–White syndrome surgical experience with 47 patients. Thorac Cardiovasc Surg 1989; 37: 299
59 Cox JL, Gallagher JJ, Cain ME. Experience with 118 consecutive patients undergoing operation for the Wolff–Parkinson–White syndrome. J Thorac Cardiovasc Surg 1985; 90: 490
60 Iva T, Tsubota M, Matsunata I, Misaki I. Surgical treatment of Wolff–Parkinson–White syndrome. Grud Serdechnososudistaia Khir 1990; 4: 21
61 Pagé PL, Pelletier LC, Kaltenbrunner W et al. Surgical treatment of the Wolff–Parkinson–White syndrome: endocardial vs epicardial approach. J Thorac Cardiovasc Surg 1990; 100: 83
62 Crawford FA Jr, Gillette PC, Zeigler V et al. Surgical management of Wolff–Parkinson–White syndrome in infants and small children. J Thorac Cardiovasc Surg. 1990; 99: 234
63 Lee AW, Crawford FA Jr, Gillette PC, Roble SM. Cryoablation of septal pathways in patients with supraventricular tachyarrhythmias. Ann Thorac Surg 1989; 47: 566
64 Ott DA, Garson A, Cooley DA, McNamara DG. Definitive operation for refractory cardiac tachyarrhythmias in children. J Thorac Cardiovasc Surg 1985; 90: 681
65 Guiraudon GM, Klein GJ, Sharma AD et al. Surgery for the Wolff–Parkinson–White syndrome: the epicardial approach. In: Zipes DP, Jalife J, eds. Cardiac electrophysiology: from cell to bedside. Philadelphia: Saunders, 1990, p 907
66 Guiraudon GM, Klein GJ, Gulamhusein S et al. Surgical repair of Wolff–Parkinson–White syndrome: a new closed-heart technique. Ann Thorac Surg 1984; 37: 67
67 Guiraudon GM, Klein GJ, Yee R et al. Surgical epicardial ablation of left ventricular pathway using sling exposure. Ann Thorac Surg 1990; 50: 968
68 Watanabe S, Koyanagi H, Endo M et al. Cryosurgical ablation of accessory atrioventricular pathways without cardiopulmonary bypass: an epicardial approach for Wolff–Parkinson–White syndrome. Ann Thorac Surg 1989; 47: 257
69 Bredikis J, Bukauskas F, Zebrauskas R et al. Cryosurgical ablation of right parietal and septal accessory atrioventricular connections without the use of extracorporeal circulation. J Thorac Cardiovasc Surg 1985; 90: 206
70 Mahomed Y, King RD, Zipes DP et al. Surgical division of Wolff–Parkinson–White pathways utilizing the closed-heart technique: a 2-year experience in 47 patients. Ann Thorac Surg 1988; 45: 495
71 Lezaun R, Brugada P, Smeets J et al. Cost–benefit analysis of medical vs surgical treatment of symptomatic patients with accessory atrioventricular pathways. Eur Heart J 1989; 10: 1105
72 Scheinman MM, Morady F, Hess DS, Gonzalez R. Catheter-induced ablation of the atrioventricular junction to control refractory supraventricular arrhythmias. JAMA 1982; 248: 851
73 Scheinman MM, Morady F. Catheter ablation for treatment of supraventricular arrhythmias. In Zipes DP, Jalife J, eds. Cardiac electrophysiology: from cell to bedside. Philadelphia: Saunders, 1990, p 970
74 Gallagher JJ, Svenson RH, Kasell JH et al. Catheter technique for closed-chest ablation of the atrioventricular conduction system: a therapeutic alternative for the treatment of refractory supraventricular tachycardia. N Engl J Med 1982; 306: 194
75 Eldar M, Griffin JC, Seger JJ et al. Catheter atrioventricular junction ablation in patients with accessory pathways. PACE 1986; 9 (6, pt 1): 810

76 Morady F, Scheinman MM, Kou WH ·et al. Long-term results of catheter ablation of a posteroseptal accessory atrioventricular connection in 48 patients. Circulation 1989; 79: 1160

77 Bardy GH, Ivery TD, Coltorti F et al. Developments, complications, and limitations of catheter-mediated electrical ablation of posterior accessory atrioventricular pathways. Am J Cardiol 1988; 61: 309

78 Warin JF. Catheter ablation of accessory pathways: technique and results in 248 patients. PACE 1990; 13: 1609

79 Scheinman MM, Evans-Bell T. Catheter ablation of the atrioventricular junction: a report of the percutaneous mapping and ablation registry. Circulation 1984; 70: 1024

80 Lemery R, Talajic M, Roy D et al. Low energy DC ablation in patients with the Wolff–Parkinson–White syndrome: clinical outcome according to accessory pathway location. PACE 1991; 14: 670 (Abstract)

81 Borggrefe M, Hindricks G, Haverkamp W et al. Radiofrequency ablation. In: Zipes DP, Jalife J, eds. Cardiac electrophysiology: from cell to bedside. Philadelphia: Saunders, 1990, 997

82 Borggrefe M, Budde T, Podczeck A et al. High frequency alternating current ablation of accessory pathway in humans. J Am Coll Cardiol 1987; 10: 576

83 Kuck KH, Schlüter M, Geiger M et al. Radiofrequency current catheter ablation of accessory atrioventricular pathways. Lancet 1991; 337: 1557

84 Borggrefe M, Hief C, Karbenn U et al. Catheter ablation of accessory pathways using radiofrequency energy: improvement of results with the use of a large tip electrode catheter. J Am Coll Cardiol 1991; 17: 109A

85 Wang X, Moulton K, Margolis D et al. Pulse duration required for radiofrequency catheter ablation of accessory pathways. Circulation 1990; 82 (Suppl III): III-719

86 Calkins H, Sousa J, El-Atassi R et al. Diagnosis and cure of the Wolff Parkinson–White syndrome or paroxysmal supraventricular tachycardias during a single electrophysiologic test. N Engl J Med 1991; 324: 1612

87 JackmannWM, Wang X, Friday KJ et al. Catheter ablation of accessory atrioventricular pathways (Wolff–Parkinson–White syndrome) by radiofrequency current. N Engl J Med 1991; 324: 1605

88 Van Hare GF, Lesh MD, Scheinman M, Langberg JJ. Percutaneous radiofrequency catheter ablation for supraventricular arrhythmias in children. J Am Coll Cardiol 1991; 17: 1613

89 Miles WM, Klein LS, Gering LE et al. Efficacy and safety of catheter ablation using radiofrequency energy in patients with accessory pathways. J Am Coll Cardiol 1991; 17: 233A

90 Swartz J, Tracy C, Fletcher R et al. A comparative study of direct current and radiofrequency atrial endocardial ablation of accessory pathways. J Am Coll Cardiol 1991; 17: 109A

91 de Buitleir M, Bove EL, Schmaltz S et al. Cost of catheter versus surgical ablation in the Wolff–Parkinson–White syndrome. Am J Cardiol 1990; 66: 189

92 de Buitleir M, Sousa J, Calkins H et al. Dramatic reduction in medical care costs associated with radiofrequency catheter ablation of accessory pathways. J Am Coll Cardiol 1991; 17: 109A

93 Klein GJ, Prystowsky EN, Yee R et al. Asymptomatic Wolff–Parkinson–White: should we intervene? Circulation 1989; 80: 1902

94 Waldo AL, Akhtar M, Benditt DG et al. Appropriate electrophysiologic atudy and treatment of patients with the Wolff–Parkinson–White syndrome. J Am Coll Cardiol 1988; 11: 1124

95 Jackman WM, Friday KJ, Fitzgerald DM et al. Use of intracardiac recordings to determine the site of drug action in paroxysmal supraventricular tachycardia. Am J Cardiol 1988; 62: 8L

96 Milstein S, Sharma AD, Klein GJ. Electrophysiologic profile of asymptomatic Wolff–Parkinson–White pattern. Am J Cardiol 1986; 57: 1097

8

Selection of pacemaker mode for the management of symptomatic bradycardia

M. Clarke

INDICATIONS FOR PERMANENT PACING

The first pacemaker implantation in 1958[1] was quickly followed by various technological and clinical developments that established single-chamber ventricular stimulation as life-saving therapy in patients with syncope due to atrioventricular (AV) block.[2] Initially, this was considered all that was required, and in the first two decades of permanent cardiac pacing scant attention was paid to those aspects of the heart's natural rhythm which are capable of enhancing the quality of a person's life, both at rest and on exercise. However, over the last ten years a large number of new features have been introduced into pacemaker designs to offer programmability, telemetry, intracardiac electrograms and various pacing modes as a routine.[3-7]

Before implanting a permanent pacemaker, the cardiologist should carefully assess the patient's general medical status as well as the specific features of the cardiac arrhythmia. Whereas at one time pacing was used solely for the treatment of AV block, the clinical indications for pacemaker implantation have now increased to include appropriate control of any symptomatic bradycardia. In 1984, a task force representing the combined opinions of the American Heart Association (AHA) and the American College of Cardiology (ACC) published guidelines for the selection of patients requiring pacemaker therapy.[8] The AHA/ACC working group has categorized potential pacemaker recipients into three groups.

Class I consists of those conditions in which there is general agreement that permanent pacemakers should be implanted. The condition should be chronic or recurrent, and not due to transient causes such as recent myocardial infarction, drug toxicity and electrolyte imbalance. If the arrhythmia fulfils these criteria, then a single episode of a relevant symptom is adequate to justify permanent pacing. The symptoms recognized as significant in this group of patients include syncope, seizure, congestive heart failure, dizziness, confusion, or limited exercise tolerance. A number of disorders are listed in this category:

1. Acquired symptomatic complete AV block

2. Congenital complete AV block with severe bradycardia and significant symptoms
3. Symptomatic Mobitz II AV block
4. Wenckebach second-degree AV block with symptoms due to haemo-dynamic instability
5. Symptomatic sinus bradycardia
6. Symptomatic sinus bradycardia related to drug therapy for which there is no acceptable alternative
7. Sinus node dysfunction, including tachycardia–bradycardia syndrome, sino-atrial block and sinus arrest
8. Sinus node dysfunction, with or without symptoms, associated with potentially life-threatening ventricular arrhythmias secondary to the bradycardia
9 Syncope due to carotid sinus syndrome and other similar entities.

Patients with complete heart block and symptoms can be paced without further documentation. In those patients with sinus node dysfunction and carotid sinus syndrome, it is recommended that correlation should be sought between the symptoms and the bradycardia. The symptoms in this group of patients should be clearly attributable to the bradycardia rather than any other cause.

Class II consists of those conditions in which permanent pacemakers are frequently used, but there is some divergence of opinion with respect to the necessity of their insertion. The use of a pacemaker in this group of patients would be acceptable if the medical history and prognosis can be documented by evidence that pacing would assist in the overall management. The following conditions are included in this group:

1. Asymptomatic acquired complete AV block
2. Congenital AV block without symptoms
3. Bifascicular and trifascicular block with syncope, providing other plausible causes of syncope have been excluded
4. Prophylactic pacemaker use after myocardial infarction where there has been transient complete or Mobitz II AV block
5. Asymptomatic Mobitz II AV block
6. Overdrive pacing in recurrent ventricular tachycardia.

Class III consists of those conditions in which there is general agreement that pacemakers are not necessary. Listed in this group are some of the following:

1. Syncope of unexplained cause
2. Sinus bradycardia without specific symptoms
3. Sinus arrest or sino-atrial block without significant symptoms
4. Asymptomatic prolonged RR intervals with atrial fibrillation
5. Bradycardia during sleep
6. Asymptomatic bifascicular block.

Atrioventricular block

AV block is defined as an impairment of the conduction of the cardiac impulse from the atrium to the ventricles, and can occur at various levels within the conducting system. AV conduction delay can be identified proximal to the AV node, within the AV node or distally in the His– Purkinje system.

First-degree heart block

This is characterized by a prolonged PR interval without failure of ventricular conduction. The PR interval is shorter in children and at faster heart rates. Values for the normal PR interval at various heart rates and differing age groups are available,[9] the range being 130–200 ms. First-degree AV block is due to delay in impulse propagation either through the atrium or the AV node. Since the conduction delay may occur in the atrium rather than the conducting system itself, the more accurate terminology for first-degree AV block used by electrophysiologists is 'prolongation of the PR interval'. As an isolated finding, first-degree AV block cannot be considered an indication for pacing.

Second-degree heart block

This occurs when there is intermittent failure of a P wave to be conducted to the ventricle. In Mobitz II second-degree AV block, the PR interval remains constant before the non-conducted P wave occurs. The presence of a wide QRS favours the site of block as being infra-His in site. Mobitz type II AV block is widely regarded as being more serious than the Wenckebach form of second-degree block. The Wenckebach form is characterized by a progressive lengthening of the PR interval until the dropped P wave occurs. The sequence is restored from the next P wave.

Although considered benign by many authorities, recent reports have suggested a more serious prognosis, even in asymptomatic patients. Shaw et al.,[10] reporting the results of the West of England Bradycardia Survey, followed 214 patients with asymptomatic second-degree AV block of various types, and reported a long-term follow-up. The five-year survival without pacing was 41%. However, the five-year survival with pacing was 78%, a figure identical to the national standard actuarial survival for non-affected controls within a similar population. Furthermore, there was no difference in survival between Mobitz II and Wenckebach patients. The AHA/ACC guidelines on pacemaker implantation categorize asymptomatic Wenckebach patients as not requiring a pacemaker. It is accepted that Wenckebach phenomenon can occur during sleep in normal individuals with a high vagal tone and such people clearly do not require treatment. However, those asymptomatic patients with second-degree AV block occurring during the majority of the 24 hours clearly ought to be considered for prophylactic pacemaker implantation,[11] as the published data have documented a reduction in life expectancy if untreated.

Complete atrioventricular block (third-degree atrioventricular block)

This indicates that there is no conduction from the atrium to the ventricle. It must be distinguished from AV dissociation, in which a subsidiary pacemaker focus in the AV junction or the ventricle is more rapid than the sino-atrial node. In AV dissociation, the QRS complexes are faster than the P waves, whereas in complete AV block the atrial rate is faster and there is no AV conduction. Acquired complete AV block occurs more commonly with ageing, either with calcification of the conducting system, or due to ischaemic heart disease.

Atrial fibrillation with a slow ventricular response, even if there are variable RR intervals, should be considered as AV block and should be paced if symptomatic.

Bifascicular and trifascicular blocks

These should be considered for pacing if intermittent AV block or syncope is present. Asymptomatic bifascicular block does not require pacing.

Sino-atrial dysfunctional

Sinus node dysfunction

This has been reported under a variety of names in the literature. Four distinct arrhythmias can occur:

1. Sinus bradycardia
2. Sinus arrest
3. Sino-atrial block
4. Tachycardia–bradycardia syndrome.

The main diagnostic doubts occur in relation to sinus bradycardia, as in some patients the bradycardia is only present at rest, and in others there is a problem on exercise. To overcome this confusion, the term 'chronotropic incompetence' has been introduced.

Chronotropic incompetence

This can be defined as an abnormal behaviour of sinus node function due to spontaneous disease or pharmacological agents, characterized by any of the following:

1. Sinus bradycardia < 50 beats/min at rest

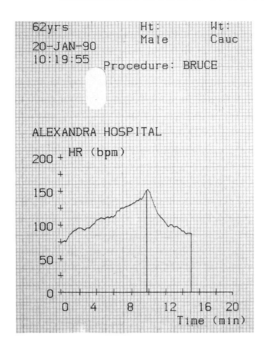

62yrs   Ht: Wt:
                     Male   Cauc
20-JAN-90
10:19:55   Procedure: BRUCE

ALEXANDRA HOSPITAL

        HR (bpm)
200 +

   +
150 +

   +
100 +

   +
 50 +

   +
  0 +
    0   4   8   12   16   20
                         Time (min)

Fig. 8.1 Exercise-induced heart rate response of a normal individual. There is a sharp rise in heart rate at the beginning of exercise, with a subsequent linear increase to peak levels. After exercise, the rate falls steadily to the resting value within 5 minutes.

2. Failure to achieve sinus rates > 120 beats/min at peak exercise
3. Sluggish initial sinus response to exercise
4. Sudden drop in sinus rate after exercise.

   Chronotropic incompetence can therefore be assessed by a combination of ambulatory ECG monitoring and exercise testing. If ambulatory ECG monitoring is unhelpful, treadmill testing using a standard protocol for maximum stress testing will frequently unmask the features described above. The normal sinus response to exercise is for the heart rate to rise fairly quickly in the first 2 minutes, and then to climb to its maximum predicted value in linear fashion (Fig. 8.1). Sluggish initial response and failure to reach a predicted heart rate on exercise are demonstrated in Fig. 8.2. A somewhat more unusual example of chronotropic incompetence is shown in Fig. 8.3, where there is a normal response to exercise, but with a sudden drop to pre-exercise levels within 90 seconds of achieving peak exercise. This patient had frequently experienced post-exercise syncope, which was controlled by cardiac pacing with a dual-chamber adaptive rate system that activated only after the completion of exercise. A step-wise response is shown in Fig. 8.4, and this frequently indicates latent sino-atrial block which has been exposed by vigorous exercise.

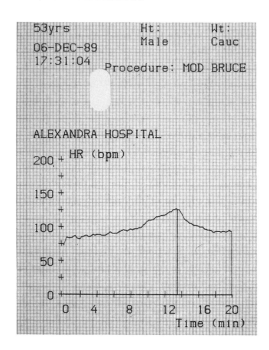

Fig. 8.2 Exercise rate response of a patient with severe chronotropic incompetence. The resting rate is slow, and there is virtually no increase in rate on exercise.

Patients with chronotropic incompetence may not experience syncope or dizziness, but will frequently describe lassitude, tiredness or poor exercise tolerance. Pacing with appropriate mode after careful assessment will be beneficial providing other causes for their symptoms are excluded first.

Carotid sinus syndrome

This is the accepted name for a disorder characterized by sudden unexplained syncope associated with a hypersensitive carotid sinus reflex. It would be more accurate to call the syndrome 'hypersensitivity of the carotid sinus reflex'.[12] Syncope occurs due to a mixture of bradycardia and hypotension in response to vagal stimulation, and contrary to popular belief compression of the neck is rarely the triggering factor. In many patients, the episodes occur spontaneously, others are related to micturition,[13] coughing[14] or swallowing (deglutition)[15] and are usually described accordingly.

The carotid sinus is innervated by the glossopharyngeal nerve and mediates its response via the vagus nerve. Cardio-inhibitory and the vasomotor responses can occur. The vasomotor response is due to profound vasodilatation, particularly in the splanchnic bed. If this response is the

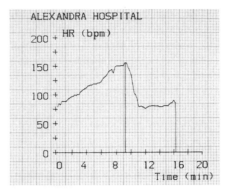

Fig. 8.3   Heart rate response in a patient with syncope due to post-exercise bradycardia. There is a good response of heart rate to exercise, but a precipitous fall of heart rate in the immediate recovery phase.

dominant feature, then cardiac pacing is not likely to be helpful.[16] Where the cardio-inhibitory features dominate, pacing with the appropriate mode is successful at controlling symptoms of syncope.[17] Carotid sinus massage

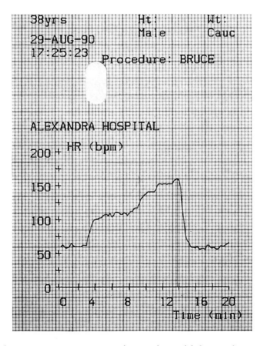

Fig. 8.4   Exercise heart rate response curve in a patient with latent sino-atrial block, showing a step-wise progression of increasing rates. There is also a sudden fall of heart rate in the immediate recovery phase. A graph of this type may identify latent sino-atrial block more accurately than a 24-hour ambulatory tape recording.

should be performed in any patient with unexplained syncope. When performing the test, the patient is recumbent and attached to an ECG monitor and recorder. The carotid arteries are palpated and auscultated to make certain there is no atheromatous disease prior to performing the test. The test is not performed if carotid arterial disease is detected. Massage (but not compression) is then performed for a period of 8 seconds. The ipsilateral temporal pulse is palpated during the massage to confirm that compression of the artery does not occur. A positive response consists of either of two features: a period of sinus arrest in excess of 3 seconds or the appearance of AV block. The vasomotor element can be determined by performing carotid sinus massage during temporary dual-chamber pacing in those patients in whom the features are suggestive of a mixed pattern. Carotid sinus massage will reveal a false positive response if performed following a recent myocardial infarction, or if the patient is taking beta-blocking agents or digitalis, and should therefore be avoided under those circumstances. When performing carotid massage, it is customary to mas-sage the right side first, and only to proceed to the left side if the former is negative. The right carotid sinus nerve exerts its influence mainly on the sino-atrial node, and the left-sided nerve on the AV node; appropriately different responses may therefore be obtained. If a patient has a very sensitive response, sinus arrest for a few seconds is likely to occur with right-sided massage, but there could be a much more prolonged episode of asystole due to AV block from left-sided massage.

Isolated vasodepressor response is uncommon, and patients with severe symptoms may have prolonged hypotension for some minutes. By contrast, the cardio-inhibitory response lasts usually only for a few seconds. Pacing is of value in cardio-inhibitory and mixed responses, but not where there is a dominant vasomotor effect.

Malignant vasovagal syncope

This is a rare disorder characterized by syncope due to a combination of bradycardia and vasodilatation, usually in response to immobility whilst in an upright posture, or related to shock or fear. It should not, however, be confused with simple vasovagal fainting spells. In malignant vasovagal syncope there is recurrent syncope, frequently without warning. A 60° tilt test will document the diagnosis.[18] The patient lies recumbent, under basal conditions, for 15 minutes, after which he is tilted feet downwards, with a footplate support, at an angle of 60°. Blood pressure recording and heart rate monitoring are undertaken. A positive response consists of marked bradycardia and hypotension occurring suddenly during the subsequent 40 minutes. Most positive tilts occur within 20 minutes. A dominant vaso-motor effect consists of a fall in blood pressure before bradycardia occurs, and this will not respond to pacing. A mixed bradycardia/hypotensive pattern in either carotid sinus syndrome or malignant vasovagal syncope

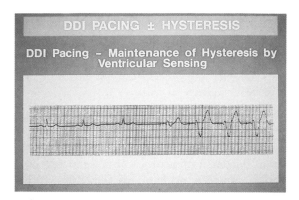

Fig. 8.5   ECG showing behaviour of a dual-chamber pacemaker (DDI mode) with programmed hysteresis. The sensing rate is 60 and the pacing rate is 80 beats/min. When the native heart rate falls below 60 beats/min, the pacemaker is activated at a pacing rate of 80 beats/min.

can be symptomatically improved by appropriate pacing with a system programmed to allow DDI mode with rate hysteresis[19] (Fig. 8.5).

PACEMAKER PRESCRIPTION FOR SYMPTOMATIC BRADYCARDIA

With the wide variety of cardiac arrhythmias and diverse haemodynamically induced symptoms described above it should be apparent that each abnormality requires a different pacing mode in order to achieve maximum symptomatic improvement. A working party of the British Pacing and Electrophysiology Group has supplemented the ACC/AHA guidelines by describing optimal modes of pacing for individual bradycardia disorders.[19] The nomenclature for pacing modes accepted for international use is the NBG (NASPE/BPEG Generic) code.[7] This is currently a code of five letters, of which the first three are used most often. (Modifications to the coding are introduced at regular intervals to accommodate newer types of pacemakers.)

The first letter indicates the chamber being *paced*:

A = Atrium
V = Ventricle
D = Dual (atrium and ventricle)
O = No pacing.

The second letter indicates the chamber being *sensed*:

A = Atrium
V = Ventricle
D = Dual (atrium and ventricle)
O = No sensing.

The third letter indicates the type of sensing that occurs:

I = Inhibited
T = Triggered
D = Dual (inhibited and triggered)
O = No sensing.

In addition, a fourth letter is designated 'R' if rate adaptation is pro-grammed. In adaptive rate (or rate-responsive) pacing, the pacing rate is modified by an algorithm which is driven by an additional sensor within the pacing system that detects a physiological or semi-physiological result of exercise or emotion. Sensing mechanisms available within pacemakers at present include oxygen saturation,[20] activity,[21] respiratory rate[22] or minute ventilation,[23] right ventricular pressure (dp/dt),[24] central venous tempera-ture[25] and evoked QT interval.[5] Although initially single-chamber systems, adaptive rate pacing has been combined with dual-chamber pacing in recent years[6] to obtain maximal haemodynamic improvement.

The fifth letter of the NBG code relates to antitachycardia function and is not relevant to bradycardia pacing.

Pacemaker prescription

The BPEG guidelines for choice of pacemaker mode are based on an attempt to produce as many of the features of normal sinus rhythm as possible within an individual patient. The general principles are:

1. The atrium should be paced/sensed unless contraindicated
2. The ventricle should be paced if there is actual or threatened AV block
3. Rate response may be used to overcome chronotropic incompetence, but is not necessary in an inactive patient
4. Hysteresis may be valuable if the bradycardia is intermittent.

Utilization of these basic principles allows the pacemaker to behave as physiologically as possible.[26] This includes restoration of AV synchrony and/or adaptive rate pacing as necessary. Benefits of the various features may be summarized as follows.

Atrioventricular synchrony

Atrial pacing for sinus node disease has been established for over 20 years,[27] but the theoretical potential benefits of maintaining normal AV synchrony in these patients have been recognized only recently.[28] Similarly, patients with AV block treated by dual-chamber atrial tracking pacemakers can be demonstrated to have improved haemodynamics compared with single-chamber ventricular pacing.[29] In patients with normal ventricles, AV synchrony maintains optimal preload, and contributes up to 30% of the cardiac output at rest. It prevents elevation of the venous pressure due to either atrial systole against a closed AV valve or ventricular systole with an open AV valve. It also avoids the mitral and tricuspid valve regurgitation which occurs with VVI pacing.[30] Furthermore, similar benefits can be demonstrated in patients with non-compliant ventricles,[29] but the total cardiac output is limited by the extent of left ventricular disease. On exercise, AV synchrony is also important, but its contribution to the total cardiac output in all groups of patients is less than at rest.

In addition to atrial contraction and maintenance of AV synchrony, the time interval between atrial and ventricular systole is important. In patients with heart block, this optimal interval varies according to pacing rate and ventricular compliance.[31] In patients with isolated sinus node disease treated by atrial pacing, the natural AV conduction is usually suitable. There are, however, some patients with atrial rate-responsive pacemakers who develop a prolonged AV conduction time with exercise, thus mimicking extreme first-degree AV block with a demonstrable fall in cardiac output due to loss of atrial transport function.[32] Such patients are best served by dual-chamber rate-responsive pacing with automatic shortening of the AV interval at faster rates. In all groups of patients treated by dual-chamber pacing, optimal adjustment of the AV interval may be achieved only by echocardiographic assessment and exercise testing in patients with borderline left ventricular function.

Rate modulation

Cardiac output depends on stroke volume and heart rate. In the majority of patients, demands for an increase in cardiac output are primarily met by increasing the heart rate. Trained athletes are the exception to this generalization, in that they are able to increase their stroke volume more proportionally. By contrast, patients with left ventricular disease due to cardiomyopathy or coronary artery disease have a very limited or absent ability to increase stroke volume. Such patients occur not uncommonly within the pacemaker population. Adaptive rate pacing with adjustment of the pacemaker rate by a sensor is now frequently employed. This results in an increase in the cardiac output in patients with AV block[21] and sinus node disease.[33] Furthermore, patients achieve higher workloads and greater exercise tolerance when treated with rate-modulated pacemakers.[21, 33]

Atrial pacing

The haemodynamic benefits of atrial pacing in patients with sinus node disease are well established, and are referred to above. More recently, however, attention has focused on the effects of the chosen pacing mode on cardiovascular morbidity and mortality.[28, 34] Rosenqvist et al.[28] followed 168 patients treated with either atrial (AAI) or ventricular (VVI) pacing for a period of four years. The two groups of patients were identical in all respects except for the mode of pacing. The following data emerged after the four years.

Permanent atrial fibrillation was more common in the VVI group: 69% compared to 9% in the AAI cohort. In patients who had no history of atrial fibrillation prior to implantation, the figures were 18% and 3%, respectively.

Congestive cardiac failure was also more common in the VVI group: 37% versus 16% in the AAI group. The difference was still significant if those patients developing atrial fibrillation were excluded.

Strokes were somewhat more common after two years in the VVI group (13%) compared with the AAI treated group (4.5%), but these figures did not achieve statistical significance.

Long-term survival was higher in those treated by AAI pacing. At four years, the mortality in the VVI group was 23% compared with 8% in the AAI group.

All of these data (with the exception of those relating to strokes), achieved statistical significance in favour of the atrial paced group of patients. The results relating to the incidence of atrial fibrillation, congestive heart failure and mortality are in keeping with numerous other reports in the literature.[35-38] The interpretation of these reports must render the use of VVI pacing in patients with sinus node disease, at its best, questionable, and at its worst, obsolete.

Atrial arrhythmias

The presence of atrial activity other than permanent atrial flutter/fibrillation generally warrants placement of an atrial lead. Paroxysmal atrial fibrillation is not a contraindication to atrial pacing[37] as this may stabilize the atrial rhythm[38] and concomitant drug therapy may be beneficial in others. Although single-chamber atrial pacing may suffice in many patients with sinus node disease,[37] the presence of minor AV conduction abnormalities, including first-degree AV block or bundle branch disease with a normal PR interval, would be better served by a dual-chamber system.[39, 40]

Pacemaker syndrome

Pacemaker syndrome can be suspected when haemodynamic symptoms not present prior to implantation occur in the presence of a normally functioning pacemaker system. In general, VVI pacing in patients with normal atrial contraction is the culprit.

Two distinct mechanisms can occur: retrograde ventriculo-atrial (VA) conduction and loss of atrial synchrony. An immediate drop in blood pressure may occur when the pacemaker overrides sinus rhythm due to loss of atrial transport (Fig. 8.6). In addition, VA conduction may result in

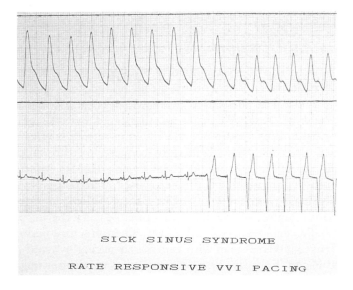

SICK SINUS SYNDROME

RATE RESPONSIVE VVI PACING

Fig. 8.6 Pacemaker syndrome – fall in arterial pressure associated with onset of ventricular (VVI) pacing.

regurgitation through the AV valves causing abnormal venous neck pulsations or dyspnoea. More importantly, VA conduction activates the stretch receptors in the walls of the atria and pulmonary veins.[41] These impulses are transmitted centrally by the vagal afferents resulting in peripheral vasodilatation. The patient may thus experience dizziness or syncope.

The incidence of pacemaker syndrome is difficult to ascertain, but it probably causes serious symptoms in 10% of patients paced in VVI mode, with a further 15% having significant impairment of life as a result.[42] The incidence is probably much higher;[43] latent pacemaker syndrome is regularly encountered when a patient receives a dual-chamber pacemaker as a routine generator change after many years of VVI pacing, with the abolition of previously unsuspected symptoms of lassitude, minor dizziness and lack of energy. Correct choice of pacemaker mode at the time of implantation will avoid this increasingly common problem.

CHOICE OF PACEMAKER MODE

The BPEG working party on pacemaker prescription has recommended optimal and alternative modes as being suitable to control symptomatic bradycardia.[19] The optimal mode will be required by the majority of patients and the alternative mode for the less active patient (Table 8.1). In the very infirm, e.g. those incapacitated by severe strokes or with terminal malignant disease, then VVI pacing will serve as a reasonable third alternative to prevent syncope.

Sinus node disease

Optimal mode AAIR – Alternative mode AAI – Inappropriate mode VVI

If there is no evidence of AV conduction problems, then the treatment of choice which maintains AV synchrony, atrial contraction and rate response is the AAIR mode. The alternative mode, which is suitable for less active patients, would be AAI. VVI is contraindicated because of the high incidence of pacemaker syndrome, and the long-term anxieties regarding the increased risks of atrial fibrillation, congestive heart failure and a reduced life expectancy. A single atrial pacing lead is inserted and a standard multiprogrammable pacemaker is used. The cost is therefore the same as for single-chamber ventricular pacing. The generator is programmed with a higher sensitivity (e.g. 1 mV) because the intracardiac P waves are smaller than ventricular R waves. The refractory period is made somewhat longer (400 ms) than with ventricular pacing to avoid sensing of the far-field R and T waves. The latter is not common, but may occur in unipolar atrial pacing systems.

Atrioventricular block

Optimal mode DDD – Alternative mode VDD – Inappropriate modes AAI/DDI

In this group of patients, normal chronotropic behaviour of the sinus node can be demonstrated but there is a partial or complete block of AV conduction. In order to maintain AV synchrony and rate response, the mode of choice is the DDD system. Two leads are required: one in the atrium and the other in the ventricle. At the lower programmed rate (which can be as low as 40–50 beats/min) the atrium will be paced. At all other rates the atrium will be sensed and this results in stimulation in the ventricle after an appropriate AV delay. At the maximum tracking rate (e.g. 120–150 beats/min) the pacemaker will not track at 1:1 but will perform a variety of manoeuvres such as 'pacemaker Wenckebach' or 'rate smoothing'. These are protective mechanisms to prevent very fast ventricular pacing should an atrial tachyarrhythmia occur.

One potential problem with the DDD mode is the possibility of 'pacemaker-mediated tachycardia'. This occurs where there is retrograde VA conduction after a ventricular event, the resulting P′ wave occurring outside the postventricular atrial refractory period (PVARP). The P′ wave is therefore detected by the atrial sensing amplifier and a ventricular stimulus is delivered. The resulting ventricular contraction results in a further retrograde P′ wave via VA conduction and an endless loop tachycardia occurs. (The mechanism is very similar to naturally occurring tachycardias such as the WPW syndrome.) The pacemaker-mediated

Table 8.1   Recommended pacemaker modes[19]

Diagnosis	Optimal	Alternative	Inappropriate
SND	AAIR	AAI	VVI VDD
AVB	DDD	VDD	AAI DDI
SND & AVB	DDDR DDIR	DDD DDI	AAI VVI
Chronic AF with AVB	VVIR	VVI	AAI DDD VDD
CSS	DDI	DDD VVI	AAI VDD
MVVS	DDI	DDD	AAI VVI VDD

AVB = atrioventricular block; SND = sino-atrial node disease; AF = atrial fibrillation or flutter; CSS = carotid sinus syndrome; MVVS = malignant vaso-vagal syndrome.

tachycardia is usually the same rate as the maximum tracking rate of the pacemaker. It can be terminated by programming the PVARP to a longer value.

An alternative mode would be VDD, which can be inserted using a special single lead which has a standard ventricular tip with a small bipole floating in the right atrium to detect P waves. This behaves in a similar fashion to the DDD mode, the difference being at the lower programmed rate. Whereas the DDD mode results in atrial pacing at this point, in the VDD mode and the pacemaker behaves as a VVI pacemaker at the lower rate. This is unsatisfactory haemodynamically, and increases the possibility of pacemaker syndrome and pacemaker-mediated tachycardia. The VDD mode has little to recommend it. The single-pass lead at best results in 98% atrial sensing, which is unsatisfactory. Furthermore, all the haemodynamic advantages of VDD are utilized by the DDD mode, which has a somewhat lower incidence of problems due to pacemaker-mediated tachycardia and more versatility.

Contraindicated modes in AV block are AAI and DDI. In the former there will be no conduction to the ventricle and in the latter there is no tracking of P waves on exercise. VVI mode is not recommended for routine pacing of complete heart block, but may be used as a back-up option to reduce symptoms in a patient with, for example, severe immobility due to a previous hemiplegia or with terminal neoplasia.

Sinus node disease with atrioventricular block

*Optimal modes DDDR, DDIR – Alternative modes DDD, DDI –
Inappropriate modes AAI, VVI*

Patients with sinus node disease and AV block will require a dual-chamber
adaptive rate system to produce AV synchrony and rate modulation.
DDDR can be used if there is intermittently normal sinus node function. If
there is persistent chronotropic incompetence, then DDIR will be more
appropriate. In the DDDR system, the pacemaker will increase its rate in
response to exercise by either tracking the native P waves or by pacing the
atrium at higher rates in response to the sensor, depending which is the
dominant.

The alternative modes for the less active patient would still require dual-
chamber pacing with either DDD or DDI programmed. AAI and VVI are
inappropriate for the reasons explained above.

Chronic atrial fibrillation with atrioventricular block

*Optimal mode VVIR – Alternative mode VVI – Inappropriate modes
AAI/DDD/VDD*

With chronic atrial fibrillation, there is no prospect of restoring AV
synchrony. Rate response will be provided by using a VVIR pacemaker.
The alternative mode would be VVI without the rate modulation. Any
pacemaker system which has atrial sensing is inappropriate and this includes AAI, DDD and VDD.

Carotid sinus syndrome

*Optimal mode DDI – Alternative mode DDD – Inappropriate modes
AAI/VDD*

There are a number of unusual features of carotid sinus syndrome which
require correction by pacing. These are:

1. Bradycardia is due to a combination of sinus arrest and AV block
2. Sinus arrest is frequently very sudden
3. AV block does not occur at normal or fast atrial rates
4. Symptoms rarely occur on exercise
5. Symptoms rarely occur when recumbent
6. Syncope is partly due to vasodilatation.

In order to satisfy these features, the most appropriate pacing mode
available at present is DDI with programmed rate hysteresis (Fig. 8.6).
This allows onset of dual-chamber pacing at a fast rate when bradycardia is
imminent, but does result in pacing during sleep or at other times of natural
bradycardia.[17] Typical programmed rates would be to have pacing at 80–90
beats/min with a hysteresis value of 35–45 beats/min.

Malignant vasovagal syndrome

Optimal mode DDI – Alternative mode DDD – Inappropriate modes AAI/VVI/VDD

The six features listed above for carotid sinus syndrome also apply to malignant vasovagal syndrome. DDI pacing with rate hysteresis is therefore the most successful way of managing this condition.[17] The high incidence of vasodilatation that occurs means that VVI pacing is contraindicated in the management of symptomatic patients with malignant vasovagal syndrome.[43]

Consequences of increased usage of sophisticated pacing systems

A VVIR generator costs about 40% more than a VVI model, and a dual-chamber system 40–100% more. A dual-chamber system requires two leads, further increasing the cost. In addition, rate-responsive systems have a shorter battery life because of their faster pacing rates. The benefit in terms of improved quality of life and better long-term survival[30, 44–47] make the choice of a sophisticated system very cost effective when compared to other medical treatments.[48]

Follow-up with VVIR and dual-chamber systems is more complex and time consuming. Additional time needs to be allocated, together with facilities to perform exercise testing and ambulatory ECG monitoring where required. Supporting staff will require additional training. When a pacemaker has been 'fine-tuned', the subsequent follow-up is less time consuming.

SUMMARY

A carefully prescribed individual pacemaker system as described above is medically sound and justifiable, resulting in measurable benefits in terms of quality of life and improved life expectancy compared with standard VVI pacing.

REFERENCES

1 Elmqvist R, Senning A. An implantable pacemaker for the heart. In: Smyth CN, ed. Medical Electronics. Proceedings of the Second International Conference on Medical Electronics. London: Illife, 1959, p 253
2 Ginks W, Siddons H, Leatham A. Prognosis of patients paced for chronic atrioventricular block. Br Heart J 1979; 41: 633–636
3 Sutton R, Citron P, Perrins J. Physiological cardiac pacing. PACE 1980; 3: 207
4 Clarke M, Allen A. Use of telemetered electrograms in the assessment of normal pacemaker function. J Electrophysiol 1987; 1: 388–395
5 Rickards A, Norman J. Relation between QT interval and heart rate: new design of a physiological adaptive pacemaker. Br Heart J 1981; 45: 56
6 Kappenberger L, Hepers L. Rate responsive dual chamber pacing. PACE 1986; 9: 987

7   Bernstein A, Camm J, Fletcher R et al. The NASPE/BPEG generic pacing code for antibradyarrhythmia and adaptive rate pacing and antitachycardia devices. PACE 1987; 10: 794–799
8   Frye RL, Collins JJ, DeSanctis RW et al. Guidelines for permanent pacemaker implantation – May 1984. A report of the joint American College of Cardiology/American Heart Association Task Force on assessment of Cardiovascular Procedures (Subcommittee on Pacemaker Implantation). J Am Coll Cardiol 1984; 4: 434–442
9   Clarke M, Keith JD. Atrioventricular conduction in acute rheumatic fever. Br Heart J 1972; 34: 472–477
10 Shaw D, Kekwick C, Veale D, Gowers J, Whistance T. Survival in second degree atrioventricular block. Br Heart J 1985; 53: 587–593
11 Campbell R. Chronic Mobitz type I second degree atrioventricular block: has its importance been underestimated? Br Heart J 1985; 53: 585–586
12 Morley C, Sutton R. Carotid sinus syndrome: editorial review. Int J Cardiol 1984; 6: 287–293
13 Haldane JH. Micturition syncope. Can Med Assoc J 1969; 101: 712
14 Hart G, Oldershaw P, Cull R, Humphrey P, Ward D. Syncope caused by cough-induced complete atrioventricular block. PACE 1982; 5: 564–566
15 Igaluer S, Swartz B. Heart block periodically induced by the swallowing of food in a patient with cardiospasm (vasovagal syncope). Ann Otol Rhinol Laryngol 1936; 45: 875
16 Morley C, Perrins E, Grant P, Chan S, McBrien D, Sutton R. Carotid sinus syndrome treated by pacing: analysis of persistent symptoms and role of atrioventricular sequential pacing. Br Heart J 1982; 47: 411–418
17 Sutton R, Ingram A, Clarke M. DDI pacing in the management of sick sinus, carotid sinus and vasovagal syndromes. PACE 1988; 11: 827
18 Fitzpatrick A, Sutton R. Tilting towards a diagnosis in recurrent unexplained syncope. Lancet 1988; 1: 658–660
19 Clarke M, Sutton R, Ward D et al. Pacemaker prescription for symptomatic bradycardia: a report of a working party of the British Pacing and Electrophysiology Group. Br Heart J 1991; 66: 185–191
20 Stangl K, Wirtzfeld A, Heinze R, Laule M. First clinical experience with an oxygen saturation controlled pacemaker in man. PACE 1988; 11: 1882–1887
21 Humen D, Anderson K, Brumwell D, Huntley S, Klein G. A pacemaker which automatically increases its rate with physical activity. In: Steinbach K, Glogard A, Laszkovicsa D, Schneibelhofer W, Weber H, eds. Cardiac pacing. Darmstadt: Steinkopff Verlag, 1983, pp 252–264
22 Rossi P, Plicchi G, Canducci G. Respiration as a reliable physiological sensor for the cardiac pacing rate. Br Heart J 1984; 51: 7–14
23 Lau C, Antoniou A, Ward D, Camm AJ. Reliability of minute ventilation as a parameter for rate responsive pacing. PACE 1989; 12: 321–330
24 Sutton R, Sharma A, Ingram A, Camm J, Lindemans F, Bennett T. First derivative of right ventricular pressure as a sensor for an implantable rate responsive VVI pacemaker. PACE 1988; 11: 487
25 Alt E, Völker R, Högl B, MacCarter D. First clinical results with a new temperature-controlled rate responsive pacemaker. Circulation 1988; 78(Suppl III): 116–124
26 Ryden L, Kruse B. Hemodynamic aspects of physiologic pacing. In: Barold SS, ed. Modern cardiac pacing. Mount Kisco, NY: Futura, 1985, pp 19–32
27 Clarke M, Evans DW, Milstein BB. Sinus bradycardia treated by long term atrial pacing. Br Heart J 1970; 32: 458–461
28 Rosenqvist M, Brandt J, Schuller H. Long-term pacing in sinus node disease: effects of stimulation mode on cardiovascular morbidity and mortality. Am Heart J 1988; 116: 16–22
29 Kruse I, Arnman K, Conradson T, Ryden L. A comparison of the acute and long-term haemodynamic effects of ventricular inhibited and atrial synchronous ventricular inhibited pacing. Circulation 1981; 65: 846–855
30 Naito M, Dreyfus L, David D, Nicholson E, Mardela T, Kmetzo J. Re-evaluation of the role of atrial systole in cardiac hemodynamics: evidence for pulmonary venous regurgitation during abnormal atrioventricular sequencing. Am Heart J 1983; 105: 295–302

31 Greenberg B, Chatterjee K, Parmley WW et al. The influence of left ventricular filling pressure on atrial contraction to cardiac output. Am Heart J 1979; 98: 742–751
32 Clarke M, Allen A. Rate responsive atrial pacing resulting in pacemaker syndrome. PACE 1987; 10: 1209
33 Rognoni G, Bolognese L, Aina F, Occhetta E, Magnani A, Rossi P. Respiratory dependent atrial pacing: management of sinus node disease. PACE 1988; 11: 1853–1859
34 Rosenqvist M, Brandt J, Schüller H. Atrial versus ventricular pacing in sinus node disease: a treatment comparison study. Am Heart J 1986; 111: 292–297
35 Santini M, Alexidou G, Porto M, Santini A, Ammirati F, Ansalone G. The sick sinus syndrome: prognosis as function of age, conduction defects and pacing mode. PACE 1989; 12: 1237
36 Bianconi L, Boccadamo R, Di Florio A et al. Atrial versus ventricular stimulation in sick sinus syndrome: effects on morbidity and mortality. PACE 1989; 12: 1236
37 Ryden L. Atrial inhibited pacing: an underused mode of cardiac stimulation. PACE 1988; 11: 1375–1379
38 Egobasti A, Gueunoun M, Saadjian A et al. Long-term follow-up of patients treated with VVI pacing and sequential pacing with special reference to VA retrograde conduction. PACE 1988; 11: 1929–1934
39 Sutton R, Kenny R. Natural history of sick sinus syndrome. PACE 1986; 9: 1110–1114
40 Rosenqvist M, Obel I. Atrial pacing and the risk for AV block: is there a time for change of attitude? 1989; 12: 97–101
41 Akhtar M. Retrograde conduction in man. PACE 1981; 4: 548–562
42 Ausubel K, Furman S. The pacemaker syndrome. Ann Int Med 1985; 103: 420–429
43 Fitzpatrick AP, Travill CM, Vardas PE et al. Recurrent symptoms after ventricular pacing in unexplained syncope. PACE 1990; 13: 619–624
44 Perrins J, Morley C, Chan S, Sutton R. Randomised controlled trial of physiological and ventricular pacing. Br Heart J 1983; 50: 112–117
45 Lau CP, Rushby J, Leigh-Jones M et al. A double blind cross-over study on the symptomatology and quality of life in patients with rate responsive pacemakers. J Am Coll Cardiol 1989; 13: 113A
46 Fitzgerald WR, Graham IM, Cole T, Evans DW. Age, sex and ischaemic heart disease as prognostic indicators in long-term cardiac pacing. Br Heart J 1979; 42: 57–60
47 Edhag O, Swann A. Prognosis of patients with complete heart block or arrhythmic syncope who were not treated by cardiac pacemakers. Acta Med Scand 1976; 200: 457–463
48 Williams A. Economics of coronary artery bypass grafting. Br Med J 1985; 291: 326–329

9

Hypertrophic cardiomyopathy: diagnosis, prognosis, management

J. T. Stewart   W. J. McKenna

Hypertrophic cardiomyopathy is defined as a heart muscle disorder of unknown origin that is characterized by hypertrophy of a non-dilated left ventricle. The first systematic description of the condition was made by the pathologist Donald Teare in 1958, from the postmortem appearances of the hearts of 9 adolescents and young adults, 8 of whom had died suddenly.[1] Soon after that description the familial pattern of the disorder was recognized. At that time hypertrophic cardiomyopathy was considered uncommon, and its association with sudden cardiac death was emphasized.

In the ensuing 30 years the incidence and natural history of hypertrophic cardiomyopathy have become better defined. Modern diagnostic methods, used in conjunction with family screening programmes, have demonstrated large numbers of asymptomatic individuals. In adults, a marker of the risk of sudden cardiac death has been identified, and there is evidence that the risk can be modified by drug therapy. Most recently, the genetic basis of hypertrophic cardiomyopathy has been identified in a number of families.

DIAGNOSIS

The diagnostic criteria of hypertrophic cardiomyopathy have changed since it was first described, and the relationship of the anatomical findings to the pathophysiology and prognosis of the condition, although better defined, remains controversial. By comparison to the diagnostic methods in common use today, those of the early 1960s were crude and insensitive; the natural history data from that era, most of which come from specialist centres, are probably inaccurate as a result. The incidence of hypertrophic cardiomyopathy, in particular, must be seen in relationship to the diagnostic methods available.

Emphasis was initially placed on the clinical findings of hyperdynamic left ventricular function and an outflow tract gradient, in patients with the classical symptoms of chest pain, dyspnoea and syncope. Invasive investigations in patients with a 'jerky' arterial pulse, an ejection systolic murmur and an active cardiac impulse demonstrated the haemodynamic correlates of these physical signs and showed that the outflow tract gradient was labile and could be influenced by a variety of pharmacological and physiological manoeuvres.[2-4] Data from this era suggested that obstruction to left ventricular emptying was the essential feature of hypertrophic cardiomyopathy. This view had to be revised following the recognition of patients with left ventricular hypertrophy but no obstruction to ventricular emptying. It is now clear that there is a resting or provokable outflow tract gradient in only about 35% of patients.[5,6]

The development of M-mode echocardiography in the 1970s permitted the visualization of the interventricular septum and the posterior left ventricular wall at mitral valve level – the thickest and the thinnest myocardial segments. M-mode echocardiography thus provided confirmation of the earlier pathological descriptions of hypertrophy predominantly localized to the septum, and led to the assertion that asymmetrical septal hypertrophy (ASH) was the pathognomonic feature of the condition.[7] While the characteristic morphological feature of hypertrophic cardiomyopathy is asymmetrical hypertrophy of the interventricular septum, large autopsy series have shown that the left ventricular free wall is also thicker than normal in most patients and, in up to 30% of cases, left ventricular hypertrophy is symmetrical.[8] Furthermore, although ASH is seen in 50–60% of patients with hypertrophic cardiomyopathy, it is also found in other patient groups.[9]

The diagnostic method of the 1980s, – cross-sectional echocardiography – is still the most sensitive technique generally available. With cross-sectional echocardiography the entire heart can be visualized, and its use has allowed the detection of many asymptomatic individuals, in the course of family screening. Reports from non-specialist centres using cross-sectional echocardiography, and the finding of hypertrophic cardiomyopathy in both symptomatic and asymptomatic elderly patients, suggest that hypertrophic cardiomyopathy may be more common, with a more benign prognosis, than has been appreciated.[10-12] Cross-sectional echocardiography has further demonstrated that left ventricular hypertrophy may have almost any distribution – asymmetrical septal, symmetrical, or predominantly involve the distal ventricle – and that, in addition, there is right ventricular hypertrophy in over one-third of patients (Fig. 9.1).[13-15]

The diagnostic criterion of unexplained left ventricular hypertrophy may itself require revision. Two families were reported recently in whom there were the characteristic histological abnormalities of myocyte disarray and an excess of loose connective tissue, in the absence of cardiac hypertrophy.[16] Ultimately, accurate diagnosis of the condition may require identification of the gene responsible or of a genetic marker which is linked to the gene locus. A recent publication reported the finding of a DNA locus on chromosome 14 which was co-inherited with familial hypertrophic cardiomyopathy in a large kindred.[17] Subsequent work has demonstrated that the abnormality resides in the gene which codes for the beta cardiac myosin heavy chain.[18-20] This advance in the understanding of the genetics of hypertrophic cardiomyopathy means that a molecular diagnosis, using a

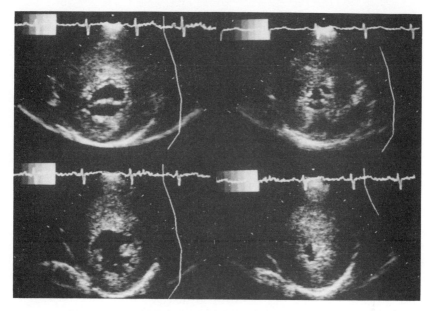

Fig. 9.1   Typical cross-sectional echocardiographic appearance in the short-axis parasternal view in a young patient with hypertrophic cardiomyopathy and ASH at mitral valve level (upper), and papillary muscle level (lower). A diastolic frame is shown on the left and a systolic frame on the right. (Courtesy of Dr P. Nihoyannopoulos)

gene probe, may ultimately replace cross-sectional echocardiography as the diagnostic test of choice (Fig. 9.2).

PROGNOSIS

The natural history of hypertrophic cardiomyopathy in adults is of slow progression of symptoms over many years, but survival data from referral centres indicate that there is also an annual disease-related mortality of 2–3% from sudden unexpected cardiac death.[21–25] Treatment of the condition may require drugs or surgery (myotomy/myectomy or mitral valve replacement) for the control of symptoms, although neither has been shown to improve prognosis, cardiac transplantation for uncontrollable symptoms (which may improve prognosis), low-dose amiodarone, regardless of symptom status, in those shown to be at high risk of sudden death, or the use of the implantable cardioverter–defibrillator. Of these, only low-dose amiodarone has been shown to improve prognosis.[24]

Treatment of the condition in childhood poses particular problems, and the natural history may be more aggressive when hypertrophic cardiomyopathy presents in the very young. In particular, when it appears for the first time in infancy hypertrophic cardiomyopathy seems to behave differently from the disease in other age groups. The diagnosis is frequently missed at

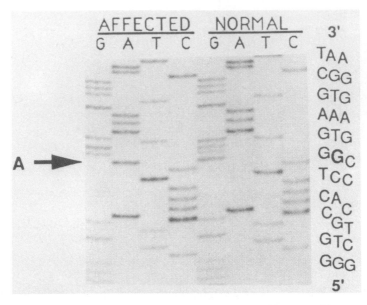

Fig. 9.2   DNA sequencing gel from a young patient with typical hypertrophic cardiomyopathy (left) and from a normal individual from the same family (right). In each of the affected individuals in this family there was a replacement of a guanine molecule by an adenine molecule on exon 13, which did not occur in any of the normal family members. The finding of this missense mutation, which causes an amino acid change in a region of beta cardiac myosin heavy chain that has been conserved through over 600 million years of evolution, provides evidence that it is the mutation responsible for hypertrophic cardiomyopathy in this family. (With permission from Cell Press)

presentation, which may be with stillbirth, sudden infant death ('cot' death), or with a systolic murmur. The correct diagnosis is likely to be made when the presenting features are heart failure and cyanosis.

Few centres have much experience of treating very young children with the disease. Maron et al. have reviewed the multicentre experience in 20 infants under the age of one year. The five-year mortality was 50%, with cardiac failure the commonest mode of death, and 9 out of the 11 infants (82%) who presented in heart failure died.[25] These data suggest that when hypertrophic cardiomyopathy is diagnosed in the first year of life the prognosis is very poor, and outcome is probably determined by left ventricular function.

In older children the presentation is more likely to be with chest pain and exertional dyspnoea, as is the case with adults. The clinical hallmark of the disorder, unexplained left ventricular hypertrophy, may develop during a growth spurt during childhood or adolescence; if already established, it may progress during a growth spurt.[26] Unfortunately the prognosis in children, while not as bad as in infants, is worse than in adults, and the annual mortality from sudden cardiac death is 4–6%.[27] Sudden death, in both children and adults, frequently occurs in patients whose symptoms are mild or who are asymptomatic.

Identification of the patient at risk of sudden death

Analysis of outcome in large series of patients indicates that those features which best predict the risk of sudden death are: diagnosis in childhood or adolescence; a family history of hypertrophic cardiomyopathy and sudden death; and syncopal episodes.[28] The predictive accuracy of the risk of sudden death of clinical, haemodynamic and angiographic characterization, including the assessment of left ventricular outflow tract gradients, is low (sensitivity 70%, specificity 68%, positive predictive accuracy 24%).

The single best marker of the high-risk adult is the identification of non-sustained ventricular tachycardia on ambulatory ECG monitoring, which is associated with a sevenfold increase in the incidence of sudden death.[29,30] In adults, the finding of non-sustained ventricular tachycardia represents a sensitive (> 70%) and specific (> 80%) marker of increased risk of sudden death. The negative predictive accuracy is high (97%), but the positive predictive accuracy is relatively low (23%), reflecting the fact that the majority of patients with non-sustained ventricular tachycardia do not die during short-term (three-year) follow-up.

Since the negative predictive accuracy of non-sustained ventricular tachycardia is high, asymptomatic adults who do not have this marker probably do not require further investigation in terms of risk assessment. The low positive predictive accuracy of this finding, however, means that some patients with non-sustained ventricular tachycardia are at higher risk of sudden death than others. Further work is required to improve risk stratification in this group. In particular, the role of electrophysiological investigation in refining the risk assessment of those patients who do have features of increased risk (syncope, 'malignant family history', exertional hypotension and non-sustained ventricular tachycardia) requires definition. Such patients should undergo assessment at referral centres with a particular interest in the condition. Electrophysiological testing should be undertaken with a view to detecting conduction tissue disease, accelerated atrioventricular conduction (either intranodal or via an accessory pathway), and inducible monomorphic ventricular tachycardia. Other electrophysiological measurements which could reflect the extent and distribution of myocardial disarray, such as dispersion of ventricular depolarization and repolarization, may aid in further risk factor stratification. Although for the moment this is speculative, such information could be particularly valuable in the young patients where the mortality is highest, and our ability to predict an adverse outcome is worst.

Mechanism of sudden death

The mechanism of sudden death in most patients is unknown, and the association with non-sustained ventricular tachycardia does not mean that this arrhythmia is the initiating mechanism. Several potential initiating mechanisms, which may be interrelated, including haemodynamic collapse and rhythm disturbances, exist, and may lead to the terminal event, which is ventricular fibrillation in most patients. For example, a supraventricular tachycardia, usually atrial fibrillation, whether or not associated with a very rapid ventricular response may lead to haemodynamic collapse and ventricular fibrillation.[32] Primary haemodynamic collapse, for which many potential mechanisms exist,[6,21,31,33–35] may produce myocardial ischaemia, arrhythmias and ventricular fibrillation. If either primary haemodynamic collapse or a supraventricular tachycardia were the initiating event, then the outcome (survival versus sudden death) might be determined by the electrical stability of the myocardium, which itself is probably a function of myocardial disarray (Fig. 9.3). Support for this hypothesis comes from the observation that there is greater cellular disarray in the hearts of adolescents who die suddenly than in adults who die suddenly. Adult patients who die of other causes have the least disarray.[21,28]

A history of recurrent syncope and a malignant family history are ominous features in the young patient with hypertrophic cardiomyopathy, but the majority of those who die suddenly do not have these markers. The incidence of sudden death in children and adolescents is higher than in adults, but the occurrence of non-sustained ventricular tachycardia on

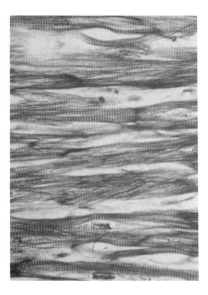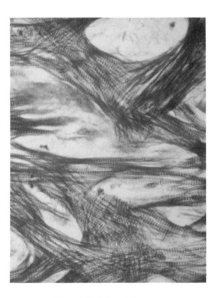

Fig. 9.3   Myofibrillar stain of myocardium from a normal heart (left) and from a young patient with hypertrophic cardiomyopathy who died suddenly (right). In contrast to the orderly arrangement of myocytes in the normal heart, there is considerable myocyte and myofibrillar disarray surrounding areas of increased loose connective tissue in the heart from the affected individual. (Courtesy of Professor M.J. Davies)

ambulatory monitoring is rare, and it is not a useful prognostic indicator.[27] It is of interest, however, that symptoms of impaired consciousness were generally absent in the younger members of a group of patients who experienced exertional hypotension during treadmill exercise.[34] The absence of warning about exertional hypotension may allow the development of regional myocardial ischaemia in such cases. It is possible that exercise hypotension may prove to be a useful marker of risk in this group, but longer follow-up studies are required to establish whether or not this is so.

MANAGEMENT OF HYPERTROPHIC CARDIOMYOPATHY

Symptomatic treatment

Where possible therapy should be chosen to treat specific symptoms. In attempting to identify the best therapy for any particular individual, it is desirable to know how important different aspects of impaired left ventricular function are to that individual, and the impact of any treatment strategy on the disordered physiology. For example, is there an important abnormality of ventricular emptying (outflow tract obstruction), and if so which drug would be most effective at reducing the gradient? Are ventricular relaxation (fall in pressure during isovolumic relaxation) or ventricular filling (diastolic compliance) the dominant abnormalities? Is there evidence of myocardial ischaemia? Are there important rhythm disturbances? There is no evidence that any of the currently available treatment regimens may cause regression of hypertrophy or alteration of the characteristic histological abnormality – myocyte disarray – therefore all symptomatic treatments are palliative, rather than curative.

Beta-blocking drugs

The greatest experience in the pharmacological treatment of hypertrophic cardiomyopathy has been with the beta-adrenergic blockers, particularly with propranolol. Obstruction to left ventricular emptying is increased by manoeuvres which increase myocardial contractility, by a reduction in impedance to left ventricular ejection (afterload reduction), or by a reduction in left ventricular size at the onset of systole (decreased left ventricular filling). Beta-blockade has the potential to reduce resistance or obstruction to left ventricular emptying by acting on all of these mechanisms. Given the importance of the effects of beta-blockade on the peripheral vasculature as well as its direct cardiac effects, it is probably better to use drugs which are not cardioselective. There is, in addition, some evidence, gained in short-term experiments in the cardiac catheter laboratory, that propranolol is more effective at reducing the outflow tract gradient than newer, cardioselective agents.[3,4,36]

Propranolol slows the heart rate at rest and blunts the rate response to exercise, thereby reducing myocardial oxygen demand (lower rate/pressure product for a given level of exercise), and can attenuate the rise in outflow tract obstruction which may accompany exercise.[37] Beta-blockade does not affect active myocardial relaxation during diastole, but by slowing the heart rate it prolongs diastole, increasing the time available for ventricular filling. It can also reduce left ventricular end-diastolic pressure and derived indices of contractility, but not the time constant of ventricular relaxation.[38] Early catheter studies of ventricular filling in hypertrophic cardiomyopathy suggested a beneficial direct effect on left ventricular compliance, in addition to the effect on heart rate,[39,40] but this remains controversial.[41]

All the previously discussed effects of beta-blockers reduce the myocardial oxygen demand, while the prolongation of diastole and the lowering of the left ventricular end-diastolic pressure should improve myocardial perfusion. Propranolol has been shown, in short-term haemodynamic and metabolic studies, to reverse the abnormalities induced by isoprenaline infusion, and to increase coronary sinus flow.[42] In clinical practice, beta-blockers are effective in controlling chest pain.

There is no evidence that beta-blocking drugs can reduce myocardial hyertrophy in hypertrophic cardiomyopathy, and there are no good controlled data on the effect of propranolol on mortality, although one non-randomized trial using very high doses of the drug showed good symptomatic control and no mortality over a five-year period.[43] Our own experience suggests that while propranolol is a useful drug for the control of symptoms, it does not prevent sudden death. During a mean follow-up of six years, 18 out of 164 patients (11%) taking a mean dose of 280 mg propranolol daily died suddenly.[44] Nevertheless propranolol is usually well tolerated, and its safety record is good.

Calcium channel blockers

The other main class of drugs used to treat the symptoms of hypertrophic cardiomyopathy is the calcium channel blockers, particularly verapamil.[45] When given acutely by intravenous bolus, verapamil slows conduction through the atrioventricular node (which is calcium dependent), and slows impulse formation in the sinus node, thus tending to slow heart rate. Its vasodilatory action in the peripheral circulation may, however, cause a reflex tachycardia.[46,47] Like propranolol, verapamil is negatively inotropic causing a reduction in the left ventricular outflow tract pressure gradient.[46,47] There is also evidence of a direct effect on delayed and incoordinate left ventricular relaxation and early diastolic filling.[48-51]

The exact mechanism by which verapamil improves ventricular relaxation is not clear. It may be related to a reduction in myocyte cytosolic calcium concentration, resulting in increased speed of relaxation, although there is some evidence that the speed of relaxation is increased by an improvement in regional asynchrony, rather than by changes in cytosolic calcium concentration.[51,52] The passive elastic properties of the left ventricular myocardium, a function of the cellular architecture of the myo-cardium, do not change.[53]

In long-term use, verapamil is associated with an improvement in functional class in most patients with symptomatic hypertrophic cardiomyo-pathy,[54] and, in high doses, verapamil has been shown to produce a significantly greater reduction in the outflow tract gradient than pro-pranolol.[6,46,47,49] There is also a profound effect on diastolic left ventricular function, and the filling characteristics of the left ventricle. During chronic verapamil usage, the distensibility of the left ventricle appears to improve, although the exact mechanism is uncertain.[55] Altered ventricular loading, negative inotropism, an improvement in the oxygen supply-and-demand relationship of the hypertrophied myocardium, or correction of abnormal myocardial cytosolic calcium transients may play a role.[45,56] There is a correlation between ventricular asynchrony, filling rate, functional class and symptom status,[57] and verapamil can improve asynchrony, increase the early diastolic filling rate and compliance, and improve symptoms.

Some workers have claimed a reduction in angiographic left ventricular mass with verapamil use,[55] but this has not been confirmed using echo-cardiography.[54] The influence of verapamil on prognosis is also de-batable.[47,53] Less is known about diltiazem, but in the short term the effect of diltiazem on symptom status and haemodynamic variables in hypertro-phic cardiomyopathy appears to be comparable to that of verapamil.[58-60]

Initial experiments with the acute administration of nifedipine showed haemodynamic effects which ought to have been beneficial. Delayed left ventricular relaxation was improved, early diastolic filling enhanced, with improved left ventricular compliance.[61,62] However, nifedipine also causes intense peripheral vasodilatation, with a reflex increase in heart rate, which may be deleterious,[61,62] and indeed in some patients there has been a substantial increase in the magnitude of the outflow tract gradient, parti-cularly if the initial resting gradient was high.[63]

Initial enthusiasm for the use of nifedipine has not been borne out by clinical practice. In a direct double-blind, placebo-controlled comparison with verapamil, nifedipine was less effective in controlling symptoms and improving exercise tolerance.[63] Overall, any increase in left ventricular compliance and improvement in diastolic function has been overshadowed by the complications of the intense peripheral vasodilatation. After an early report of the possible beneficial effect obtained by using a combination of nifedipine and propranolol, this regimen was evaluated in 15 patients whose response to verapamil had been suboptimal. Over a mean follow-up period of 18 months, symptomatic improvement was seen in only 2 patients, and in the majority there was frank deterioration.[64] This com-bination cannot be recommended.

Adverse effects are seen more commonly with calcium channel blockers than with propranolol, although discontinuation of the drug has been required infrequently. The vasodilatory action of the calcium channel blockers, particularly nifedipine and diltiazem, has the potential to increase the outflow tract gradient, and increase obstruction to left ventricular ejection. A 7% incidence of pulmonary oedema, and some deaths, with verapamil use have been reported by one group.[65] The exact cause is not clear, but is probably a combination of the effect of reduced afterload with increased outflow tract obstruction, and negative inotropism. Verapamil, in particular, may unmask pre-existing but unsuspected conduction tissue disease. In 120 patients treated with oral verapamil, profound sinus brady-cardia with junctional escape rhythm was seen in 11%, second-degree atrioventricular block occurred in 4%, and there was sinus arrest in 2%.[65]

Cardiac surgery

The use of cardiac surgery for the relief of symptoms, and to improve prognosis, is contentious. Cardiac surgery for this condition developed in the era when it was believed that the primary abnormality in hypertrophic cardiomyopathy was hyperdynamic systolic function, and that intraventri-cular pressure gradients, particularly of the outflow tract, were responsible for symptoms. Experience of surgical treatment is limited in most centres, although over 1000 cases have been reported world wide. The first oper-ations were designed to 'relieve' hypertrophy of the subaortic portion of the muscular septum. Beginning with the simple transaortic ventriculotomy of Cleland and Morrow,[66-68] the technique employed has become more complex and extensive, and usually consists of myotomy/myectomy of the interventricular septum (removal of a segment of the upper anterior septum), with or without replacement of the mitral valve via a transaortic, transventricular, or left transatrial approach. Early surgical results sug-gested that myotomy/myectomy alone could improve the degree of mitral regurgitation,[69] but later surgeons have advocated mitral valve replacement as well, and in some cases mitral valve replacement without myectomy.[70] Good results for mitral valve replacement have been obtained in the relatively small number of patients whose condition is complicated by severe mitral regurgitation.

The majority of patients submitted to surgery have not responded to medical therapy, or have had deteriorating symptoms and impaired exer-cise tolerance after showing a good initial response to either beta-blockade or to calcium channel blockers. Because of the significant morbidity and mortality of surgery, most centres require that patients are at least in New York Heart Association functional class III, despite medical therapy, before surgery will be considered. Usually the patients will have a signifi-cant resting or provokable left ventricular outflow tract pressure gradient as well.

In one of the centres with the largest experience of the surgical manage-ment of hypertrophic cardiomyopathy, the stated aims of surgery are: geometric correction of left ventricular cavity angulation by subvalvar septal myectomy (performed by the transaortic approach), leading to enlargement of the outflow tract, and abolition or significant reduction of the resting or provokable outflow tract gradient.[71] This is claimed to improve diastolic function as well, and to reduce the degree of mitral regurgitation.

To ensure optimal results, these workers perform a detailed haemodynamic assessment when the patient is on the operating table with the chest open, but before cardiopulmonary bypass has been instituted. A deep intraventricular myectomy is performed via an aortotomy, and any fibrous connections of the papillary muscle apparatus to the ventricular wall are excised. The meticulous haemodynamic assessment is repeated before the chest is closed after discontinuation of bypass.

Between 1963 and 1988, 248 patients with hypertrophic cardiomyopathy complicated by refractory symptoms and outflow tract obstruction, and 6 patients with relatively little functional impairment but a malignant family history of sudden death and/or recurrent syncope and cardiac arrest, underwent such surgery. In the 1960s, early postoperative mortality was 25%; this had fallen to 2.7% by the 1980s. The improved mortality rates are related to better patient selection (no patients in NYHA functional class IV in the 1980s), and improved surgical technique. The commonest mode of death in the early postoperative period was intractable cardiac failure; surgical mortality was increased by additional procedures, particularly mitral valve replacement (27.8% early mortality).

The reduction in left ventricular outflow tract gradient and pulmonary artery pressure was impressive, and most of those who survived the operation had an improvement in symptom status of at least one functional class, which seemed to be maintained during follow-up for a mean of 4.5 years. Their uncontrolled results also seem to demonstrate an improvement in survival over patients treated medically, with a disease-related mortality of 1.1% per annum, although excluded from analysis are patients dying from myocardial infarction.

As these results, and others like them, show there is no doubt that myotomy/myectomy can significantly improve symptoms in some patients who are difficult to manage medically, but abolition of the outflow tract gradient is not necessarily the explanation of its success. An influence on myocardial innervation, vascular reflexes, the effect of pericardiotomy, and the negatively inotropic effect of cardiopulmonary bypass may all profoundly influence symptoms. These results also demonstrate that the early surgical mortality is still higher than for other types of cardiac surgery. Notwithstanding the most recent results of the Dusseldorf group, the overall perioperative mortality of myotomy/myectomy is 5–10%.[72] A recent report of the use of intraoperative echocardiography to direct surgery suggests that the perioperative mortality can be reduced by this technique.[73] The transventricular approach carries a particularly high risk of late death due to cardiac failure.

Cardiac transplantation has been advocated in hypertrophic cardiomyopathy both for the treatment of intractable symptoms, and in situations where the risk to the individual of sudden cardiac death is very high. Provided that severe and irreversible changes in the pulmonary vascular bed secondary to left ventricular dysfunction have not occurred, transplantation may be a very useful treatment option.

Arrhythmias and anti-arrhythmic drug therapy

Supraventricular arrhythmias

Approximately 5% of patients have established atrial fibrillation at the time of diagnosis, and an additional 10% will develop this arrhythmia during the subsequent five years.[74-76] Invasive haemodynamic studies during atrial fibrillation and after the restoration of sinus rhythm, and isolated case reports, indicated that its acute onset was poorly tolerated, and potentially fatal,[32,76] and a poor prognosis after the development of atrial fibrillation has often been assumed. Existing natural history studies have provided little support for this pessimistic view, and we have recently published a retrospective review of outcome in patients with hypertrophic cardiomyopathy and atrial fibrillation.[77] The outcome in 52 patients with atrial fibrillation was compared to that in a matched group of patients who remained in sinus rhythm. Symptomatic deterioration, usually new or worse chest pain and dyspnoea, associated with the acute onset of atrial fibrillation, were seen in patients with impaired left ventricular function, but the majority of such patients were restored to their previous functional class by treatment, even if they remained in atrial fibrillation. Thus, after the development of acute atrial fibrillation, symptoms are common and are related not only to the ventricular response, but also to impairment of left ventricular systolic and diastolic function. Furthermore, the development of atrial fibrillation did not adversely affect prognosis in this study.[77]

Short episodes of paroxysmal atrial fibrillation, or other supraventricular tachycardia, do not warrant treatment, as the patients are usually unaware of them and their prognostic significance is uncertain. Sustained paroxysms (30 seconds or longer) of atrial fibrillation may cause a rapid ventricular response and are associated with an important risk of embolization as well as haemodynamic collapse.[32,76,77] Such patients should be fully anticoagulated.

Class I agents, in particular disopyramide and propafenone, have been used with success to control the heart rate in atrial fibrillation, and to produce 'chemical cardioversion' back to sinus rhythm. Their role in maintaining sinus rhythm has not been systematically assessed. Amiodarone has proved itself a useful drug in the context of sustained paroxysms of atrial fibrillation. It is effective in preventing the episodes and, if breakthrough does occur, it will attenuate the ventricular rate response. It has now been shown that the use of amiodarone to treat paroxysmal atrial fibrillation may retard the development of sustained atrial fibrillation.[77]

The adverse effects of amiodarone are generally seen with plasma amiodarone concentrations in excess of 2 mg/l.[78] Fortunately there is now evidence that the suppression of supraventricular arrhythmias in hypertrophic cardiomyopathy can be obtained with plasma concentrations of 0.5–1.5 mg/l.[79] Significant adverse effects are seldom seen at these levels. The role of this drug in the prevention of sudden cardiac death in hypertrophic cardiomyopathy, and the potential mechanisms of this action, will be discussed later.

Usually atrial fibrillation develops because of atrial distension, a consequence of raised filling pressure in a stiff, hypertrophied left ventricle, and provided that the ventricular rate is controlled its development may have little effect on the patients' functional status. In such patients there will have been a gradual reduction in the contribution made by atrial systole to stroke volume, as ventricular compliance has diminished and atrial distension has increased with time. Thus, by the time atrial fibrillation develops, atrial transport will have ceased to be of much haemodynamic importance.

In a minority, however, atrial fibrillation may develop in the absence of atrial distension and with normal filling pressures, because of involvement of atrial tissue in the disease process. Such patients may depend on atrial transport for a considerable fraction of their stroke volume, and the restoration and maintenance of sinus rhythm in such individuals is very important. In them every effort should be made to restore sinus rhythm by cardioversion, supported by treatment with amiodarone.

If sinus rhythm cannot be restored, either chemically or by DC cardioversion, or if it cannot be maintained, digoxin is an appropriate agent for the control of the ventricular rate, as it is in atrial fibrillation of other causes. One should perhaps be cautious in its use in patients with hyperdynamic systolic left ventricular function and a significant outflow tract gradient, because it may possibly worsen obstruction to left ventricular emptying. Most patients in atrial fibrillation, however, have impaired systolic function and do not suffer any deleterious haemodynamic consequences as a result of digoxin use.

Ventricular arrhythmias

Clinical sustained monomorphic ventricular tachycardia is rare in hypertrophic cardiomyopathy, with only a handful of cases reported in the literature.[80,81] In a study published recently, 51 patients, out of more than 200, had ventricular tachycardia detected by ambulatory monitoring, but sustained ventricular tachycardia (> 30 beats at $\geqslant 120$ beats/min), associated with symptomatic deterioration, was seen in only 2.[81] In both patients the relatively rare finding of a left ventricular aneurysm in the presence of normal epicardial coronary arteries was demonstrated by angiography.

Inducible monomorphic ventricular tachycardia is also uncommon. In a series of 7 consecutive patients investigated because of syncope, sustained monomorphic ventricular tachycardia was induced at electrophysiological study in 3, but spontaneous ventricular tachycardia was not documented.[82] In our own experience, 2 of 17 (12%) patients investigated because of syncope had sustained monomorphic ventricular tachycardia at electrophysiological study; monomorphic ventricular tachycardia had previously been documented as the cause of syncope in one. In 17 controls without syncope there were no cases of spontaneous sustained monomorphic ventricular tachycardia, and none could be induced at electrophysiological study, although non-sustained polymorphic ventricular tachycardia was induced in 4 patients and ventricular fibrillation was induced in 1.

Fananapazir et al. included programmed ventricular stimulation (PVS) in their electrophysiological evaluation of 155 patients.[84] PVS produced non-sustained ventricular tachycardia (3–30 beats at a rate of $\geq$ 120 beats/min) in 14% and sustained ventricular tachycardia (defined as a tachycardia > 30 beats, or a tachycardia that requires termination because of haemodynamic instability) in 43%. The significance of these findings is uncertain because the stimulation protocol was very aggressive (up to 3 premature stimuli in 2 right ventricular sites and 1 left ventricular site, with 3 different paced ventricular drive-cycle lengths of 600, 500, and 400 ms), and sustained monomorphic ventricular tachycardia was seen in only 16 of the 155 patients (10%). In the other 50 patients (32% of the total or 76% of those inducible), the response (polymorphic ventricular tachycardia in 48 and ventricular fibrillation in 2) would be considered non-specific and uninterpretable in patients with other cardiac diseases, such as coronary artery disease. In the group studied there was an association between inducibility of sustained ventricular arrhythmia and clinical presentation; it was more common in those with cardiac arrest, syncope, or presyncope than in those who were asymptomatic.

The combined European experience is in general agreement with the incidence of induced ventricular arrhythmias in relation to the aggressiveness of the stimulation protocol. What is different is that the patients with inducible polymorphic ventricular tachycardia have not experienced the adverse outcome which the NIH study would have predicted for them.[85,86]

In those rare cases with clinical sustained ventricular tachycardia, the approach to therapy should be the same as the approach to the treatment of ventricular tachycardia in other conditions. Although such patients may be difficult to resuscitate from arrhythmias which cause haemodynamic embarrassment, treatment should be guided by electrophysiological study, and a 'stepped' approach to therapy can be taken. If drug therapy fails, electrophysiologically guided surgical resection of the aneurysm would be appropriate. In the event of failure of surgery, the patient could be fitted with an automatic implantable cardioverter–defibrillator.

Non-sustained ventricular tachycardia, on the other hand, is common in hypertrophic cardiomyopathy, and can be detected in about 25% of adult patients.[29,74] This arrhythmia may appear benign; it is invariably asymptomatic, and the rate is usually slow (the mean heart rate in more than 400 episodes in 52 patients was 142 beats/min). Non-sustained ventricular tachycardia frequently follows a period of relative bradycardia, and is not associated with ST segment changes or alteration in the QT interval. Analysis of different episodes in the same patients has shown considerable variation in the QRS morphology, suggesting multiple sites of origin,[28] which is in keeping with a disease process which is diffuse and generalized.

As discussed earlier, the importance of non-sustained ventricular tachycardia is that it has been demonstrated, in work from two independent centres, that it is the single best predictor of risk of sudden death in adult patients.[29,30] Treatment of these patients with low-dose amiodarone significantly improves survival in the short term,[83] and the indications are that this benefit is sustained during long-term therapy. This will be amplified in the next section.

Prevention of sudden death

There is no good evidence that symptomatic therapy with propranolol or verapamil can influence the prognosis in hypertrophic cardiomyopathy. The enthusiasm of the proponents of a surgical approach to therapy, and the possibility that in patients with significant left ventricular outflow tract obstruction who survive the operation of myotomy/myectomy, survival may be greater than in patients with obstruction who do not undergo surgery, must be tempered by the perioperative mortality, and the knowledge that patients with significant obstruction are a minority. Most of those who die suddenly do not have left ventricular outflow tract obstruction; indeed many, particularly among children and adolescents, have no symptoms beforehand.

Some centres have begun implanting the automatic cardioverter–defibrillator in patients with recurrent syncope or others perceived to be at high risk of sudden death. The use of this device in such patients has not yet been justified. In most cases the initiating mechanism of syncope is not clear (conduction disturbance, supraventricular arrhythmia, myocardial ischaemia, peripheral vasodilatation, or acute obstruction of the left ventricular outflow tract are all potential mechanisms in an individual), and the rationale for defibrillation is uncertain. The device might restore sinus rhythm (if this were not the rhythm anyway), without restoring cardiac output.

Even in patients with one episode of out-of-hospital ventricular fibrillation, the use of the automatic implantable cardioverter–defibrillator may be controversial. A series of 33 survivors of cardiac arrest was reported recently.[87] The 18 patients with a resting or provokable left ventricular outflow tract gradient underwent surgery (septal myotomy–myectomy in 17, and mitral valve replacement in 1), and all but 2 received antiarrhythmic therapy with a class I agent postoperatively; the remaining 17 received medical therapy alone (a class I agent in 11, and amiodarone in 4). Five patients survived more than 1 cardiac arrest, 4 of whom were in the medical group, and there were 11 deaths (8 disease related) during follow-up for a mean of seven years. Four patients, 2 in each group, died suddenly and 4, all in the surgical group, died of progressive heart failure. Actuarial survival for the whole group was 97% at one year, 74% at five years, and 61% at ten years, which is not significantly different from survival for a group of patients with hypertrophic cardiomyopathy who have not experienced cardiac arrest.

Thus, aborted episodes of sudden death may not carry the same ominous prognosis with which they are associated in coronary artery disease, but such patients represent a difficult management problem, and more information about them is needed. The projected availability of the automatic implantable cardioverter–defibrillator with ECG monitoring capability may provide the follow-up data in this group which would help to decide whether or not all such patients should have the device implanted.

Non-sustained ventricular tachycardia is not usually associated with symptoms, so treatment is not required on symptomatic grounds, but treatment with low-dose amiodarone significantly improves survival in the short and medium term.[83] No such marker has been identified in children, and there is a natural reluctance to commit children to an indefinite period of treatment with amiodarone because of the potential side effects. Nevertheless encouraging results have been seen in an uncontrolled study with very low doses of amiodarone (plasma concentration 0.5 mg/l), in a group of high-risk children with an expected annual mortality of at least 8%. Although confirmation of benefit is required, no deaths occurred over a three-year period in a cohort of 15 patients.[75]

A clinical study of the use of high-dose amiodarone in patients with refractory symptoms and arrhythmias reported several sudden deaths, particularly during a prolonged high-dose loading period.[88] The mode of action of amiodarone in preventing sudden death at low dose, particularly in the absence of sustained spontaneous arrhythmias, is speculative. Prevention of primary arrhythmias, supraventricular tachycardias in particular, raising the threshold for ventricular fibrillation, or an effect on the control of peripheral blood flow may all be relevant.

Summary of treatment options

When dyspnoea is the dominant symptom in patients who show slow filling throughout diastole, prolongation of the filling time by slowing the heart rate, with either propranolol or verapamil, is appropriate. Where there is dyspnoea in association with definite outflow tract obstruction (50% or more of the left ventricular stroke volume within the ventricular cavity at the onset of the gradient), very high-dose verapamil may be effective in reducing both the degree of obstruction and the symptoms. If this fails, myotomy – myectomy may produce an improvement in haemodynamic indices and improvement in symptom status and functional class.

With disease progression there may be gradual reduction in left ventricular systolic performance. Treatment of congestive symptoms in such patients aims to reduce pulmonary and systemic venous pressure, but because the left ventricular diastolic pressure–volume curve in hypertrophic cardiomyopathy is steep, a small change in volume can produce a large change in pressure. It is important, therefore, to avoid excessive preload reduction as this may lead to systemic hypotension. On the whole, diuretics are best avoided in hypertrophic cardiomyopathy, unless there is frank pulmonary oedema. If preload reduction is deemed necessary, then nitrates are probably the best agents and have the added advantage of their anti-ischaemic effect.

Although systolic anterior movement of the mitral valve and the resulting outflow tract gradient are usually associated with some degree of mitral regurgitation, this is rarely severe in volume terms. Rarely, the degree of mitral regurgitation may be sufficiently severe to cause dyspnoea in its own right. Mitral valve replacement is obviously appropriate in such patients, but meticulous assessment of mitral regurgitation is necessary before proceding to surgery. An elevated pulmonary capillary wedge pressure with a prominent 'v' wave may be seen in the absence of severe regurgitation, if the atria are themselves diseased and non-compliant.

Chest pain in the presence of normal epicardial coronary arteries probably represents ischaemia in the majority of patients, and usually responds to treatment with verapamil or propranolol. When choosing between them, propranolol is the safer drug, but patients with severe or refractory symptoms may not respond to it. Though verapamil may be effective in this group, it is precisely these patients who are most at risk from its adverse effects. In such cases therapy with verapamil should be initiated slowly, and in hospital.

If chest pain is related to a definite outflow tract gradient, and is refractory to medical therapy, myectomy may be useful. Coronary arteriography should be performed in patients over the age of 40 who complain of chest pain. Atherosclerotic coronary artery disease can co-exist with hypertrophic cardiomyopathy, and the results of coronary artery bypass surgery combined with myectomy are good.[89] In the last resort, cardiac transplantation should be considered for intractable symptoms.

Symptomatic tachycardias should be treated in the same way as in other forms of cardiac disease. Troublesome ventricular or supraventricular ectopic activity may respond to simple therapy, such as low-dose propranolol. Paroxysmal or sustained atrial fibrillation carries a substantial risk of systemic thromboembolism, and patients with such rhythm disturbances should be anticoagulated. Perhaps the best drug for converting atrial fibrillation to sinus rhythm, and maintaining sinus rhythm, is amiodarone.

Patients with hypertrophic cardiomyopathy who have outflow tract turbulence or mitral regurgitation are at high risk of infective endocarditis. Vegetations usually form on the anterior mitral leaflet, which is frequently thickened and abnormal, at the point where it strikes the interventricular septum, or on the septum itself. If there is mitral regurgitation or turbulent flow in the outflow tract, patients should receive antibiotic prophylaxis for dental work, and other procedures likely to cause bacteraemia.

REFERENCES

1 Teare RD. Asymmetrical hypertrophy of the heart in young adults. Br Heart J 1958; 20: 1–8
2 Braunwald E, Morrow AG, Cornell WP, Augen MM, Hilbish TF. Idiopathic hypertrophic subaortic stenosis: clinical, hemodynamic, and angiographic manifestations. Am J Med 1960; 29: 924–945
3 Braunwald E, Lambrew CT, Harrison DC, Morrow AG, The hemodynamic effects of circulatory drugs in patients with idiopathic subaortic stenosis. In: Cardiomyopathies. Ciba Found Symp 1964; 81: 172–188
4 Goodwin JF, Shah PM, Oakley CM, Cohen J, Yipintsoi T, Pocock W. The clinical pharmacology of hypertrophic obstructive cardiomyopathy. In: Cardiomyopathies. Ciba Found Symp 1964; 81: 189
5 Braunwald E, Lambrew C, Rockoff S, Ross J, Morrow AG. Idiopathic hypertrophic subaortic stenosis. I. Description of the disease based upon an analysis of 64 patients. Circulation 1964; 29 (Suppl 4): III-3–119
6 Maron BJ, Bonow RO, Cannon RO III, Leon MB, Epstein SE. Hypertrophic cardiomyopathy: interrelations of clinical manifestations, pathophysiology and therapy. (Parts 1 and 2). N Engl J Med 1987; 316: 780–789, 844–852
7 Henry WL, Clark CE, Epstein SE. Asymmetric septal hypertrophy: echocardiographic identification of the pathognomonic anatomic abnormalities of IHSS. Circulation 1973; 47: 225–233
8 Roberts CS, Roberts WC. Hypertrophic cardiomyopathy: morphologic features. In: Zipes DP, Rowlands DJ, eds. Progress in Cardiology 2/2. Philadelphia: Lea & Febiger, 1989
9 Maron BJ, Epstein SE. Hypertrophic cardiomyopathy. Recent observations regarding the specificity of three hallmarks of the disease: asymmetric septal hypertrophy, septal disorganisation and systolic anterior motion of the anterior mitral leaflet. Am J Cardiol 1980; 45: 141–154
10 Shapiro LM, Zezulka A. Hypertrophic cardiomyopathy: a common disease with a good prognosis. Five year experience of a district general hospital. Br Heart J 1983; 50: 530–553
11 Wahedra D, Gunnar RM, Scanlon PJ. Prognosis in hypertrophic cardiomyopathy with asymmetric septal hypertrophy. Postgrad Med J 1985; 61: 1107–1109
12 McKenna WJ, Kleinebenne A. Hypertrophic cardiomyopathy in the elderly. In: Coodley EL, ed. Geriatric heart disease. Littleton: John Wright, PSG, 1985, pp. 260–268
13 Maron BJ, Gottdiener JS, Epstein SE. Patterns and significance of distribution of left ventricular hypertrophy in hypertrophic cardiomyopathy: a wide angle, two dimensional echocardiographic study of 125 patients. Am J Cardiol 1981; 48: 418–428
14 Shapiro LM, Kleinebenne A, McKenna WJ. The distribution of left ventricular hypertrophy in hypertrophic cardiomyopathy: comparison to athletes and hypertensives. Eur Heart J 1985; 6: 967–974
15 McKenna WJ, Kleinebenne A, Nihoyannopoulos P, Foale RA. Echocardiographic

measurement of right ventricular wall thickness in hypertrophic cardiomyopathy: relation to clinical and prognostic features. J Am Coll Cardiol 1988; 11: 351–358

16 McKenna WJ, Stewart JT, Nihoyannopoulos P, McGinty F, Davies MJ. Hypertrophic cardiomyopathy without hypertrophy: 2 families with myocardial disarray in the absence of increased myocardial mass. Br Heart J 1990; 62: 287–290

17 Jarcho JA, McKenna W, Pare JAP et al. Mapping a gene for familial hypertrophic cardiomyopathy to chromosome 14q1. N Engl J Med 1989; 321: 1372–1378

18 Solomon SD, Geisterfer-Lowrance AAT, Vosberg H-P et al. A locus for familial hypertrophic cardiomyopathy is closely linked to the cardiac myosin heavy chain genes. CRI-L436, and CRI-L329 on chromosome 14 at q11–q12. Am J Hum Genet 1990; 47: 389–394

19 Tanigawa G, Jarcho JA, Kass S et al. A molecular basis for familial hypertrophic cardiomyopathy: an α/β cardiac myosin heavy chain hybrid gene. Cell 1990; 62: 991–998

20 Geisterfer-Lowrance AAT, Kass S, Tanigawa G et al. A molecular basis for familial hypertrophic cardiomyopathy: a β cardiac myosin heavy chain gene missense mutation. Cell 1990; 62: 999–1006

21 Loogen F, Kuhn H, Krelhaus W. The natural history of hypertrophic cardiomyopathy and the effect of therapy. In: Kaltenbach M, Loogen F, Olsen EGJ, eds. Cardiomyopathy and myocardial biopsy. New York: Springer-Verlag, 1978, pp 268 299

22 Maron BJ, Lipson LC, Roberts WC, Savage DD, Epstein SE. 'Malignant' hypertrophic cardiomyopathy: identification of a subgroup of families with unusually frequent premature death. Am J Cardiol 1978; 41: 1133–1140

23 Maron BJ, Roberts WC, Epstein SE. Sudden death in hypertrophic cardiomyopathy: a profile of 78 patients. Circulation 1982; 65: 1388–1394

24 McKenna WJ, Oakley CM, Krikler DM, Goodwin JF. Improved survival with amiodarone in patients with hypertrophic cardiomyopathy and ventricular tachycardia. Br Heart J 1985; 53: 412–416

25 Maron BJ, Tajik AJ, Ruttenberg HD et al. Hypertrophic cardiomyopathy in infants: clinical features and natural history. Circulation 1982; 65: 7–17

26 Maron BJ, Spirito P, Wesley Y, Arce J. Development and progression of left ventricular hypertrophy in children with hypertrophic cardiomyopathy. N Engl J Med 1986; 315: 610–614

27 McKenna WJ, Deanfield JE. Hypertrophic cardiomyopathy: an important cause of sudden death. Arch Dis Child 1984; 59: 971–975

28 McKenna WJ, Alfonso F. Arrhythmias in the cardiomyopathies and mitral valve prolapse. In: Zipes D, Rowlands D, eds. Progress in cardiology. Philadelphia: Lea and Febiger, 1988, pp 59–75

29 McKenna WJ, England D, Doi YL, Deanfield JE, Oakley CM, Goodwin JF. Arrhythmia in hypertrophic cardiomyopathy. 1. Influence on prognosis. Br Heart J 1981; 46: 168–172

30 Maron BJ, Savage DD, Wolfson JK, Epstein SE. Prognostic significance of 24 hour ambulatory electrocardiographic monitoring in patients with hypertrophic cardiomyopathy: a prospective study. Am J Cardiol 1981; 48: 252–257

31 McKenna WJ. The natural history of hypertrophic cardiomyopathy. In: Brest AN, Shaver JA, eds. Cardiovascular clinics. Philadelphia: Davis, 1988, pp 135–148

32 Stafford WJ, Trohman RG, Bilsker M, Zaman L, Castellanos A, Myerburg RJ. Cardiac arrest in an adolescent with atrial fibrillation and hypertrophic cardiomyopathy. J Am Coll Cardiol 1986; 7: 701–704

33 McKenna WJ, Harris L, Deanfield J. Syncope in hypertrophic cardiomyopathy. Br Heart J 1982; 47: 177–179

34 Frenneaux MP, Counihan PJ, Caforio ALP, Chikamori T, McKenna WJ. Abnormal blood pressure response during exercise in hypertrophic cardiomyopathy. Circulation 1990; 82: 1995–2002

35 Counihan PJ, Frenneaux MP, Webb DJ, McKenna WJ. Abnormal vascular responses to supine exercise in hypertrophic cardiomyopathy. Circulation 1991; 84: 686–696

36 Swanton RH, Brooksby IAB, Jenkins BS, Webb-Peploe MM. Haemodynamic studies of beta-blockade in hypertrophic obstructive cardiomyopathy. Eur J Cardiol 1977; 5(4): 327–341

37 Cohen LS, Braunwald E. Amelioration of angina pectoris in idiopathic hypertrophic subaortic stenosis with beta-adrenergic blockade. Circulation 1967; 35: 847–851

38 Thompson DS, Wilmshurst P, Juul S et al. Pressure-derived indices of left ventricular relaxation in patients with hypertrophic cardiomyopathy. Br Heart J 1983; 49: 529–567

39 Webb-Peploe MM, Oakley CM, Croxson RS, Goodwin JF. Cardio-selective beta-adrenergic blockade in hypertrophic obstructive cardiomyopathy. Postgrad Med J 1971; 47 (Suppl): 93–97

40 Webb-Peploe MM. Management of hypertrophic obstructive cardiomyopathy by beta-blockade. In: Hypertrophic obstructive cardiomyopathies. Ciba Found Symp 1974; 37: 103–112

41 Speiser KW, Krayenbuhl HP. Reappraisal of the effect of acute beta-blockade on left ventricular filling dynamics in hypertrophic obstructive cardiomyopathy. Eur Heart J 1981; 2: 21–29

42 Cuccurullo F, Mezzetti A, Lapenna D et al. Mechanism of isoproterenol-induced anginal pectoris in patients with obstructive hypertrophic cardiomyopathy and normal coronary arteries. Am J Cardiol 1987; 60: 667–673

43 Frank MJ, Abdulla AM, Canedo MI, Saylors RE. Long-term medical management of hypertrophic obstructive cardiomyopathy. Am J Cardiol 1978; 42: 993–1001.

44 McKenna WJ, Deanfield J, Faruqui A, England D, Oakley CM, Goodwin JF. Prognosis in hypertrophic cardiomyopathy: role of age, and clinical, electrocardiographic and hemodynamic features. Am J Cardiol 1981; 47: 532–538

45 Lorell BH. Use of calcium channel blockers in hypertrophic cardiomyopathy. Am J Med 1985; 78 (Suppl 2B): 43–54

46 Rosing DR, Kent KM, Borer JS, Seides SF, Maron BJ, Epstein SE. Verapamil therapy: a new approach to the pharmacologic treatment of hypertrophic cardiomyopathy. I. Hemodynamic effects. Circulation 1979; 60: 1201–1207

47 Rosing DR, Kent KM, Maron BJ, Epstein SE. Verapamil therapy: a new approach to the pharmacologic treatment of hypertrophic cardiomyopathy. II. Effects on exercise capacity and symptomatic status. Circulation 1979; 60: 1208–1213

48 Hanrath P, Mathey DG, Siegert R, Bleifeld W. Left ventricular relaxation and filling patterns in different forms of left ventricular hypertrophy: an echocardiographic study. Am J Cardiol 1980; 45: 15–23

49 Bonow RO, Rosing DR, Bacharach SL et al. Effects of verapamil on left ventricular systolic function and diastolic filling in patients with hypertrophic cardiomyopathy. Circulation 1981; 64: 787–796

50 Hasin Y, Lewis BS, Lewis N, Weiss AT, Gotsman MS. Long-term effect of verapamil in hypertrophic cardiomyopathy. Int J Cardiol 1982; 1: 243–251

51 Hess OM, Murakami T, Krayenbuehl HP. Does verapamil improve left ventricular relaxation in patients with myocardial hypertrophy? Circulation 1986; 74: 530–543

52 Bonow RO, Vitale DF, Maron BJ, Bacharach SL, Frederick TM, Green MV. Regional left ventricular asynchrony and impaired global left ventricular filling in hypertrophic cardiomyopathy: effect of verapamil. J Am Coll Cardiol 1987; 9: 1108–1116

53 Hess OM, Grimm J, Krayenbuehl HP. Diastolic function in hypertrophic cardiomyopathy: effects of propranolol and verapamil on diastolic stiffness. Eur Heart J 1983; 4 (Suppl F): 47–56

54 Rosing DR, Condit JR, Maron BJ et al. Verapamil therapy: a new approach to the pharmacologic treatment of hypertrophic cardiomyopathy. Effects of long-term administration. Am J Cardiol 1981; 43: 545–553

55 Kaltenbach M, Hopf R, Kober G, Bussmann WD, Keller M, Petersen Y. Treatment of hypertrophic obstructive cardiomyopathy with verapamil. Br Heart J 1979; 42: 35–42

56 Bonow RO, Ostrow HG, Rosing DR et al. Effects of verapamil on left ventricular systolic and diastolic function in patients with hypertrophic cardiomyopathy: pressure–volume analysis with a nonimaging scintillation probe. Circulation 1983; 68: 1062–1073

57 Bonow RO, Dilsizian V, Rosing DR, Maron BJ, Bacharach SL, Green MV. Verapamil-induced improvement in left ventricular diastolic filling and increased exercise tolerance in patients with hypertrophic cardiomyopathy: short- and long-term effects. Circulation 1985; 72: 853–864

58 Suwa M, Hirota Y, Kawamura K. Improvement in left ventricular diastolic function during intravenous and oral diltiazem therapy in patients with hypertrophic cardiomyopathy: an echocardiographic study. Am J Cardiol 1984; 54: 1047–1053

59 Toshima H, Koga Y, Nagata H, Toyomasu K, Itaya K, Matoba T. Comparable effects of

oral diltiazem and verapamil in the treatment of hypertrophic cardiomyopathy. Jpn Heart J 1986; 27: 701–715

60 Iwase M, Sotobata I, Takagi S, Miyaguchi K, Jing HX, Yokotu M. Effects of diltiazem on left ventricular diastolic behaviour in patients with hypertrophic cardiomyopathy: evaluation with exercise pulsed Doppler echocardiography. J Am Coll Cardiol 1987; 9: 1099–1105

61 Lorell BH, Paulus WJ, Grossman W, Wynne J, Cohn PF. Modification of abnormal left ventricular diastolic properties by nifedipine in patients with hypertrophic cardiomyopathy. Circulation 1982; 65: 499–507

62 Paulus WJ, Lorell BH, Craig WE, Wynne J, Murgo JP, Grossman W. Comparison of the effects of nitroprusside and nifedipine on diastolic properties in patients with hypertrophic cardiomyopathy: altered left ventricular loading or improved muscle inactivation? J Am Coll Cardiol 1983; 2: 879–886

63 Rosing DR, Cannon RO, Watson RM, Kent KM, Lakatos E, Epstein SE. Comparison of verapamil and nifedipine effects on symptoms and exercise capacity in patients with hypertrophic cardiomyopathy (abstract). Circulation 1982; 66 (Suppl II): 24

64 Hopf R, Thomas J, Klepzig H, Kaltenbach M. Behandlung der hypertropischen Kardiomyopathie mit Nifedipin und Propranolol in Kombination. Z Kardiol 1987; 76: 469–478

65 Epstein SE, Rosing DR. Verapamil: its potential for causing serious complications in patients with hypertrophic cardiomyopathy. Circulation 1981; 64: 437–441

66 Goodwin JF, Hollman A, Cleland WP, Teare D. Obstructive cardiomyopathy simulating aortic stenosis. Br Heart J 1960; 22: 403–414

67 Morrow AG, Brockenbrough EC. Surgical treatment of idiopathic subaortic stenosis: technique and hemodynamic results of subaortic ventriculotomy. Ann Surg 1961; 154: 181–189

68 Cleland WP. The surgical management of obstructive cardiomyopathy. J. Cardiovasc Surg 1963; 4: 489–491

69 Brauwald E, Lambrew CT, Rockoff DS, Ross J, Morrow AG. Idiopathic hypertrophic subaortic stenosis. Circulation 1964; 30 (Suppl IV): 1–119

70 Cooley DA, Wukasch DC, Leachman RD. Mitral valve replacement for idiopathic subaortic stenosis: results in 27 patients. J Cardiovasc Surg 1976; 17: 380–387

71 Schulte HD, Bircks W, Losse B. Surgical treatment of hypertrophic obstructive cardiomyopathy (HOCM): early and late results. In: Zipes DP, Rowlands DJ, eds. Progress in cardiology 2/2. Philadelphia: Lea & Febiger, 1989, pp 195–215

72 Maron BJ, Merrill WH, Freier PA et al. Long-term clinical course and symptomatic status of patients after operation for hypertrophic subaortic stenosis. Circulation 1978; 57: 1205–1213

73 McIntosh C, Maron BJ. Current operative treatment of obstructive hypertrophic cardiomyopathy.Circulation 1988; 78: 487–495

74 Savage DD, Seides SF, Maron BJ, Myers DM, Epstein SE. Prevalence of arrhythmia during 24 hour electrocardiographic monitoring and exercise testing in patients with obstructive and non obstructive hypertrophic cardiomyopathy. Circulation 1979; 59: 866–875

75 McKenna WJ, Franklin RCG, Nihoyannopoulos P, Robinson KR, Deanfield JE. Arrhythmia and prognosis in infants, children and adolescents with hypertrophic cardiomyopathy: J Am Coll Cardiol 1988; 11: 147–153

76 Glancy DL, O'Brien KP, Gold HK, Epstein SE. Atrial fibrillation in patients with idiopathic hypertrophic subaortic stenosis. Br Heart J 1970; 32: 652–659

77 Robinson K, Frenneaux MP, Stockins B, Karatasakis G, Poloniecki JD, McKenna WJ. Atrial fibrillation in hypertrophic cardiomyopathy: a longitudinal study. J Am Coll Cardiol 1990; 15: 1279–1285

78 Harris L, McKenna WJ, Rowland E, Krikler DM. Side effects of long-term amiodarone therapy.Circulation 1983; 67: 45–51

79 McKenna WJ, Harris L, Rowland E et al. Amiodarone for long-term management of patients with hypertrophic cardiomyopathy. Am J Cardiol 1984; 54: 802–810

80 Geibel A, Brugada P, Zehender M, Stevenson W, Waldecker B, Wellens HJJ. Value of programmed electrical stimulation using a standardized ventricular stimulation protocol in hypertrophic cardiomyopathy. Am J Cardiol 1987; 60: 738–739

81 Alfonso F, Frenneaux M, McKenna WJ. Clinical sustained monomorphic ventricular tachycardia in hypertrophic cardiomyopathy: association with left ventricular apical aneurysm. Br Heart J 1989; 61: 178–181

82 Kowey PR, Eisenberg R, Engel TR. Sustained arrhythmias in hypertrophic obstructive cardiomyopathy. N Engl J Med; 310: 1566–1569

83 McKenna WJ, Oakley CM, Krikler DM, Goodwin JF. Improved survival with amiodarone in patients with hypertrophic cardiomyopathy and ventricular tachycardia. Br Heart J 1985; 53: 412–416

84 Fananapazir L, Tracy C, Leon MB et al. Electrophysiologic abnormalities in patients with hypertrophic cardiomyopathy: a consecutive analysis of 155 patients. Circulation 1989; 80: 1259–1268

85 Kuck K-H, Kunze K-P, Schluter M, Nienaber CA, Costard A. Programmed electrical stimulation in hypertrophic cardiomyopathy: results in patients with and without cardiac arrest or syncope. Eur Heart J 1988; 9: 177–185

86 Borgreffe M, Podczeck A, Breithardt G. Electrophysiologic studies in hypertrophic cardiomyopathy (abstract). Circulation 1986; 74 (Suppl II): 1922

87 Cecchi F, Maron BJ, Epstein SE. Long-term outcome of patients with hypertrophic cardiomyopathy successfully resuscitated after cardiac arrest. J Am Coll Cardiol 1989; 13: 1283–1288

88 Fananapazir L, Leon MB, Bonow RO, Tracy CM, Cannon RO, Epstein SE. Sudden death during empiric amiodarone therapy in symptomatic hypertrophic cardiomyopathy. Am J Cardiol 1991; 67: 169–174

89 Cokkinos DV, Krajcer Z, Leachman RD. Coronary artery disease in hypertrophic cardiomyopathy. Am J Cardiol 1985; 55: 1437–1438

10

Conservative surgery for mitral valve disease

D. J. M. Keenan

Mitral valve repair is not a new technique but one which dates from the beginning of open heart surgery.[1,2] It was because of the equivocal results obtained that it fell into disrepute, especially when reliable prosthetic valves were introduced. Ironically, however, when these valves themselves were shown, one by one, to have their own drawbacks and hazards, this, together with the increasing awareness of the cumulative effects of a lifetime of anticoagulant therapy, led to a reappraisal of the alternatives to valve replacement in the treatment of mitral valve disease. It is particularly to Carpentier that we are indebted. He has set about systematically analysing the aetiology and pathophysiology of mitral regurgitation and has used this information to form a rational basis for the surgical treatment of the condition.[3]

AETIOLOGY

Mitral valve disease is commonly due to rheumatic fever, degeneration (floppy valve syndrome), myocardial ischaemia, infective endocarditis and congenital malformation. Rheumatic valve disease generally affects the commissures, with resultant fusion. The leaflets become thickened and later calcified and the chordae become shortened and fused with eventual adherence of the leaflets, especially the posterior leaflet, to the papillary muscles.

The degenerative diseases are classified by Carpentier[4] into three groups: Barlow's disease, fibroelastic deficiency and Marfan's syndrome affecting the mitral valve. Barlow's mitral valve is characterized by gross excess of valve tissue, with thickened leaflets, a dilated annulus and elongated and ruptured chordae. In contrast the fibroelastic diseased valve has no excess of tissue but, rather, very thin cusps with elongated chordae which are very frequently ruptured. In Marfan's syndrome the valve tissue is stretched, with thin cusps and distended annulus, together with some elongation of the chordae which are rarely ruptured.

The mechanisms for ischaemic regurgitation are as follows:

1. If the myocardium underlying a papillary muscle is fibrotic the muscle

fails to move or moves paradoxically during systole, and regurgitation occurs.

2. Ischaemia of the papillary muscle and supporting myocardium can lead to transient regurgitation, a situation which can be corrected by revascularization. The posteromedial papillary muscle is more frequently involved by virtue of its more precarious blood supply.

3. Fibrosis of a papillary muscle is a common sequel of ischaemia and can lead to elongation, causing prolapse of the related part of the valve.

4. Complete papillary muscle rupture is rare and leads to acute massive regurgitation, whilst rupture of one of the heads of the muscle, which is more common, leads to severe regurgitation, the tolerance of which will depend on left ventricular function.

5. Left ventricular dilatation leads to lateral displacement of the papillary muscles with failure of the leaflets to meet, causing central regurgitation.

PATHOPHYSIOLOGY

Carpentier[3] has emphasized the need for classifying mitral disease according to the functional disturbance of the motion of the leaflets and has divided it into three: I, normal leaflet motion; II, leaflet prolapse; III, leaflet restriction. Type I dysfunction is caused by annulus dilatation, secondary to left ventricular dilatation, or a leaflet perforation. Type II dysfunction is caused by rupture or elongation of either papillary muscles or chordae, as occurs in the degenerative diseases or myocardial ischaemia. Type III dysfunction is caused by fusion of chordae or commissures, which classically occurs following rheumatic fever.

Congenital valvular lesions can be represented in all of the three types of leaflet dysfunction. Mitral valve repair in children follows the same principles as in adults, with a detailed functional analysis of the deformity and a repair. However the underlying lesions are more complex and there are frequently associated congenital lesions.[5] There is much advantage in avoiding a prosthetic valve in a child, with the attendant problems of life-long anticoagulation and premature tissue calcification.[6]

PREOPERATIVE INVESTIGATION

The assessment of mitral valve disease relies primarily on two-dimensional and Doppler echocardiography. The functional classification of mitral leaflet motion into three types is used directly in describing the echocardiographic features of the leaking valve, with the definition of prolapse being a 2-mm projection of any portion of the mitral leaflet past the plane of the annulus. An assessment of thickening of the leaflets can be made and calcification identified. Mitral valve area can be calculated. Using Doppler and colour flow imaging an assessment of the regurgitation can be made and the direction of the jet can be determined, this being opposite to the leaking leaflet. When a central jet is present the problem is usually one of restricted movement (type III). Left ventricular function can be assessed using echocardiography and measurements made of ventricle and atrium. Finally, any congenital anomalies can be demonstrated and assessed.

The technique of transoesophageal echocardiography provides enhanced pictures which more closely resemble the naked eye appearances of the valve and this affords more accurate preoperative planning of the repair procedure. This technique is invaluable in the operating theatre, where it can be used before commencing cardiopulmonary bypass, and particularly after cessation of bypass, to test the adequacy of the repair, whilst the chest is still open, with the possibility of carrying out a further procedure in the event of a poor echocardiographic result.

Cardiac catheterization is rarely required in the preparation of patients for mitral valve repair, although coronary angiography is frequently carried out to complete the detailed preoperative investigation.

INDICATIONS FOR SURGERY

Mitral valvotomy, the simplest conservative operation, remains the procedure of choice for purely stenotic valves with non-calcified, pliable leaflets. These are seen primarily in younger patients in developing countries. One might expect such a patient to be suffering from moderate symptoms (NYHA class II) or to have had one episode of paroxysmal nocturnal dyspnoea or pulmonary oedema. It is widely believed that mitral valvotomy carried out under direct vision (open mitral valvotomy), whilst on cardiopulmonary bypass, is a better operation than that performed via a left thoracotomy (closed valvotomy), with a much more accurate split of the two commissures being possible. In the West appropriate patients are exceedingly rare and might be better managed by percutaneous balloon dilatation, whilst in developing countries, in practice, cost precludes open valvotomy as does it preclude balloon dilatation of stenotic valves.[7]

The decision and timing of a mitral valve repair procedure for mitral regurgitation remains a very difficult problem. This is because, unlike mitral stenosis, mitral regurgitation leads to deterioration of left ventricular function if left too long. It has been shown, in a medically treated group, that the natural history of mitral regurgitation is poor due to progressive left ventricular dysfunction[8] and this has also become apparent when analysing the causes of late death following successful mitral valve replacement, where myocardial failure and its sequelae predominate.[9-13] It must be said that patients with mitral regurgitation are usually referred later rather than earlier for surgery. The onset of atrial fibrillation is vitally important in this respect. One of the chief advantages of a repair operation is that anticoagulant therapy can be discontinued two or three months postoperatively. However, if chronic atrial fibrillation is present then life-long anticoagulation is required and an important benefit in avoiding a prosthetic valve has been lost. The repair operation should be performed before or very shortly after the onset of atrial fibrillation and, post-operatively, energetic steps should be taken to re-establish sinus thythm so that anticoagulants can be discontinued.

The timing of surgery depends also on the likelihood of being able to effect a repair, in contradistinction to having to carry out a replacement, as one is more likely to operate early and thus avoid the small but finite morbidity associated with a prosthetic valve and anticoagulants. In general terms, however, patients should not be allowed to progress to functional class III or beyond, and a careful watch must be kept on medical therapy lest the physician be lulled into complacency by the use of increasing diuretics and afterload-reducing drugs. Serial echocardiographic assessments must be made of left ventricular dimensions so that enlargement is quickly identified. The same caveat applies to the left atrium. Any patient demonstrated to have increasing left ventricular dysfunction should be operated on, regardless of symptoms.

Finally, in the decision-making analysis it should be remembered that it is nearly impossible to effect a repair of a calcified valve. Such patients require a valve replacement.

Mitral regurgitation is frequently caused by myocardial ischaemia but it is rare to have to repair a valve in such a setting because the regurgitation is frequently too mild to warrant surgery. The indications for intervention are modulated by the requirement of surgery for other reasons (e.g. coronary artery bypass grafting). If a patient with moderate regurgitation requires revascularization then it would be reasonable, at the same time, to repair the regurgitant valve and, in such circumstances, usually only an annuloplasty ring is required. If, in the presence of moderate regurgitation, revascularization is not needed, serial echocardiography is used, as before, to arrive at a decision based on left ventricular and atrial size. The situation is much easier in the case of acute massive incompetence, due to either papillary muscle rupture or to rupture of one of the heads of a papillary muscle. With such a patient, automatically in NYHA class IV, there is clearly an indication for urgent repair, which involves suturing the ruptured papillary muscle to an appropriate (non-ischaemic) area of the ventricle or, if only one of the heads has gone, suturing it to an adjacent papillary muscle.[14] When an acute infarct gives rise to lesser degrees of regurgitation there is a lot to be gained by not proceeding to early repair but rather persisting with medical therapy and performing serial echocardiography.

Finally, minor degrees of regurgitation noted incidentally require no intervention, even if such a patient is going forward for myocardial re-vascularization.

OPERATIVE TECHNIQUE

The operation is carried out on standard cardiopulmonary bypass with hypothermia. Carpentier emphasizes the need to carry out a perioperative assessment of the valve under direct vision and this involves the same principles as before, with assessment of anterior and posterior leaflet prolapse and restriction involving an evaluation of the chordae and papillary muscles, together with assessment of annular dilatation (Fig. 10.1).

For type I mitral insufficiency, where there is simple annular dilatation with no subvalvular lesions, the placement of a prosthetic ring in the annulus is sufficient to sustain permanent remodelling of the annulus. The annulus normally has a longer transverse than anteroposterior diameter. With dilatation the opposite is true and the prosthetic ring reverses this. The base of the anterior leaflet, between the two commissures, remains constant in all situations because the fibrous skeleton of the heart does not allow this area to lengthen, whereas the base of the posterior leaflet does stretch. Therefore the ring is placed so that the fixed anterior leaflet distance is equal to the upper portion of the ring, but the dilatation which occurs around the posterior leaflet is gathered in and held rigid by the ring, restoring the normal geometry and preventing later recurrence of regurgitation by preventing secondary dilatation after repair (Fig. 10.1C, D).

The repair of leaflet prolapse depends on whether the anterior or posterior leaflet is prolapsing and whether or not the chordae are ruptured or elongated. Ruptured chordae to the posterior leaflet are repaired by excising a quadrantic wedge of leaflet (Fig. 10.1A) but no more than half of the posterior leaflet may be excised in a repair procedure. Ruptured chordae to the anterior leaflet are treated by chordal transposition, which necessitates movement of chordae, and a small piece of the posterior leaflet, anteriorly. Such an area of posterior leaflet is usually made available by concomitant repair of the posterior leaflet. If the posterior leaflet is not to be repaired then it is still possible to sacrifice a small area of the posterior leaflet to carry out an anterior repair by transposition. Chordal elongation is treated by either shortening the relevant papillary muscle or, if more severe, by implanting the chordae in the body of the papillary muscles (Fig. 10.2).

Restrictive movement, when due to commissural fusion, is treated by direct cutting and separation of the commissures. When restriction is due to papillary muscle dysfunction, then a portion of the papillary muscle can be reimplanted into an area with viable myocardium. This is done by cutting a trench in the myocardium and suturing the portion of the papillary muscle into the trench, with closure of the trench over this.

A ring is placed in nearly all repairs. A situation where it is not used is when simple open mitral commissurotomy has been performed. Likewise, it is not placed when there is no dilatation of the annulus such as occurs with papillary muscle rupture due to ischaemia, or if there has been perforation of a cusp related to bacterial endocarditis. One attempts to avoid a ring in a growing child.

The repair is usually tested by injecting a volume of cold saline into the ventricular cavity and assessing the valvular competency. Following the

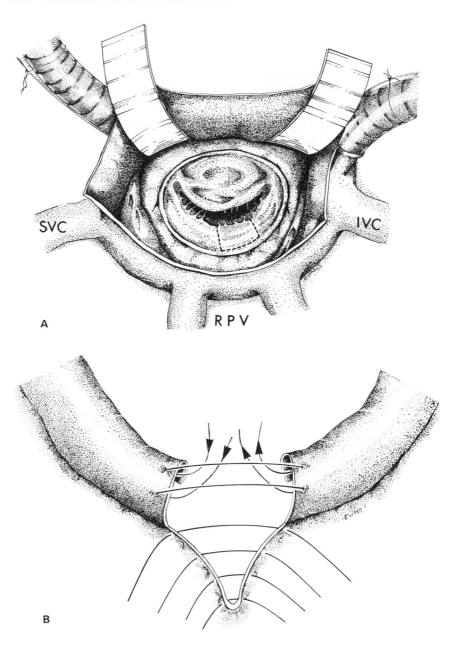

cessation of cardiopulmonary bypass, detailed assessment can be carried out by intraoperative, transoesophageal echocardiography. At this point if there remains important mitral regurgitation, a decision must be made as to whether or not this will be easily repaired or whether the repair procedure should be abandoned and a mitral valve replacement performed.

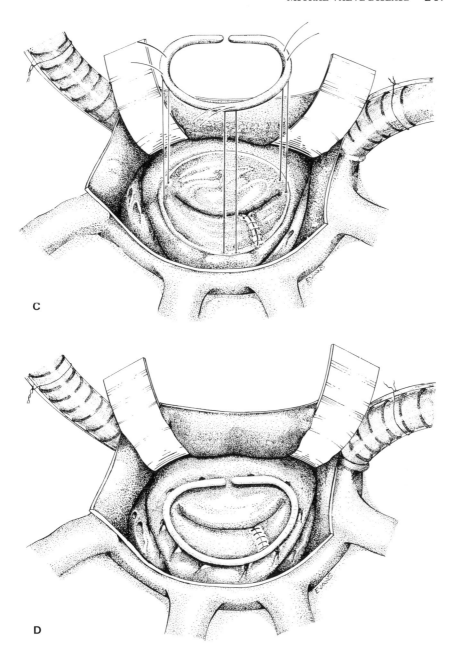

Fig. 10.1 **A** View of the mitral valve which has been exposed by opening the left atrium superior to the right pulmonary veins (RPV). Cannulae, for cardiopulmonary bypass, have been placed in the superior vena cava (SVC) and the inferior vena cava (IVC). A quadrantic area of the posterior leaflet (indicated) is to be excised. **B** Method of repair of the excised quadrant of the posterior leaflet. **C** A Carpentier annuloplasty ring is being placed using interrupted sutures. **D** The completed repair with the ring in place.

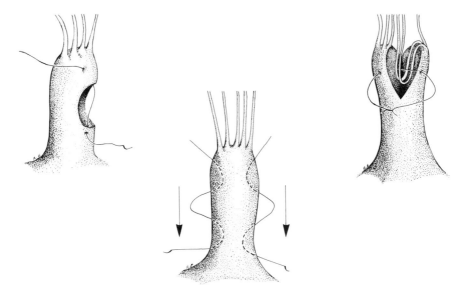

Fig. 10.2   Three methods to shorten chordae and treat leaflet prolapse. The chordae can be shortened by burying them in the papillary muscle or the muscle itself shortened.

Additionally, the presence of a gradient between the left ventricular cavity and the aorta can be sought and if present might also necessitate a revision of the repair.[15-17]

RESULTS

The results of mitral repair, particularly the late results, must be superior to the results currently obtained by mitral valve replacement. Several large series have confirmed that the procedure can be performed with a low operative risk and good long-term result.[11,12,19-21]

Operative mortality

The operative mortality usually being quoted varies between 0% and 5%, with an average of 3.5%. A comparative study carried out in the Cleveland Clinic[14] which, though uncontrolled, compared the mortality between repaired and replaced valves revealed that the respective mortalities were 1% and 4.1% ($p = 0.0006$). This trend towards lower mortality with repaired valves is consistent in the literature although criticism voiced about non-comparability of groups is probably justified. In order to compare two groups Craver et al[18] looked at 65 consecutive valve repairs and compared them with an equal group of controls obtained by computer-matching algorithms and from a database. The early mortality for the two groups was 1.5% and 4.6%, respectively.

Survival

It is only with the passage of time that the late survival of patients with prosthetic valves in situ has become commonplace, with the ten-year survival in Starr's series[22] at 56%. Cohn et al[13] reported results in 1985 with actuarial survival rates at nine years of 60% and Bloomfield et al[10] have recently reported the results of a 12-year comparative study in which the mitral valve was replaced by either a Bjork–Shiley or a porcine bio-prosthetic valve in which 44% and 40%, respectively, of patients were alive. The relatively poor survival figures after mitral valve replacement may be related not only to preoperative left ventricular dysfunction in patients with mitral regurgitation, but also to impaired left ventricular function consequent upon removal of the papillary muscles. Goldman et al[23] have shown in a study comparing left ventricular function pre- and post-bypass, in two groups having either a mitral valve repair or replacement, that repaired hearts had a lower pulmonary capillary wedge pressure, maintained their ejection fraction and did not suffer from regional ventricular dysfunction, unlike the 'replaced group'.

In the Starr series[22] 50% of late deaths were due to cardiac disease, with an additional 16% related to the valve. These valve-related deaths were due to embolization, endocarditis, bleeding complications and prosthetic valve thrombosis. More recent series put these figures higher, with Cohn et al[13] stating that 63% of all survivors of mitral valve replacement died of a cardiac cause, 18% of a valve-related problem and 7% of a non-cardiac cause but, worryingly, 12% had unknown causes of death. Bloomfield et al[10] report, for mitral valve replacement, 64% dying of a cardiac cause, 16% of a possible cardiac cause, 18.5% of a non-cardiac cause and 1.5% unknown.

Long-term survival results of mitral valve repair are now available. In Carpentier's series[21] the five-, ten- and 15-year survival figures are 92%, 85% and 73%, respectively. Survival is better in patients with a rheumatic aetiology (81% at 15 years) compared to those with a degenerative aetiology (71%). Carpentier attributes this to the older age of the latter group. In Spencer's shorter series[20] the five-year survival was 90%. Thus, in the medium to long term the survival figures for mitral valve repair are good. In Carpentier's series[21] there were 36 late deaths, of which 20 (56%) were related to cardiac disease, 14 (39%) were unrelated and 2 (6%) unknown.

Reoperation

It is important to ensure that the repair is durable and, again in Carpentier's long series,[21] 12% needed reoperation up to 15 years, giving a linearized rate of 1% per patient-year. During follow-up, reoperation was more likely in those whose prime aetiology was rheumatic rather than degenerative. Of the 23 patients having a reoperation, 10 were within the first two years, suggesting that the primary operation was flawed. Four of the 10 benefited from a further repair, whilst all of the late failures, due to progression of the disease, needed a replacement. Other series show a similar number requiring a further procedure within the first year (3%).[19] These figures compare favourably with the figures for prosthetic valves, where there is an incidence of valve replacement for endocarditis, thrombosis and malfunction. There is also a higher reoperation rate for tissue valve replacements when these start to degenerate.

In Kirklin's series,[11] where a comparison was made between the results of valve repair and replacement for mitral incompetence, there was no significant difference in the numbers of patients requiring reoperation following the two procedures (8% versus 6%). The hazard function of reoperation being required is different between the two groups, with valve repair having a low constant risk, and valve replacement having an early peak of hazard at six months and then a rise in the late phase.

Valve-related morbidity

The problems of endocarditis, thromboembolism and anticoagulant-related haemorrhage are all much less in patients with repaired valves versus replaced valves. The incidence of endocarditis on repaired valves is very low. In a North American series of 244 patients,[14] the incidence was recorded as 0%, an identical figure coming from Sand et al,[11] whose comparable figure for prosthetic mitral valve endocarditis was 2.8% (medium follow-up of 54 months). In his series of repaired valves, Carpentier[21] reported an incidence of 5% in a follow-up over 15 years of 189 patients, giving a linearized rate of 0.2% per patient-year.

Again, the incidence of thromboembolism following repair is low, compared with valve replacement. Cosgrove et al[19] have reported an incidence of 1.6% per patient-year with repaired valves. Cohn et al[13] have compared the incidence and, over a three-year follow-up period, found that the incidence was 0% with repair and 12% with valve replacement.

Anticoagulant-related haemorrhage can be a significant problem and all patients with mechanical prostheses incur such hazards. The risk of a significant bleeding complication is 1–2% per patient-year.[24] The majority of patients with repaired valves are not maintained on anticoagulants after the first three months unless atrial fibrillation persists. If atrial fibrillation persists, despite cardioversion, the level of anticoagulation required is less than that needed for a prosthetic valve[25] and should place the patient at less risk of haemorrhage.[26]

Functional results

Finally, the functional results of the repair procedure must be equal or superior to those of valve replacement. In Spencer's series,[20] at mean follow-up of 26 months, 85.2% of patients were in NYHA class I or II (88.6% in class III or IV preoperatively). Carpentier's results[21] at 15 years were 74% in NYHA class I or II and 24% in class III (3% in class II and 97% in class III and IV preoperatively). In his series 69% were in sinus rhythm at this point.

CONCLUSION

Mitral regurgitation is not a benign condition; the majority of patients succumb to progressive cardiac failure. Mitral valve replacement with a prosthetic valve has been, until recently, the accepted mode of treatment but the increasing awareness of the imperfections of artificial valves and the hazards of long-term anticoagulation have led to a search for an alternative approach. Mitral valve repair, which has been pioneered by Carpentier, has been shown to have a low operative risk with good long-term results and a much reduced morbidity. Thus, mitral repair should be considered earlier in the course of the disease than has been usual for valve replacement, in order to preserve left ventricular function. The technique should be considered in the surgical treatment of all non-calcified leaking mitral valves.

KEY POINTS FOR CLINICAL PRACTICE

1. Mitral regurgitation is not a benign condition, with the majority of patients dying of congestive cardiac failure.
2. There is no perfect prosthetic valve. They all incur to a greater or lesser degree the risks of embolization, endocarditis, valve thrombosis and structural deterioration.
3. In patients with mechanized prosthetic valves, anticoagulant-related haemorrhage occurs at a rate of 1–2% per year.
4. Patients with mitral regurgitation should be followed up by echocardiography and should be referred before significant enlargement of atrium or ventricle occurs.
5. Mitral regurgitation can be effectively treated by mitral valve repair. All non-calcified leaking valves should be repaired. The operation has a low mortality and a durable result, better than valve replacement.
6. The development of atrial fibrillation is critical. If a valve is repaired at this point, then postoperative cardioversion is usually successful and long-term anticoagulation is not required.

REFERENCES

1 Lillehei CW, Gott VW, DeWall RA, Vario RL. Surgical correction of pure mitral insufficiency by annuloplasty under direct vision. Lancet (Minneapolis) 1957; 77: 446–449

2 Merendino KA, Bruce RA. One hundred and seventeen surgically treated cases of valvular rheumatic heart disease: with preliminary report of two cases of mitral regurgitation treated under direct vision with the aid of a pump oxygenator. JAMA 1957; 164: 749–755

3 Carpentier A. Cardiac valve surgery: the 'French correction'. J Thorac Cardiovasc Surg 1983; 86: 323–337

4 Carpentier A. Valve reconstruction in predominant mitral valve incompetence. In: Duran C, Angell WW, Johnson AD, Oury JH, eds. Recent progress in mitral valve disease. London: Butterworth, 1984, pp 265–274

5 Carpentier A. Mitral valve reconstruction in children. In: Anderson RH, Macartney FJ, Shinebourne EA, Tynan M, eds. Paediatric cardiology 5. Edinburgh: Churchill Livingstone, 1983, pp 361–368

6 Solymar L, Rao PS, Mardini MK et al. Prosthetic valves in children and adolescents. Am Heart J 1991; 121: 557–568

7 Turi ZG, Reyes VP, Raju BS et al. Percutaneous balloon versus surgical closed commissurotomy for mitral stenosis: a prospective, randomised trial. Circulation 1991; 83: 1179–1185

8 Ramanathan KB, Knowles J, Connor MJ et al. Natural history of chronic mitral insufficiency: relation of peak systolic pressure/end systolic volume ratio to morbidity and mortality. J Am Coll Cardiol 1984; 3: 1412–1416

9 Jamieson WRE, Allen P, Miyagishima RT et al. The Carpentier–Edwards standard porcine bioprosthesis. J Thorac Cardiovasc Surg 1990; 99: 543–561

10 Bloomfield P, Wheatley DJ, Prescott RJ, Miller HC. Twelve-year comparison of a Bjork–Shiley mechanical heart valve with porcine bioprosthesis. N Engl J Med 1991; 324: 573–579

11 Sand ME, Naftel DC, Blackstone EH, Kirklin JW, Karp RB. A comparison of repair and replacement for mitral valve incompetence. J Thorac Cardiovasc Surg 1987; 94: 208–219

12 Perier P, Deloche A, Chauvaud S et al. Comparative evaluation of mitral valve repair and replacement with Starr, Bjork, and porcine valve prostheses. Circulation 1984; 70 (Suppl I): I-187–I-192

13 Cohn LM, Allred MS, Cohn LA et al. Early and late risk of mitral valve replacement. J Thorac Cardiovasc Surg 1985; 90: 872–881

14 Cosgrove DM, Stewart WJ. Mitral valvuloplasty. Curr Probl Cardiol 1989; 14(7): 353–416

15 Gallerstein PE, Berger M, Rubenstein S, Berdoff RL, Goldberg E. Systolic anterior motion of the mitral valve and outflow obstruction after mitral valve reconstruction. Chest 1983; 83: 819–820

16 Schiavone WA, Cosgrove DM, Lever HM, Stewart WJ, Salcedo EE. Long term follow up of patients with left ventricular outflow tract obstruction after Carpentier ring mitral valvuloplasty. Circulation 1988; 78 (Suppl 1): I-60–I-65

17 Mihaileanu S, Marino JP, Chauvaud S et al. Left ventricular outflow obstruction after mitral valve repair (Carpentier's technique): proposed mechanisms of disease. Circulation 1988; 78 (Suppl 1): I-78–I-84

18 Craver JM, Cohen C, Weintraub WS. Case-matched comparison of mitral valve replacement and repair. Ann Thorac Surg 1990; 49: 964–969

19 Cosgrove DM, Chavez AM, Lytle BW et al. Results of mitral valve reconstruction. Circulation 1986; 74 (Suppl I): I-82–I-86

20 Galloway AC, Colvin SB, Baumann G et al. Long term results of mitral valve reconstruction with Carpentier techniques in 148 patients with mitral insufficiency. Circulation 1988; 78 (Suppl I): I-97–I-105

21 Deloche A, Jebara VA, Relland JYM et al. Valve repair with Carpentier techniques: the second decade. J Thorac Cardiovasc Surg 1990; 99: 990–1002

22 Teply JF, Grunkemeier GL, Sutherland HD, Lambert LE, Johnson VA, Starr A. The ultimate prognosis after valve replacement: an assessment of 20 years. Ann Thorac Surg 1981; 32: 111–119

23 Goldman ME, Mora F, Guarino T, Fuster V, Mindich BP. Mitral valvuloplasty is superior to valve replacement for preservation of left ventricular function: an intraoperative two-dimensional echocardiographic study. J Am Coll Cardiol 1987; 10: 568–575

24 Grunkemeier GL, Rahimtoola SH. Artificial heart valves. Ann Rev Med 1990; 41: 251–263

25 Poller L. Laboratory control of anticoagulant therapy. Semin Thromb Hemost 1986; 12: 13–19

26 Altman R, Rouvier J, Gurfinkel E et al. Comparison of two levels of anticoagulant therapy in patients with substitute heart valves. J Thorac Cardiovasc Surg 1991; 101: 427–431

11

Aortic dissection: recognition, investigation and management

D. J. M. Keenan

RECOGNITION

Aortic dissection is characterized by a sudden tear in the aortic intima. Blood tracks within the aortic wall, separating the media into two:[1] it can track proximally or distally and may or may not involve the entire circumference of the wall. If the adventitia of the aorta ruptures, it usually does so very proximally, thus producing cardiac tamponade, or into the left chest or, more rarely into the abdomen, leading to death. It may, however, reenter the aortic lumen, creating a false channel.

The origin of dissection is thought to be a primary rupture of the intima with the passage of luminal blood into the wall, although a minority view is that haemorrhage occurs in the wall from rupture of the vasa vasorum and that it is this haemorrhage which is the dissecting force.[1] Although a dissection may originate anywhere in the aorta, the two most common sites of tear are just above the aortic valve, and distal to the left subclavian artery, reflecting the torsional forces which exist at these points. There is general agreement that the basic process behind aortic dissection is one of a degeneration of the aortic media, the strength of which depends on the elastic lamellar units and the smooth muscle cells.[2] In younger people degeneration of the elastic tissue is thought to lead to dissection, whilst in the older group cellular abnormality of the smooth muscle is thought responsible. Either of these degenerative processes leads to medial accumulation of mucopolysaccharide, giving rise to 'cystic medial necrosis'. Certain conditions predispose to aortic dissection, most notably Marfan's syndrome and the Ehlers–Danlos syndrome. These are thought to be due to loss of elastic tissue. Hypertension is an associated factor, again related to accelerated medial degeneration.

Dissection is seen more commonly in men, with the obvious exception of the group occurring in the last trimester of pregnancy. There are a host of conditions with which aortic dissection is associated: bicuspid aortic valve, Turner's syndrome, Noonan's syndrome, coarctation and congenital arteritis. Finally, dissection can occur following cardiac catheterization or cardiac surgery and, in the latter case, areas in the ascending aorta which had been used for cannulation or proximal anastomosis for aorto-saphenous vein grafting have been implicated.

Aortic dissection is classified as acute if it is seen within two weeks of inception, and after this it is described as chronic. It can involve any structure in the aorta, so that proximal dissection can disrupt the origin of a coronary artery causing infarction, or the head or spinal vessels leading to stroke or paraplegia. Other important organs to be affected are the kidneys and gastrointestinal tract, with reports of sudden loss of the circulation to a limb being well recognized. Aortic regurgitation occurs very commonly in ascending aortic dissection. It occurs for a variety of reasons: prolapse of the intimal flap into the aortic valve orifice, prolapse of the aortic wall supporting the valve and dilatation of the aortic annulus supporting the valve, leading to failure of coaption of the leaflets.

De Bakey divided the process into three (Fig. 11.1): type I dissection involves the entire aorta, while type II is confined to the ascending aorta and type III is isolated to the thoracic aorta (from the left subclavian artery distally).[3] Types I and II are grouped together as most of the considerations for these are common.

The natural history of aortic dissection is that 40% of patients survive 24 hours from the initiation, 25% survive for one week and 10% survive for three months.[4] Ascending aortic dissection is much more common than descending, but many of the former group die immediately and do not

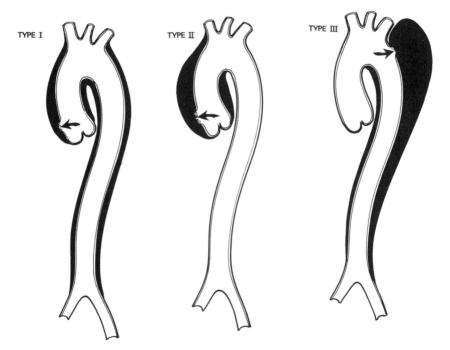

Fig. 11.1   The De Bakey classification of aortic dissection. Types I and II (sometimes referred to as type A) are grouped together as they are treated similarly.

present for treatment. The prognosis for ascending aortic dissection is significantly worse than descending.

Clinical features

Patients with aortic dissection present with a myriad of symptoms, and unless a high index of suspicion is maintained then many patients will die undiagnosed. The most common time of presentation for ascending aortic dissection is in the fifth decade and for the descending aorta the sixth decade. Severe, sudden chest pain is the classical symptom. It is usually excruciating and maximal at its onset with radiation to the neck, back and jaw. It may be described as 'tearing' and may be accompanied by sweating, vomiting and syncope. The patient may attempt to move about to dissipate it; it is unlike the pain of myocardial infarction. A neurological presentation may occur, with stroke or paraplegia, or there may be left heart failure due to acute aortic regurgitation. Cardiac tamponade may also be a cause of shock, while occlusion of a coronary artery may lead to myocardial infarction. In a recent review, despite almost all patients presenting with severe pain, over half were misdiagnosed, mostly as suffering from acute myocardial infarction, although angina, stroke and acute limb ischaemia were the provisional diagnoses made.[5]

Some signs are helpful. The patient may have the stigmata of Marfan's syndrome (tall and thin, lenticular dislocation, high arched palate, arachnodactyly and chest deformity). There may be evidence of shock with hypovolaemia or tamponade. There may be signs of aortic regurgitation and hypertension may be present. The blood pressure may differ in the two arms and any of the pulses may be absent.

INVESTIGATION

Laboratory tests are not usually helpful. There may be evidence of renal dysfunction or anaemia. The ECG usually shows left ventricular hypertrophy but does not show acute changes. The enzymes are normal unless there is frank myocardial infarction. A chest radiograph is usually helpful, showing widening of the aortic shadow and/or the presence of a left pleural effusion. These features are non-specific.

The definitive diagnosis, which previously could be made only by direct aortography, can now be made by a plethora of tests (Table 11.1), and much debate exists as to which test is the most valuable. This problem may be approached in two ways. First, an investigation is required which can be easily and quickly performed, preferably in a non-invasive way, to distinguish aortic dissection from other causes of chest pain and thus rapidly allow active treatment. Second, an investigation is required which delineates the extent of the process so that surgery, if deemed appropriate, can be planned. The ideal investigation would be one that could combine these

Table 11.1   The investigative procedures capable of diagnosing aortic dissection. Direct aortiography used to be regarded as the 'gold standard' but is invasive and is now no longer required in diagnosing aortic dissection or in planning the surgical treatment of it. Intravenous digital subtraction angiography may not have enough definition to accurately diagnose aortic dissection and help plan surgery. Echocardiography with a transoesophageal probe has advantages over the other non-invasive techniques in that it can be quickly performed at the bedside and is very accurate. Currently it is the procedure of choice in making the diagnosis and planning surgery

Echocardiography: transthoracic
                   transoesophageal
Computed tomography
Nuclear magnetic resonance imaging
Direct aortography
Intravenous digital subtraction angiography

two functions, but it cannot be overstated that the main requirement is to include aortic dissection as a differential diagnosis in the large variety of patients presenting urgently with apparent medical (myocardial infarction, unstable angina, stroke) and surgical (abdominal pain, ischaemic limb) problems and to have a rapidly and easily available test which can identify or exclude a dissection. This is even more important now that acute myocardial infarction is being actively treated with thrombolytic agents and there are reports of death from misdiagnosed, ruptured dissections treated in this way.[6] Thus, any patient presenting with pain suggestive of an infarct but without the ECG changes should be viewed with suspicion. This, in fact, is an oversimplification as either coronary ostium can be occluded by a dissection, thus bringing about ECG changes. A high index of suspicion must be maintained in possible cases as generally the pain of dissection does not conform to the usual pain reported with infarction. Which investigation is decided upon will depend on the institution involved and the interests of the various physicians encountering the acute admissions, but it must be readily available for 24 hours per day.

Screening investigation

All investigations, other than direct aortography, are in this category. Echocardiography (Fig. 11.2), with colour flow mapping, has the advantage of being increasingly readily available in most hospitals and is transportable, so that the investigation can be performed at the bedside. Further, sick patients are not given contrast medium, which helps preserve renal function. Simultaneously aortic regurgitation can be accurately assessed

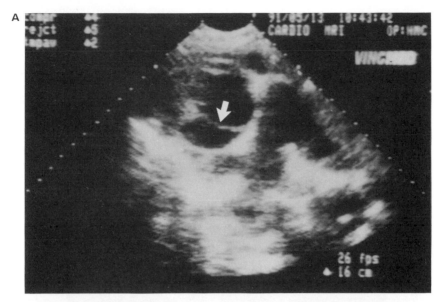

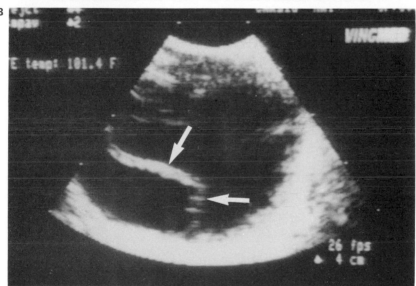

Fig. 11.2 Transthoracic (**A**) and transoesophageal (**B**) echocardiograms of an aortic dissection. The flap is arrowed.

and visualization of the ascending aorta is usually good, although limitations occur in patients with poor acoustic windows (e.g. the obese and those with emphysema). With the addition of transoesophageal echocardiography the diagnostic yield rises to nearly 100% as there is no acoustic window impedance.[7-11] Very little inconvenience is caused to the patient

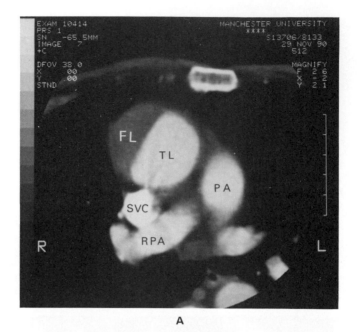

A

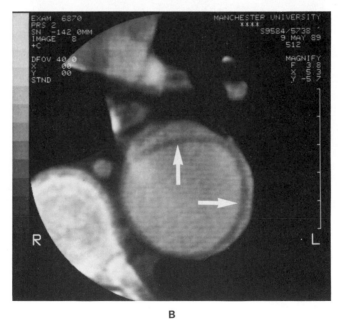

B

Fig. 11.3 CT scan. **A** Magnified scan in which contrast has been given intravenously. The dissection in the ascending aorta divides it into two (the true lumen (TL) and the false lumen (FL)). (PA, pulmonary artery; RPA, right pulmonary artery; SVC, superior vena cava). **B** Magnified scan of the descending thoracic aorta in which an intimal flap can clearly be seen.

by the passage of the oesophageal probe and accurate information concerning both the ascending and descending aorta and the coronary ostia is found.[10] The actual intimal tear was identified in half the cases in one series and in 87% in another series.[9, 11] The aortic arch is not well visualized by echocardiography but this technique undoubtedly qualifies as both a screening test and a test on which to plan definitive therapy.

Computed tomography (CT) (Fig. 11.3) has a high diagnostic yield and gives excellent definition, so that the intimal flap can be identified throughout the entire thoracic aorta.[9,12 – 15] The definition in the transaxial plane is, however, somewhat limited. The study is enhanced by the addition of intravenous contrast and shows differential opacification of the two channels. Widening of the aorta and the presence of a haematoma surrounding the aorta may be clearly seen. It is probably fair to say that CT scanning is as accurate as direct aortography in diagnosing acute dissection,[12] but it gives no information concerning the presence or degree of aortic regurgitation, or left ventricular function. It can be used as a screening test if it is readily available but, obviously, the patient has to be moved to have the examination. As a screening test this may not be a great inconvenience but, with severely ill patients, as many with acute dissection are, this will be an important limiting factor.

Magnetic resonance (MR) imaging (Fig. 11.4) is exceedingly accurate in diagnosing aortic dissection, giving very good definition of all the aortic structures, with further information concerning the major blood vessels in addition.[14, 18, 19] The intimal flap can be clearly identified and usually the intimal tear also. No contrast medium is required, although again no information is obtained concerning aortic regurgitation. Experience with this technique is required for accurate interpretation.[20] Patients who have pacemakers or intracerebral aneurysm clips must be excluded and again the patient must be transported to the machine. Whilst monitoring of the patient is limited during the study, one can at least monitor oxygen saturation. The pictures obtained with MR are superb. In the future, MR imaging will undoubtedly be readily available and at that point limitation will be a function of transportation of an ill patient.

Intravenous digital subtraction angiography has been claimed[21, 22] to be as accurate as direct aortography in identifying aortic dissection, although that has not been my experience. My impression has been that it is not accurate enough to use as a screening test.

Definitive investigation

Direct aortography (Fig. 11.5) has been regarded as being the 'gold standard' in diagnosing aortic dissection but, of late, closer scrutiny and comparison with other techniques has shown this to be no longer the case.[10, 13] However, it has the advantage that it usually visualizes the flap

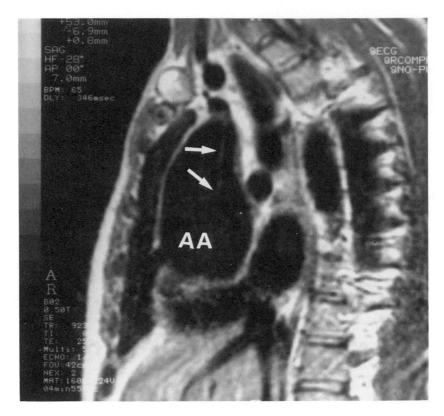

Fig. 11.4   MR image. This is an ECG-gated spin echo (SE 923/25) image of a patient with annulo-aortic ectasia who has massive enlargement of the ascending aorta and aortic root. There is an ascending aortic dissection. The intimal flap is arrowed (AA, ascending aorta).

and differential opacification is obtained in the aorta. Further, aortic regurgitation can be observed and the left ventricle accurately outlined. Knowledge of coronary artery stenoses can be gained only by this technique. However, the procedure is highly invasive, requiring a catheter to be passed up an already compromised aorta, and coronary angiography can be difficult, and therefore dangerous, in the presence of an intimal tear and aortic regurgitation. A balance must be achieved: on the one hand a complete knowledge of the coronary anatomy is required so that bypass grafts can be applied, and on the other hand there should be minimal delay in starting the operation. It should be emphasized that the operation for aortic dissection is usually carried out to save life.

The other available investigations have already been discussed under the screening investigations. Surgery can be planned using echocardiography with an oesophageal probe, CT scanning, MR imaging and direct aortography. Surgically, two decisions must be made: does the patient need a surgical procedure, and if so what approach should be used? This latter

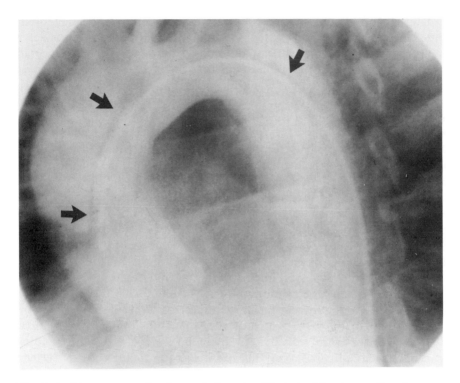

Fig. 11.5   Direct aortography of a type I dissection. The intimal flap (arrowed) can be seen
ascending to descending aorta.

question is important because ascending aortic dissections are approached
via a median sternotomy incision, while descending thoracic aortic procedures are approached via a left thoracotomy.

All ascending aortic dissections require repair unless the situation is
hopeless, i.e. profound stroke, gross debility or short life expectancy from
some other illness. This is because death inevitably occurs due to rupture of
the aorta, most commonly the ascending aorta. Usually, ascending aortic
dissections give rise to severe aortic regurgitation which also requires
urgent treatment. Descending aortic dissection, i.e. De Bakey type III, is
not generally regarded as necessitating urgent surgery, surgery in this
group being reserved for the complications of the dissection, i.e. loss of a
renal artery or acute limb ischaemia, or paraparesis. However, Miller et al
advocate urgent surgery for this group also and have produced better
results, so the matter is not yet resolved.[23]

The definitive diagnostic test therefore must discern whether the dissection is in the ascending aorta or not. If it is, surgery is indicated, and if not,
knowledge of the renal status is required, knowledge of lower limb perfusion and paraparesis being best gained clinically. Renal status is probably
best assessed by MR imaging.[14]

Thus it can be seen from the above that most patients can be diagnosed, and surgery planned, using one investigation; this is all to the good, as delay is largely responsible for reducing the number of patients surviving to go forward for surgery. All hospitals admitting emergency patients, i.e. most hospitals, must have either an echocardiographic service (including a transoesophageal probe) or a CT scanning facility. Thus, patients who on admission are thought to be suffering from myocardial infarction and whose symptoms do not 'add up', or have been heard to have an early diastolic murmur, can be screened for aortic dissection, especially before any active thrombolytic therapy is commenced. If neither of the above facilities is available then there must be a very low threshold for referring such patients to a cardiac surgical facility. Cardiologists, for their part, must desist from replicating investigations so that a patient is not investigated by echocardiography, CT scan and finally direct aortography, with the obvious consequences in terms of timing. However, if there is a strong clinical suspicion of dissection, not borne out by the first investigation, there should be no hesitation in performing an additional investigation to increase one's chance of obtaining a positive result.[8, 13, 14, 18]

Coronary angiography remains the final problem. Perhaps this should be reserved for patients with clear indications, such as a history of angina, ECG evidence of old infarction, left ventricular regional wall abnormalities on echocardiography or several important risk factors for coronary artery disease.

MANAGEMENT

Early management

Immediately the diagnosis is suspected or confirmed the stress in the aortic wall should be reduced by using beta-blocking drugs to reduce the systemic blood pressure. This necessitates admitting the patient to a unit where blood pressure can be carefully controlled whilst intravenous beta-blocking agents are administered. Labetalol can be given intravenously in 10-mg increments, bringing the systolic blood pressure to 100 mmHg (mean greater than 60 mmHg). A urinary catheter is useful so that hourly urine output can be monitored. Oxygen therapy can be instituted in such a unit. The diagnostic tests can be performed in and from this unit and when the diagnosis has been confirmed the patient can be transferred for surgery, if this is required.

Definitive correction

Ascending aorta.   The aim of surgery for ascending aortic dissection is to prevent death from aortic rupture and to restore flow to vital organs, if this has been compromised. The repair does not require the removal of the intimal tear, not does it attempt to remove all, or even most, of the dissected aorta. The repair is directed at the ascending aorta because this is the area most likely to rupture, because aortic regurgitation requires treatment and because repair in this area is most likely to restore normal forward flow in the true distal aortic lumen, through the graft which has been interposed. All operations are carried out on cardiopulmonary bypass with femoral artery and right atrial cannulation. Hypothermia is used, which may be profound if the aortic clamp is to be removed and the circulation stopped. The operation consists of longitudinally opening the ascending aorta: this involves opening the false and then the true lumen, transecting the two walls of the aorta above the aortic valve and resuspending the aortic valve.[22] The transected aorta, which consists of one tube inside the other, is sewn back together. This is facilitated by placing Teflon felt both inside and outside to enable the friable tissues to hold the sutures, and by placing biological glue to hold the tissues together.[24] Closure of the two walls prevents blood from tracking outside the wall where the valve is suspended and allows normal aortic valve geometry to be restored. The aorta is again transected proximal to the brachiocephalic artery and the two walls sewn back in continuity in the same fashion. A Dacron tube graft is then interposed between the two repaired ends of the aorta (the interposition technique).[25] When the distal anastomosis is nearly complete the cross-clamp, if one has been applied, is released and the site of retrograde flow from the bypass circuit via the femoral artery is noted. If flow comes up the true lumen the anastomosis is completed in the usual way with the confidence that flow has been confirmed between the graft, and therefore the left ventricle, the true lumen in the aortic arch, and the femoral artery in which the bypass cannula lies. However, if on the release of the clamp flow is seen to come from the false lumen, then there must be a distal re-entry site supporting retrograde flow from the femoral artery. If the anastomosis is completed in the usual way, on definitive release of the cross-clamp or on resumption of full flow, the coronary arteries will not be supplied and ischaemia will ensue. Thus, a side arm must be taken from the arterial inflow and placed in the graft to supply the heart until such time as it is ready to take over the circulation again. One's hope at this point is that forward flow through the true lumen in the aortic arch and the aorta will be sufficient to collapse the false lumen, which is no longer fed with forward flow. This is probably over-optimistic as many of these false lumina persist afterwards.[26] However, the operation is to remove the pending site of rupture and treat regurgitation and this will be accomplished.

In patients with Marfan's syndrome or annulo-aortic ectasia who dissect, the surgery required is more complicated. In such patients the coronary artery orifices are normally displaced distally, so that if the operation already described were to be performed, a long segment of aorta, from aortic valve to above the coronary orifices, would remain. It has been shown that this segment of aorta continues to dilate with time and eventually becomes aneurysmal.[27] Thus in such patients a composite graft containing an aortic prosthesis at one end is used.[24, 28] The aortic valve is excised and the composite graft sewn in to the aortic annulus. The orifices of the coronary arteries are then sewn into two holes made in the side of the graft and the distal anastomosis completed as for the interposition technique, sewing the distal end of the graft to the transected and repaired dissected aorta, just proximal to the brachiocephalic artery. Previously, the graft which was to be placed in the aorta was sewn in using an inclusion technique, whereby the graft was placed leaving the aorta in continuity, but this technique led to complications, with the possibility of a false aneurysm developing between the graft and the native wall, compressing the graft; therefore the 'interposition' technique is now more commonly used. Thus the entire area of the aortic root is excluded from the circulation.[29]

Various subtle changes have occurred in the past decade, making the operation less risky. There have been improvements in oxygenator design, and better understanding and application of myocardial protection. The Dacron grafts have steadily improved, so that now one rarely sees bleeding through the interstices of the graft. The recent rediscovery of aprotinin as a haemostatic agent has transformed these operations in terms of bleeding. Aprotinin is thought to stabilize platelets and if given in large doses throughout the operation total blood loss is much reduced.[30]

Descending thoracic aorta.   Surgery for dissection in this area is generally performed only for complications, as the survival with medical treatment is good (80% one-year survival).[31] Such patients have aggressive and prolonged hypotensive therapy. Surgery is indicated for persisting pain, limb ischaemia, paraparesis (not paraplegia), acute renal failure and haemothorax. However, the Stamford group advocates near-routine surgical treatment for all acute dissections, with good results, although this viewpoint has not gained widespread acceptance.[22] Patients with Marfan's syndrome, presenting with distal dissection, are regarded by all as exceptions and are brought forward for urgent surgery, with or without complications, because of the high instance of aneurysm formation, following dissection in this group.[32]

The operation, when it is required, consists of performing a left thoracotomy and exposure of the left femoral vessels. Support of the distal circulation is achieved either using a bypass circuit, with blood removed from the femoral vein, oxygenated and pumped into the femoral artery (femoro-femoral bypass, with heparinization), or a Gott shunt, which is a heparin-bonded tube placed between either the left ventricular apex, left atrium or ascending aorta, and the femoral artery. This shunt relies on the left ventricle and lungs for its forward velocity and oxygenation, respectively. The upper descending thoracic aorta is mobilized and clamped. The aorta is opened longitudinally and inspected. Sometimes it is possible to sew the proximal end of the Dacron graft to the undissected proximal aorta. If not, and always at the distal end, the two aortic lumina are reapproximated and a graft sewn as in the interposition technique. An intraluminal, sutureless prosthesis, which is a Dacron tube graft with a felt cover and metal spool at each end, can sometimes be used.[33] This is fixed in position by placing nylon tapes around the aorta, just beyond the aortotomy, and tying these onto the metal spools which are in the lumen.

Aortic arch.   Dissection involving the aortic arch is rare and has the highest mortality, and tends therefore not to be brought forward for surgery.[32] When surgery is embarked upon, as for impending rupture, profound hypothermia with circulatory arrest is used.[34, 35] The arch may have to be replaced by a tube graft with reimplantation of a cuff of aorta from which the head and neck vessels take origin. The exact procedure varies with each patient presenting as occasionally only the concave surface of the aorta needs to be replaced, thus leading to a much less complex operation.[35]

The early mortality following surgery depends on the site of the dissection, with proximal dissections incurring a mortality of between 8% and 40%.[22, 35-39] The results for distal aortic dissection (type III) depend upon the indications for surgery. In uncomplicated cases the Stamford group have reported a 13% mortality.[22] A similar result has been reported by Crawford et al.[40] However, in complicated cases the mortality can be up to 50%.[41]

Late management

Long-term survival following repair of dissection has been relatively good, with 60% of survivors surviving ten years.[42] Multi-varied analysis has shown that stroke, chronic renal failure and myocardial infarction predict a poor long-term survival.[42] The site of dissection does not appear to influence the survival.

Late follow-up of all patients with aortic dissection is very important, as the commonest cause of late death is rupture of an aneurysm of the aorta (29% over 20 years).[43] Haverich et al have reported a reoperation rate of 13% at five years and 22% at ten years.[42] The most important determinant is the persistence of the false channel post-repair rather than the site of the dissection. If the false channel persists following the repair there is a predisposition to aneurysm formation. Patients with Marfan's syndrome are particularly prone to late aneurysm formation as they are prone to the development of a further dissection. Hypertension is obviously an important risk factor which must be controlled in all patients. Following resuspension of the aortic valve, aortic regurgitation might persist necessitating aortic valve replacement based on the usual criteria. Thus all patients should be kept under long-term review with aggressive and close monitoring of blood pressure. Serial chest radiographs should be taken to watch for aneurysm formation, and also ultrasound examination of the abdominal aorta periodically performed. As a long-term screening technique, when it is more readily available, MR imaging, which requires no radiation, will be ideal for periodic assessment. Late development of aneurysm is an indication for further surgery to replace the aneurysmal portion of the aorta or great vessel prior to its rupture.

CONCLUSION

Aortic dissection is a condition which masquerades under a variety of symptoms and presentations. Classically, there is acute chest pain which is unlike that of a myocardial infarct and which radiates to the back. However, in a recent series half the patients were initially misdiagnosed, and thus a high index of suspicion must be maintained. Recent developments have taken place in non-invasive diagnosis with echocardiography, including transoesophageal echocardiography, CT and nuclear magnetic imaging all vying to be the investigation of first choice. At present transoesophageal echocardiography is the favoured technique because of its accuracy, ready availability, its ease of transport and its speed. Direct aortography is no longer required, as surgery can be planned around the non-invasive studies. The role of surgery is now better understood and, with the availability of less porous grafts and of haemostatic agents, results are improving. Death occurs due to rupture and surgery is directed primarily at averting this.

Urgent surgery is advised for all ascending aortic dissections because of the very grave prognosis if left untreated. Hypotensive therapy is maintained while investigating the patient and while awaiting surgery. Surgery consists of replacing the ascending aorta with a Dacron tube graft and resuspending the aortic valve, in the process of closing off the dissection proximal to the graft. The distal end of the graft is sewn to the repaired distal aorta. Descending thoracic aortic dissections are usually treated medically (hypotensive therapy) unless there are complications such as persistent pain, bleeding or loss of flow to a vital organ or limb, as medical therapy gives good short-term results.

Long-term follow-up is vital as there is a high incidence of aneurysm formation, and rupture of such aneurysms is the commonest cause of late death. Hypotensive therapy must be maintained over the long term.

REFERENCES

1 Wheat MW. Pathogenesis of aortic dissection. In: Doroghazi RM, Slater EE, eds. Aortic dissection. New York: McGraw-Hill, 1983, pp 85–90
2 Hirst AE, Gore I. The aetiology and pathology of aortic dissection. In: Doroghazi RM, Slater EE, eds. Aortic dissection. New York: McGraw-Hill, 1983, pp 13–54
3 De Bakey ME, McCollum CH, Crawford ES et al. Dissection and dissecting aneurysms of the aorta: 20 year follow up of 527 patients treated surgically. Surgery 1982; 92: 1118–1134
4 Hirst AE Jr, Johns VJ Jr, Kime SW Jr. Dissecting aneurysm of the aorta: a review of 505 cases. Medicine 1958; 37: 217–279

5 Butler J, Ormerod OJM, Giannopoulous N et al. Diagnostic delay and outcome in surgery for type A aortic dissection. Q J Med 1991; 289: 391–396

6 Butler J, Davies AH, Westaby S. Streptokinase in acute aortic dissection. Br Med J 1990; 300 (6723): 517–519

7 McLeod AA, Monaghan MJ, Richardson PJ et al. Diagnosis of acute aortic dissection by M-mode and cross-sectional echocardiography: a five year experience. Eur Heart J 1983; 4: 196–202

8 Taams MA, Gussenhoven WJ, Schippers LA et al. The value of transoesophageal echocardiography for diagnosis of thoracic aortic pathology. Eur Heart J 1988; 9: 1308–1316

9 Erbel R, Eugerding R, Daniel W et al. Echocardiography in diagnosis of aortic dissection. Lancet 1989; i (8636): 457–461

10 Ballal RS, Nanda NC, Gatewood R et al. Usefulness of transoesphageal echocardiography in assessment of aortic dissection. Circulation 1991; 84: 1903–1914

11 Adachi H, Omoto R, Kyo S et al. Emergency surgical intervention of acute aortic dissection with rapid diagnosis by transoesophageal echocardiography. Circulation 1991; 84 (suppl III): III-14–III-19

12 Oudkerk M, Overbosch E, Dee P. CT recognition of acute aortic dissection. AJR 1983; 141: 671–676

13 Singh H, Fitzgerlad E, Ruttley MST. Computed tomography: the investigation of choice for aortic dissection? Br Heart J 1986; 56: 171–175

14 Anderson MW, Higgins CB. Should the patient with suspected acute dissection of the aorta have MRI, CAT scan or aortography as the definitive study? Cardiovasc Clin 1990; 21 (1): 293–304

15 Walters NA, Thompson KR. Acute dissection of the aorta: which test? Aust NZ J Surg 1989; 59: 617–620

16 Vasile N, Mathieu D, Keita K et al. Computer tomography of thoracic aortic dissection: accuracy and pitfalls. J Comput Assist Tomogr 1986; 10: 211–215

17 Morgan JM, Oldershaw PJ, Gray HH. Use of computed tomographic scanning and aortography in the diagnosis of acute dissection of the thoracic aorta. Br Heart J 1990; 64: 261–265

18 Barentsz JO, Ruijs JHJ, Heystraten FMJ, Buskens F. Magnetic resonance imaging of dissected thoracic aorta. Br J Radiol 1987; 60: 499–502

19 Dinsmore RE, Wedeen BJ, Miller SW et al. MRI of dissection of the aorta: recognition of the intimal tear and differential flow velocities. AJR 1986; 146: 1286–1288

20 Kersting-Sommerhoff BA, Higgins CB, White RD et al. Aortic dissection: sensitivity and specificity of MR imaging. Radiology 1988; 166: 651–655

21 Lyons J, Gershlick A, Norell M et al. Intravenous digital subtraction angiography in the diagnosis and management of acute aortic dissection. Eur Heart J 1987; 8: 186–189

22 Miller DC. Surgical management of aortic dissection: indications, peri-operative management and long term results. In: Doroghazi RM, Slater EE, eds. Aortic dissection. New York: McGraw-Hill, 1983: pp 193–243

23 Miller DC, Mitchell RS, Oyer PE et al. Independent determinant of operative mortality for patients with aortic dissection. Circulation 1984; 70 (Suppl I): I-153–I-164

24 Cabrol C, Pavie A, Mesnildrey P et al. Long term results with total replacement of the ascending aorta and reimplantation of the coronary arteries. J Thorac Cardiovasc Surg 1986; 91: 17–25

25 Eagle KA, De Sanctis RW, Aortic dissection. Curr Probl Cardiol 1989; 14 (5): 231–278

26 Guthaner DF, Miller DC, Silverman JF et al. Fate of the false lumen following surgical repair of aortic dissection: an angiographic study. Radiology 1979; 133: 1–8

27 Svensson LG, Crawford ES, Coselli JS et al. Impact of cardiovascular operations on survival in the Marfan patient. Circulation 1989; 80 (Suppl I): I-233–I-242

28 Bentall H, De Bono A. A technique for complete replacement of the ascending aorta. Thorax 1968; 23: 338–339

29 Crawford ES, Svensson LG, Coselli JS et al. Surgical treatment of aneurysm and/or dissection of the ascending aorta, transverse aortic arch, and ascending aorta and transverse aortic arch. J Thorac Cardiovasc Surg 1989; 98: 659–674

30 Bidstrup B, Royston D, Sapsford R, Taylor K. Reduction of blood loss and blood use after cardiopulmonary bypass with high dose aprotinin. J Thorac Cardiovasc Surg 1989; 97: 364–372

31 Lindsay J Jr, Hurst JW. Clinical features and prognosis in dissection aneurysm of the aorta: a reappraisal. Circulation 1967; 35: 880–888

32 De Sanctis RW, Doroghazi RM, Austen WG, Buckley MS. Aortic dissection. N Engl J Med 1987; 317 (17): 1060–1067

33 Lemole GM, Strong MD, Spagna PM, Karamilowicz NP. Improved results for dissecting aneurysms: intraluminal sutureless prosthesis. J Thorac Cardiovasc Surg 1982; 83: 249–255

34 Graham JM, Stinnett DM. Operative management of acute aortic arch dissection using profound hypothermia and circulatory arrest. Ann Thorac Surg 1987; 44: 192–198

35 Heinemann M, Laas J, Jurmann M et al. Surgery extended into the aortic arch in acute type a dissection. Circulation 1991; 84 (Suppl III): III-25–III-30

36 Cachera PJ, Vouhe PR, Loisance DY et al. Surgical management of acute dissections involving the ascending aorta. J Thorac Cardiovasc Surg 1981; 82: 576–584

37 Borst H-G, Laas J, Frank G, Haverich A. Surgical decision making in acute aortic dissection type a. Thorac Cardiovasc Surg 1987; 35: 134–135

38 Ikonomidis JS, Weisel RD, Mouradian MS et al. Thoracic aortic surgery. Circulation 1991; 84 (Suppl III): III-1–III-6

39 Fradet G, Jamieson WRE, Janusz MT et al. Aortic dissection. Am J Surg 1988; 155: 697–700

40 Crawford ES, Svensson LG, Coselli JS et al. Aortic dissection and dissecting aortic aneurysms. Ann Surg 1988; 208: 254–273

41 Kirklin JW, Barrett-Boyes BG. Acute aortic dissection. In: Cardiac surgery. New York: Wiley, 1986, pp 1471–1491

42 Haverich A, Miller DC, Scott WC et al. Acute and chronic aortic dissections: determinants of long term outcome for operative survivors. Circulation 1987; 72 (Suppl II): II-22–II-34

43 Wolfe WG, Oldham HN, Rankin JS, Morgan JF. Surgical treatment of acute ascending aortic dissection. Ann Surg 1983; 197: 738–742

Long term management of patients with prosthetic heart valves

G. J. Grötte   D. J. Rowlands

INTRODUCTION

Annually in the health service hospitals throughout the UK between 4600 and 4700 patients have prosthetic heart valves implanted. A total of 5000 to 5200 valves are inserted in the aortic, mitral and tricuspid positions.

The cost of a prosthetic heart valve varies between £1500 and £2000, and the present total annual valve expenditure for the health service is therefore in the region of £10 000 000. The cost of the valve is of course an added expense to the cost of an open heart operation itself. In 1989 the cost of an open heart operation at Manchester Royal Infirmary was calculated at £3428 (excluding the cost of a valve), and this figure is obviously already out of date.[1] Based on the above figures the total annual cost of valve surgery in the UK is at present in the region of £25 000 000.

The in-hospital mortality following valve surgery is approximately 6% on average, and this leaves about 4400 hospital survivors annually. These patients are discharged into their own community, and it is the responsibility of General Practitioners, General Physicians, Cardiologists and Cardiac Surgeons to ensure that the long term postoperative management is optimal. Considering the vast financial investment, 'value for money' can only be obtained if there is the most meticulous after care.

HISTORICAL BACKGROUND

The modern era of cardiac surgery started in 1953 when Dr John Gibbon repaired an atrial septal defect in an 18-year-old female using extracorporeal circulation.[2] This had a successful outcome after 22 years of experimentation.

Attempts to correct valvular heart lesions go back to 1914 when Tuffier digitally dilated stenotic aortic valves through the aortic wall.[3] In 1952 Bailey carried out transventricular dilatations of the aortic valve,[4] and in 1953 Hufnagel and Harvey inserted a plastic ball valve in the descending aorta in an attempt to correct aortic regurgitation.[5] Mitral valve surgery goes back to 1923 when Cutler and Levine made a bold effort to treat mitral stenosis.[6] In 1925 Souttar performed a digital mitral commissurotomy, but it was not until 1948 that Harken[7] and Bailey in 1949[8] demonstrated the value of digital commissurotomy. Subsequently a more extensive commissurotomy was performed after a mitral valve dilator was developed (patented by Tubbs, Logan and Turner in 1959).[9]

The modern era of heart valve replacement started 30 years ago. In 1961 an article appeared in the *Annals of Surgery* that was destined radically to alter the surgical therapy of valvular heart disease. It was not a report of the first case of valve replacement, nor was it a description of the new valve model. It was simply a report of long term survival of 6 of 8 patients with a mitral prosthetic valve.[10] Since then well over 50 different prosthetic designs have been evaluated and today only a few have stood the test of time and this includes the modified version of the original Starr–Edwards valve.

AVAILABLE TYPES OF PROSTHETIC HEART VALVE

In addition to the caged ball valve, different types of mechanical heart valves were developed and tissue valves also soon became available. The two main classes of prosthetic heart valve are (a) mechanical (non-biological) valves and (b) tissue valves.

(a) Mechanical valves

1. The tilting disc valve 1969.[11]
2. The hinged bileaflet valve 1979.[12]

(b) Tissue valves

1. The aortic homograft 1962.[13]
2. Stent mounted porcine xenograft 1965.[14]
3. Bovine pericardial valve 1970.[15]

Summary

Prosthetic heart valves have been inserted for the last 30 years. Many designs have been evaluated, few have stood the test of time.

INDICATIONS FOR HEART VALVE SURGERY

During the last 30 years there have been enormous advances made in prosthetic valve design, extracorporeal perfusion techniques, myocardial protection and postoperative management. Today an elective heart valve operation is usually relatively safe and effective.

However, this does not mean that all patients with valvular heart disease should be subjected to surgery. Patients with mild valve disease are better left alone as the long term risk of heart valve replacement exceeds that of their native disease.[16] The patients who will benefit are those with moderate or severe valve disease.

Mitral stenosis

For patients with this condition surgery should be recommended when the patient is significantly symptomatic and these symptoms are backed up by echocardiographic and cardiac catheterization findings.[17] Surgical treatment for mitral stenosis does not usually involve valve replacement. In the past many patients were successfully treated with closed mitral valvotomy although most surgeons perform this operation today using cardio-pulmonary bypass.

Mitral regurgitation

Mitral regurgitation presents a somewhat more complicated problem than pure mitral stenosis. There are several causes of which the commonest are rheumatic heart disease, ischaemic malfunction of the papillary muscles, chordal rupture and myxoid degeneration of the valve leaflets (the so-called 'floppy valve'). In the case of chronic mitral regurgitation surgery should be considered for patients in New York Heart Association (NYHA) classes 3 and 4, although some patients with few symptoms should also be operated on if there is evidence of severe regurgitation and progressive left ventricular dysfunction.[18] Mitral valve replacement is not an entirely satisfactory procedure for several reasons. Optimal timing of the operation is difficult to achieve, left ventricular function may deteriorate after the procedure (as a result of an increased afterload consequent upon the abolition of the low impedance valve leak) and there is a long term risk of thrombosis and thrombo-embolism with non-biological prosthetic valves and of mechanical deterioration with biological prostheses. The current tendency is to attempt mitral valve repair when circumstances permit.

Aortic stenosis

In the adult aortic stenosis is usually the end result of thickening and calcification in a congenital bicuspid aortic valve. The rheumatic process can also attack a normal tricuspid aortic valve and the end result is often fusion of the commissures and calcification leading to severe stenosis. Of all valve lesions aortic stenosis is the most lethal (Fig. 12.1),[19] and when symptoms appear the average survival is less than 5 years.[20]

Aortic regurgitation

Chronic aortic regurgitation has a protracted course causing little disability for many years. Eventually, however, cardiac decompensation ensues. Surgi-

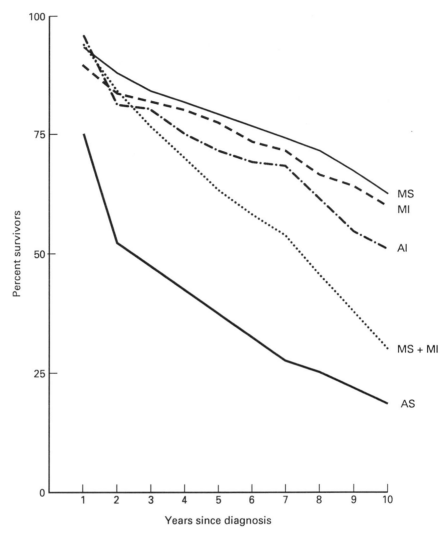

Fig. 12.1   Survival of patients with valvular heart disease treated medically. Reproduced with permission from Rapaport 1975.

cal intervention is indicated sooner rather than later if there is evidence of significant incompetence and left ventricular dysfunction, although symptoms may be mild or absent as long term survival following valve replacement is poor in patients with advanced left ventricular dysfunction.[21]

Tricuspid valve disease

Organic tricuspid valve disease is uncommon in the UK today although this may not be so in the developing world. The most common lesion seen is functional tricuspid incompetence, usually due to long-standing mitral valve disease and pulmonary hypertension. If surgical treatment is necessary an annuloplasty rather than valve replacement is indicated. If valve replacement is mandatory mechanical valves should be avoided because of high incidences of thrombotic complications and valve dysfunction.[22] Bioprosthetic valves in the tricuspid position, although not ideal, ensure a better long term result.[23, 24]

Summary

Patients with valvular heart disease who have significant symptoms should be subjected to surgery. Valve repair and reconstruction is possible in some patients particularly in the mitral and tricuspid positions. The most lethal valve condition is severe aortic stenosis.

CHOICE OF VALVULAR PROSTHESIS

A prosthetic heart valve is not a normal valve and heart valve replacement is clearly not a cure for valvular heart disease. Patients receiving prosthetic heart valves are exchanging native valve disease for prosthetic valve 'disease'.

The 'ideal' prosthetic valve should have the following characteristics:

1. *Adequate haemodynamics* (no pressure gradients, no leaks)
2. *Durability* (should not deteriorate within a human life span)
3. *Resistance to thrombosis* (should not require anticoagulants)
4. *Biocompatibility* (should not induce trauma to blood, rejection by host)
5. *Ease of insertion*
6. It should be quiet in operation, safe and cheap.

Needless to say no prosthetic valves have ever fulfilled these 'ideal' valve requirements.

Advantages and disadvantages of mechanical valves

The pioneers of cardiac valve surgery developed and used various distinct different types of valves. The mechanical valves were made of metal, plastic (later pyrolitic carbon) and some form of cloth material. Soon tissue valves which were at least partially made of biological tissue were developed and used. Nearly 30 years later both types of valve are still in widespread use.

(a) Caged ball valve

These valves are less often used today than formerly. They were popular in the 1960s but they have major drawbacks. Their design has a high valve profile. This can be troublesome if either the left ventricular outflow tract

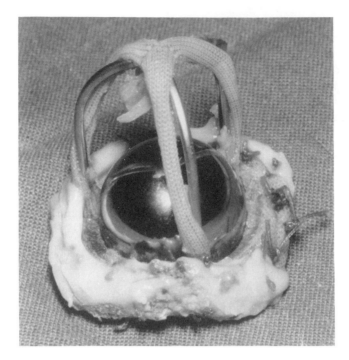

Fig. 12.2   This patient had a cloth covered Starr–Edwards valve inserted in the aortic position in 1974. Nine years later it was removed due to a paraprosthetic leak and also mild–moderate haemolysis. Note gross destruction of cloth. (Reproduced with permission from the University of Medical Illustration, Royal Infirmary, Manchester)

or the ascending aorta is small. If the physical build of the patient requires the use of a small valve size this type of valve does not perform well haemodynamically and often recreates 'native' valve stenosis. These valves also have significant embolization rates and produce haemolysis in some patients. In later models the struts were covered with cloth in the belief that neo-intima would form over the cloth and therefore produce a 'non thrombogenic' valve. In practice the cloth was destroyed producing unacceptable embolization and haemolysis rates (Fig. 12.2).

(b)   Tilting disc valve

The concept of a free floating tilting disc retained by struts was introduced in 1967 by Kaster.[25] Within two years both the Lillihei Kaster and the Bjork–Shiley tilting disc valves were in clinical use. In the mid 1970s another tilting disc valve was developed by Hall Kaster.[26, 27] This valve is now marketed under the name Medtronic/Hall valve and has gained widespread popularity throughout the world.

Compared with a caged ball valve, the low profile tilting disc valves in general have a lower embolization rate, and a better haemodynamic performance, but are more liable to complete valve thrombosis, jamming of the disc in the closed position due to impingement of suture or tissue and fracture of struts at the site of welds.

(c) Hinged bileaflet valve

In 1965 attempts were made to construct a hinged bileaflet valve.[28] This valve was implanted in patients but it soon became clear that there was a tendency for clot formation at the site of the hinges. The design was abandoned only to be revived years later with an improved hinge mechanism. Today it is marketed as the St Jude valve and has gained worldwide popularity.

The most commonly used non-biological prosthetic valves in the USA are the St Jude Medical bileaflet valve, the Medtronic Hall tilting disc valve and (decreasingly) the Starr-Edwards caged ball valve.

Advantages and disadvantages of tissue valves

Following the development of intracardiac mechanical valves, investigation into the use of tissue valves was intensified in an attempt to imitate the natural valve more closely. The homograft was developed in 1962,[13] and soon allogenic fascia lata valves were developed.[29] These latter valves initially appeared to be very promising whilst xenogenic (heterograft) tissue valves were decreasingly used.[30] In a relatively short time, however, it became apparent that there were significant problems with the fascia lata valves (poor durability and a risk of infection).[31]

Xenogenic valves were developed in 1965.[14] The aortic valve of a pig seemed a logical choice because of its physical similarity to a human valve. A substance used by the shoe industry as a tanning agent (glutaraldehyde) was known to produce stable collagen cross-linking. It was used by Carpentier and results were reported in 1970.[30] Later on buffered glutaraldehyde was introduced and this preserved collagen adequately in vivo. Bovine pericardial valves were made commercially available in 1976.[32]

Thromboembolism is a problem with both mechanical and tissue valves. However tissue valves have the advantage of a lower incidence of thromboembolism, and in the majority of patients the tissue valves do not require anticoagulation.

The main reservation about using a tissue valve is the durability. Compared with a mechanical valve, when a tissue valve fails it does so gradually and re-operations can therefore be carried out on relatively fit patients with low operative mortality. This is not true with mechanical valve failure which can be sudden and catastrophic.

Summary

Mechanical tilting and bileaflet valves are the most popular designs today. Tissue valves usually do not require anticoagulation but will eventually degenerate and fail usually 10 years after insertion. Mechanical valve failure can be catastrophic.

PRE- AND INTRAOPERATIVE MANAGEMENT OF HEART VALVE PATIENTS

The most important aspects of this topic are:

1. The full, detailed clinical and investigative assessment of the patient's need for and suitability for, valve replacement;
2. The exclusion of, or eradication of, any sources of infection (especially dental);
3. The use of prophylactic antibiotics in relation to the surgical procedure;
4. The control of bleeding in the immediate postoperative period;
5. The prevention of thrombosis and thromboembolism;
6. The immediate arrangement for long term aftercare.

Preoperative assessment of suitability for valve replacement

It would not be appropriate in this chapter to discuss the preoperative assessment in detail. It is axiomatic that a full clinical and haemodynamic assessment is essential and that alternative strategies (e.g. medical management, mitral valvotomy or mitral valve repair) have been ruled out.

Elimination of sources of infection

It is essential to eradicate any source of sepsis that could lead to bacteraemia during surgery. All patients should have a thorough dental examination and any dental treatment required must be carried out before heart surgery.

Antibiotic cover during surgery

The valve replacement procedure must be carried out in a dedicated cardiac surgical theatre. All patients receive prophylactic antibiotic cover. Our routine is to give gentamicin 80 mg i.v. 8-hourly and flucloxacillin 500 mg i.v. 6-hourly. In uncomplicated cases intravenous antibiotics can be discontinued on the second postoperative day. Oral flucloxacillin is given for a further 5 days.

Control of bleeding

Postoperative bleeding should not be a problem following a properly executed operation. Bleeding can be a problem in redo operations. The drug aprotinin (Trasylol) is extremely useful in reducing intraoperative and postoperative bleeding. The infusion of the drug is started as soon as the patient is anaesthetized.

Initiation of anticoagulant therapy

Oral anticoagulation with warfarin is started on the afternoon of the fist day after the operation. Discharge from the hospital usually occurs at 8 to 10 days after the operation, by which time stable control of the anticoagulant regime has usually been achieved.

Immediate arrangement for long term after-care

The patient and all his medical attendants and advisers need to be informed immediately of the critical importance of permanent, meticulous supervision. A handwritten discharge letter is given to the patient on discharge to be given to the General Practitioner (GP). A full typewritten discharge letter is sent to the GP and any other physicians and/or cardiologists involved within a week of discharge. The patient is subsequently reviewed in a surgical follow-up clinic 4–5 weeks after discharge. Following the visit to the surgical clinic the patient is referred back to the cardiologist for long term follow up, initially every 6 months for a year and then yearly. If the patient comes from far away he is referred back to his local cardiologist/physician.

MANAGEMENT OF PATIENTS FOLLOWING DISCHARGE FROM HOSPITAL

The long term management of patients with prosthetic heart valve has two major aspects:

1. Preventing, recognizing and treating valve-related complications
2. Dealing with clinically related problems (e.g. atrial fibrillation, myocardial dysfunction, ischaemic heart disease, diseases of the aorta, etc.).

The successful approach to long term care depends on the application of the following principles:

1. Education of the patient
2. Education of the general practitioner
3. Routine clinical checks
4. Immediate and optimal management of any problem revealed.

Education of the patient and of his attendant doctors

Education of the patient and of his medical attendants is the most important principle in the long term care of valve replacement patients. Both of these processes should be initiated prior to the discharge of the patient. In our hospital the cardiac surgery liaison sister spends about half an hour with the patient and his or her relatives explaining the importance of proper dental hygiene, meticulous anticoagulant control and the prevention of, or adequate treatment of, any infection.

The cause of death in patients with prosthetic heart valves has been studied by several authors.[33-37] Approximately 50% of deaths were cardiac in origin and not valve related. An additional 30% died from non-cardiac valve-related problems. Valve-related complications caused approximately 20% of the deaths, and the risk of death from a valve-related complication is about 1% per year.

VALVE-RELATED PROBLEMS

The main valve-related problems are:

1. Embolism
2. Valve thrombosis
3. Infective endocarditis
4. Anticoagulant related haemorrhage
5. Bland periprosthetic leaks
6. Haemodynamically significant valve dysfunction
7. Structural valve failure
8. Miscellaneous (haemolysis, valve recall, pregnancy, etc.)

Embolism from prosthetic valves

Most systemic emboli pass undetected. Small emboli to peripheral vascular beds may produce no symptoms or be misinterpreted. The incidence of embolism is therefore likely to be significantly underestimated. The incidence appears to be unrelated to the type of non-biological valve implanted.[38] It seems likely that conditions such as atrial fibrillation, enlargement of the left atrium, the presence of left atrial thrombus and severe depression of left ventricular function will predispose to systemic embolism but reports vary about the significance of these features.[39, 40] It has to be remembered that when a patient with a prosthetic heart valve develops a systemic embolus it does not necessarily follow that it is the valve, or even the heart, which is the source of the embolus. What is clear is that it is the adequacy of the anticoagulant regime which is the most important factor in preventing emboli. For non-biological prosthetic valves the INR reading should be kept within the range 3.0 to 4.5 at all times (and if possible between 3.5 and 4.5). This is a much stricter degree of anticoagulant control than is necessary for other indications and it is important that the patient, his GP and the consultant in charge of the anticoagulant laboratory should all be aware of this. Omission, poor control or withdrawal of coumarin anticoagulation substantially increases the incidence of thromboembolism in patients with mechanical valves.[41] Antiplatelet drugs alone do not protect against embolism.[42] The incidence of systemic embolism is generally greater with mitral than with aortic prosthetic valves and is greater still with double (mitral and double) valve replacement. In one large series giving a 10 year experience of users of the Medtronic Hall valve the rate of thromboembolism for patients with aortic, mitral and double (aortic and mitral) valve replacement (all patients being fully anticoagulated) was 1.3, 1.3 or 1.8%/years respectively.[43]

Valve thrombosis

This is a serious and often fatal complication of prosthetic heart valve replacement. Thrombosis of a mechanical valve can carry a mortality as high as 60% to 80%.[37] Prosthetic valve thrombosis (PVT) is unusual with tissue valves, and is more likely to occur with a tilting disc value or a hinged bileaflet valve than in a caged ball valve. Despite improvement in valve design and in prosthetic material all prosthetic valves carry a risk of thrombosis which may be as high as 0.5 to 6.0%.[39, 44, 45] The highest incidence of thrombosis occurs with tricuspid valve prosthesis where the incidence can be as high as 20%,[46] and for this reason tissue valves are usually used when tricuspid replacement is necessary. Mitral prostheses are more liable to thrombosis than aortic prostheses.[47]

Because of the high likelihood of valve thrombosis in the absence of anticoagulant therapy and of the gravity of this complication there is general agreement that anticoagulation is mandatory in all patients with mechanical prosthetic heart valves. In situations where it has proved unacceptable to use anticoagulant therapy alternative treatment with antiplatelet drugs (aspirin and dipyridamole) has been tried. Even in the least thrombogenic prosthesis antiplatelet drugs are insufficient to prevent thrombosis even in patients in sinus rhythm.[48]

The final clinical presentation of PVT is that of pulmonary oedema, arrhythmias and cardiogenic shock. However, there is no reason to believe that PVT occurs suddenly. Valves removed at surgery often show layers of thrombus which grow and gradually interfere with disc movement, and early symptoms can therefore be very vague and non specific. On auscultation the valve sounds (opening and closing clicks) are often faint or may even be absent. New murmurs are also audible. The diagnosis is confirmed by echocardiography and/or cineradiography (valve screening). Most prosthetic disc valves have a radio-opaque marker in the disc and by screening the valve it is easy to determine whether the disc opens and closes fully. Echocardiography especially in the mitral position can be quite specific.[49]

Management

Thrombosis on a mechanical prosthetic valve is a grave emergency. Most patients with this condition require urgent or semi-urgent surgery. This will either mean removal of the thrombosis or replacement of the valve, depending on the findings at the time of surgery. The operative mortality rate is high.[50]

The use of fibrinolysis has been considered in an attempt to avoid the high morbidity and mortality risks of emergency surgery in a desperately ill patient. Treatment has generally consisted of streptokinase in a loading dose of 250 000–500 000 u followed by 100 000 u hourly. Rapid improvement in the clinical state has been seen within 6 hours of starting treatment and in the majority of patients (60%) fibrinolytic therapy is all that may be required with an overall survival rate of 80–90%. The combination of fibrinolytic therapy and semi-elective or elective surgery seems to be safer than emergency surgery alone.[51]

As with the use of thrombolysis to dissolve left ventricular mural thrombosis, however, there is great concern about the potential for systemic embolization after partial dissolution of thrombotic material. In the largest available series (26 patients) thrombolytic intervention was successful in 21 cases (81%).[52] Fibrinolysis is the preferred treatment for patients with thrombosis of tricuspid valve prosthesis. In general, patients with thrombosis of mechanical aortic or mitral prostheses should go forward for surgery unless it is clearly contraindicated. If surgery is not possible or is contraindicated thrombolysis should be used and the risk of systemic embolism then has to be accepted.

Infective endocarditis

Prosthetic valve endocarditis (PVE) is a very serious complication of prosthetic valve replacement. In the early days of prosthetic valve replacement a 10% incidence was reported in patients who received no prophylactic antibiotic cover.[53] PVE is classified as *early* or *late*. The infection is classified as early if it occurs within 2 months of surgery. Late infection develops as part of a continuing long term risk and the infecting organisms are similar to those found in patients with native valve endocarditis. In early infection it is assumed that contamination occurred at the time of surgery either through an infected sternal wound or contaminated intravenous drip lines. The use of prophylactic antimicrobial therapy in patients undergoing heart valve replacement has substantially reduced the incidence of early onset infection to less than 1%, and late onset infection to just over 1%.[54–56] Most early onset infections are caused by organisms isolated from operating room equipment such as cardiopulmonary bypass tubings or from postoperative wound infections.

In late onset infection the portal of entries is assumed to be the same as that for native valve endocarditis such as bacteraemia caused by dental treatment, skin infection and deep-seated infections. There is no clear evidence that mechanical prostheses are more likely to become infected than heterografts.

The organisms involved in early onset infection are usually staphylococci (*Staph. epidermidis* and *Staph. aureus*) and gram negative bacilli, but fungi and other organisms can also be found. In late onset infection streptococci are the most common organisms but staphylococci and gram negative bacilli can also be responsible.

The clinical presentation in late onset infection is similar to that of native valve infections. However, in early onset infection the diagnosis of prosthetic valve endocarditis may be more difficult especially in patients with pneumonia, wound infections and urinary tract infections and in the presence of these infections the possibility of early PVE must always be borne in mind. The development of new regurgitant murmurs and conduction abnormalities in these ill patients strongly suggests early PVE.

Diagnoses

Because of the seriousness of the diagnosis, a high index of suspicion concerning the diagnosis of endocarditis must be maintained in relation to all patients with prosthetic valves (non-biological or biological). The presence of pyrexia, a raised sedimentation rate, unexplained anaemia or leucocytosis, splenomegaly, petechiae, clubbing or systemic emboli in a patient with a prosthetic valve should alert the attending doctor to the possibility of PVE. Antibiotics must not be given without careful consideration and certainly not before 3–6 blood cultures have been taken and haemoglobin, white cell count, ESR and the C-reactive protein level checked.

Management

Any patient with a prosthetic heart valve and suspected of PVE should be admitted immediately to the cardiology or cardiac surgical unit. Antibiotic treatment should be initiated immediately after 3–6 blood cultures have been taken wherever there are reasonable clinical grounds for suspecting PVE.

The possible need for elective or emergency re-replacement of the valve must be kept in mind at all times and for this reason the patient should be under the joint care of the cardiologist and cardiac surgeon. Those cases most likely to be cured medically are the late onset cases in which the infecting organism is a streptococcus. Those cases most likely to require urgent replacement are the early cases in which the infecting organism is a staphylococcus.

The major indications for surgery are:

1. Prosthetic valve dysfunction

2. Prosthetic valve dehiscence
3. Uncontrolled infection
4. Moderate aortic regurgitant and congestive heart failure in PVE
5. Recurrent relapse of infection
6. Persistently positive blood cultures despite appropriate antibiotic treatment
7. Myocardial or valve ring abscesses.

With early PVE surgery is almost invariably necessary. The infecting organism is often a staphylococcus. A common organism is *Staphylococcus epidermidis*, 80% of which organisms are methicillin resistant. Another common organism is *Staphylococcus aureus*. Each of these infecting organisms is best handled surgically.

The destructive effect of infection is particularly great around the sewing ring of the valve with destruction of the annulus, valve dehiscence, abscess formation and even rupture into cardiac chambers. Surgery must be radical involving total removal of the infected valve. There is no question of just placing additional sutures along areas of valve dehiscence. Abscesses must be evacuated and all infected tissue removed. In the worst cases valved dacron grafts may have to be used. Antibiotic treatment should be continued for a minimum of 6 weeks after surgery.

The optimal antibiotic regime will depend upon the relevant bacteriological information, but large doses of appropriate bactericidal antibiotics are necessary. For *methicillin resistant organisms* the use of (a) vancomycin 30 mg/kg/24 h i.v. (given in 3 equally divided doses) + (b) rifampicin 300 mg 8-hourly by mouth + (c) gentamicin 1 mg/kg i.v. 8-hourly is appropriate. Serum levels of vancomycin and of gentamicin should be monitored carefully and the dosage adjusted accordingly. The vancomycin and rifampicin should be continued for a minimum of 6 weeks and the gentamicin for 2 weeks. For *methicillin sensitive organisms* flucloxacillin 3 g 6-hourly i.v. should be used in place of vancomycin + rifampicin + gentamicin given as detailed above.

Once the above regime has been instituted (modified as appropriate in the light of detailed bacteriological information) it is essential not to lose sight of the fact that re-replacement of the prosthesis is likely to be necessary and that whilst a medical cure is possible it is unlikely. Surgery should be undertaken immediately there is evidence of significant haemodynamic deterioration or of failures to control the infection.

In the case of late onset PVE, especially where the infecting organism is a streptococcus, medical care is more often possible. The criteria for surgery remain the same and in the case both of early and of late PVE the reason for recommending immediate admission to the joint care of the cardiologist and cardiac surgeon is because the need for urgent re-operation continues to be a possibility. For infection caused by enterococci or viridans streptococci a combination of aqueous crystalline penicillin G and gentamicin in doses required to provide adequate inhibitory serum levels (guided by the bacteriology) is appropriate. In general a suitable starting dose of gentamicin is 1 mg/kg i.v. 8-hourly and a total of 20 million units of penicillin G given in 3 divided doses over 24 hours seems appropriate.

Prophylaxis

For patients with prosthetic heart valves prophylaxis with 3 g oral amoxycillin is inadequate and a much more stringent regime is required. Prophylaxis is necessary for any dental procedure which either definitely will or might possibly give rise to intra-oral bleeding (including extractions, scaling and root fillings), for childbirth and for any other surgery in which transient bacteraemia is possible (e.g. various forms of instrumentation). Appropriate cover consists of amoxycillin 1 g i.v. + netilmicin 200 mg i.v. one hour prior to the procedure, followed by amoxycillin 500 mg orally 6 hours later. For patients with penicillin allergy vancomycin 1 g i.v. over 60 minutes prior to the procedure should be used instead of the amoxycillin. It is fully understood that these are not *convenient* regimes but they are *appropriate*.

Anticoagulant-related haemorrhage

The potential risks of valve thrombosis, embolism and bleeding associated with anticoagulation therapy may deter the surgeons from implanting any type of mechanical valve. In the case of bleeding it is clear that the incidence of this complication will vary with the quality and range of anticoagulation control.[57] The level of anticoagulation is measured by the International Normalized Ratio (INR) which is defined as the thrombin time ratio measured with a thromboplastin that has been calibrated against a World Health Organization international standard reagent by an internationally acceptable method. The INR is not universally accepted in the USA although it is in Europe and Australasia. The intensity of anticoagulation can be divided into 3 groups 'low' (INR 2.0–3.5), 'medium' (INR 3.0–4.2) and 'high' (INR 3.9–5.0). In general, patients with non-biological prosthetic valves should strive to achieve the INR reading consistently within the range 3.0–4.5.

Bland paraprosthetic leaks

Minor degrees of leakage in relation to non-biological and biological prosthetic heart valves are not uncommon. These variously present with the finding of an apical systolic murmur (mitral prosthesis) or an early diastolic murmur (aortic prosthesis) or they may be discovered on routine echocardiographic assessment. They are usually present from the time of surgery and freshly developed or diagnosed leaks should always be regarded with suspicion. The leak should never be of haemodynamic significance (as judged clinically, on a chest X-ray or at echocardiographic assessment). Apart from slightly increasing the degree of haemolysis the finding of an old established, non-changing, haemodynamically insignificant leak in a patient with no suggestion of endocardial infection need not give rise to concern.

Haemodynamically significant valve dysfunction

Whenever a patient with a prosthetic heart valve has a haemodynamically significant leak through or around that valve the problem is potentially serious and re-assessment by the cardiologist and cardiac surgeon is essential. The first step is to exclude infective endocarditis. Subsequently full haemodynamic assessment is necessary to determine whether or not re-replacement (usually not a higher risk than the initial procedure) is appropriate. Occasionally the occurrence of severe haemolysis in relation to a paraprosthetic leak contribute to the need for re-operation. If re-operation is not considered necessary initially continued vigilance must be maintained [clinical, radiological (chest X-ray and valve screening) and echocardiographic assessment—all undertaken periodically].

Structural valve failure

Mechanical valve failure

Mechanical valve failure can be catastrophic although with modern valves it is extremely rare if cases of valve thrombosis are excluded. All types of mechanical valves have suffered sudden mechanical failure from poppet escape in caged/ball valves, strut fracture and disc escape in tilting disc valves and leaflet escape in bileaflet valves.

In recent years the Bjork–Shiley 60° convexo concave valve has received much publicity. This valve was designed to decrease thrombo-embolic complications and was introduced into clinical use in 1976. However, soon reports of outlet strut fracture with resulting embolization of the occluded disc appeared and the valve was withdrawn from the market in 1986. Two-thirds of all cases reported have been fatal. The risk of strut fracture varies depending on size of the valve and when it was manufactured. The lowest risk (in small valves) is 0.021% per year and the highest risk (in large-sized valves manufactured between February 1982 and June 1982) is estimated to be 0.31% per year. Generally the risk of strut fracture is not regarded to be high enough to warrant elective replacement of these valves.[58]

In the early 1980s 160 of these valves were inserted at Manchester Royal Infirmary. We know of 7 cases of strut fracture all in the mitral position. Three patients died before they could reach hospital. One patient was admitted to hospital with a diagnosis of 'subarachnoid haemorrhage'. He lived for 5 hours, and retrospective analysis of chest X-ray on admission clearly showed the presence of a minor strut in the left ventricle and the occluder disc impacted in the abdominal aorta. The remaining 3 patients were diagnosed immediately and had emergency surgery, and all 3 are well and alive today.

Tissue valve failure

The durability of tissue valves is limited by spontaneous degeneration. Tissue valves also have a tendency to calcify especially so in younger patients and in patients in renal failure on dialysis. In porcine glutaraldehyde-treated bioprosthesis the freedom from valve dysfunction due to primary tissue failure at 12 years has been reported to be 69% for aortic valves and 61% for mitral valves[59] It is possible that some of the newer valves (second-generation tissue valves) will have better durability as slightly different methods of preservation and fixation are being used today. A tissue valve usually fails slowly and diagnosis of valve failure can be made at an early stage and re-operation carried out before the patient is in gross heart failure. However, the mode of failure in pericardial xenograft valves can be more dramatic particularly so in the Ionescu Shiley pericardial valve which is no longer being manufactured. Gross incompetence can occur due to leaflets tearing away from the valve mounting structure.

The following case report illustrates the problem. A 21-year-old female patient had an aortic valve replacement for congenital aortic stenosis. A 21 mm Ionescu–Shiley pericardial xenograft was used. Two years later a regurgitant murmur was noted although the patient remained well. At 6 years she presented with severe breathlessness and also severe haemolytic anaemia. No cause for the haemolytic anaemia could be found and one had to assume it was valve related. Angiography also showed severe aortic incompetence. A re-operation was carried out and the pericardial valve was replaced by a 23 mm Medtronic Hall valve. One of the leaflets of the pericardial valve had 'disappeared' altogether, the remaining 2 were calcified and rigid (see Fig. 12.3).

Miscellaneous

Heart valve replacement in children

The number of children subjected to valve replacement will vary considerably in different parts of the world. In developing countries the prevalence of rheumatic fever remains a source of concern. In the western world valve replacement in children is a much rarer occurrence and is usually done for congenital aortic and mitral valve disease.

It was once thought that the porcine bioprosthesis was the best valve substitute in these young patients. However, it soon became clear that these

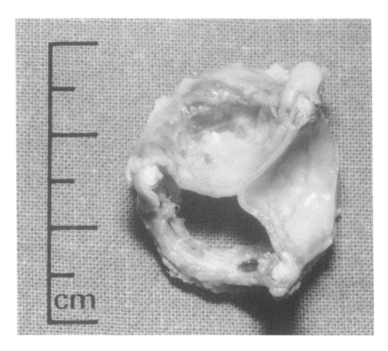

Fig. 12.3   Pericardial xenograft 6 years after implantation. The patient had severe aortic incompetence. One of the three leaflets is absent. (Reproduced with permission from the University of Medical Illustration, Royal Infirmary, Manchester)

valves were prone to very early calcification leading to severe valve stenosis and the degeneration rate in these young patients has been reported to be as high as 22.4% per patient year compared with 4.0% per patient year in older patients.[60] A mechanical prosthesis therefore seems to be the only acceptable device for valve replacements in children. Although children with implanted mechanical valves have been managed without anti-coagulation it is still advisable to anticoagulate all children with mechanical prostheses provided the anticoagulation can be monitored. If this is im-practicable they should be given aspirin and dipyridamole.

Prosthetic valve replacement in children should be avoided if at all possible. If a valve replacement is mandatory a mechanical valve should be used even though re-replacement with a larger prosthesis may be necessary subsequently in adulthood.

Prosthetic valves and pregnancy

All patients with mechanical heart valves and patients with tissue valves who are not in regular sinus rhythm ideally need anticoagulation for life. It is this aspect which presents problems in relation to pregnancy in patients with prosthetic valves. In pregnant women there exists a state of hyper-coagulability which further reinforces the need for anticoagulation. Oral anticoagulants, however, cross the placenta and can cause teratogenic lesions in the first trimester. Discontinuing anticoagulation during pregnancy even temporarily can cause disastrous thrombotic complications.[61]

There is no ideal solution to the problem of non-biological prosthetic heart valves in pregnancy. Ideally females who are likely to need valve replacement should complete their pregnancies before the prosthesis is inserted provided it is haemodynamically safe for pregnancy to proceed in the presence of the underlying native valve lesion. If the woman has aortic valve disease and cannot complete her required pregnancies before valve replacement is called for, consideration should be given to initial replacement with a biological prosthesis. Pregnancies may then proceed without any requirement for anticoagulation and therefore without significant additional risk but this course of action makes it inevitable that re-replacement (with a mechanical valve) will be necessary some 10–15 years later when the biological valve calcifies and degenerates.

For patients with mechanical prostheses in the aortic or mitral positions, the ideal method of anticoagulation during pregnancy is uncertain. The use of warfarin carries a risk of abortion and of the development of the severe warfarin embryopathy. Heparin is a large molecule which does not cross the placenta and can therefore have no teratogenic or anticoagulation effect on the fetus. It has been suggested that heparin should be given subcutaneously during the first trimester to avoid the dangers of oral anti-coagulation.[57] However there are numerous reports of systemic emboli and (even more seriously) of valve thrombosis occurring in pregnant subjects with non-biological prosthetic valves given heparin subcutaneously in place of warfarin during pregnancy. It is *possible* that heparin given sub-cutaneously could effectively prevent thrombosis and embolism during pregnancy in patients with mechanical prosthetic valves *if the drug is given in sufficient dosage and at frequent enough intervals* but no successful trial of such a regime has been reported. The frequent recommendation to use heparin in the first trimester of pregnancy is based on a desire to avoid warfarin embryopathy. The efficacy of heparin is not proven. The choice lies between maximal maternal safety (warfarin continued throughout pregnancy until 36 weeks) and maximal fetal safety (warfarin avoided throughout pregnancy). The mother must know this. There is no risk-free course of action. The commonly made recommendation to use moderate doses of subcutaneous heparin undoubtedly exposes the mother to the risk of embolic or valve thrombosis. For example Vitali et al[62] reported on 85 pregnancies in patients with mechanical prosthetic valve. In 76 cases coumarin therapy was continued until term or until 3 weeks before delivery. Of the remaining 9 cases, 4 received dipyridamole only during pregnancy, 3 received no anticoagulant and 2 received subcutaneous heparin during pregnancy. There were 9 cases of maternal thromboembolic problems including two maternal deaths related to thrombosis of the prosthesis. The deaths occurred in the two patients receiving subcutaneous heparin.

The authors have experience of a mutual patient presenting a major thrombotic problem in pregnancy. A 24-year-old female patient had a prosthetic aortic valve inserted in February 1988. On the 10th August 1989 oral anticoagulation (Sinthrome) was stopped (not by us) as she had decided to become pregnant. She was put on subcutaneous heparin 6500 units twice a day. On the 22nd November 1989 when she was 6 weeks pregnant she developed chest pain, felt dizzy and on admission to hospital the valve clicks were muffled and a loud diastolic murmur was audible. Valve screening (Fig. 12.4) showed the occluder disc to be stuck in a half-open position (disc opened fully but did not close). It was clear that she had suffered prosthetic valve thrombosis and that urgent surgery was indicated. This was carried out the following day. The small orifice of the Medtronic Hall valve was partially filled with thrombus severely impeding movement of the occluder. The valve was thrombectomized and the patient was kept on a full intravenous dose of heparin for 3 days and then restarted on warfarin. Ultrasound of the abdomen confirmed a live fetus 8 days later. At 36 weeks of pregnancy she was admitted to hospital, her Sinthrome was stopped and she was put on intravenous heparin. Four days later labour was induced and she delivered a healthy baby. Except for a postpartum haemorrhage on the 12th day she made an uneventful recovery.

The best approach is to avoid pregnancy whenever possible in patients with prosthetic heart valves. If pregnancy cannot be avoided the mother should be given the full facts about the material risks of discontinuing warfarin and of the fetal risks of continuing the drug. The safest course of action for the mother is to continue warfarin until the 36th week and then to substitute full doses of intravenous heparin until delivery. If the mother insists on maximal fetal safety subcutaneous heparin can be used but none of the regimes described so far has proved entirely safe for the mother and she must know this.

CONCLUSION

In 1896 Paget stated 'Surgery of the heart has probably reached the limit set by nature to all surgery, no new method, and no new discovery can overcome the natural difficulties that attend wound of the heart.'[63]

Paget's predictions were not true, but we should also bear in mind Galetti's statement in 1988, 'Without the unavoidable accidents entailed in a trial and error process, researchers cannot make safer, more effective implants a reality. We must not delude ourselves into thinking that perfect devices will soon be available; even the most ardent promoters of the artificial heart do not expect widespread application before the year 2000.[64]

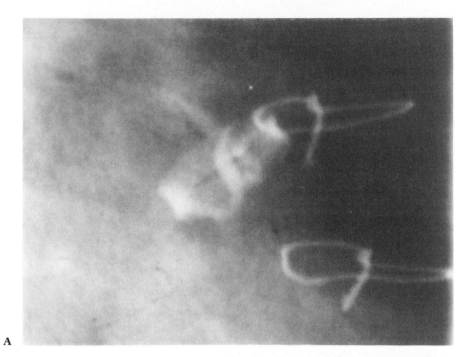

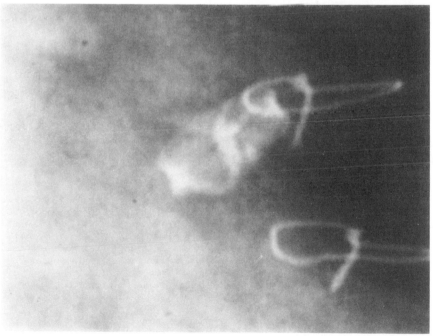

Fig. 12.4 Thrombus interfering with closure of the disc of a Medtronic Hall valve. **A** During systole the valve disc is fully open (seen at about 80° to the plane of the valve ring). **B** During diastole the valve disc is incompletely closed. Instead of lying in the plane of the valve ring it is still at about 30° to the ring. At surgery the disc could be seen to be held open by thrombus.

REFERENCES

1 Deloitte, Haskins, Sells. Management consultancy division. Costing of cardiac procedures for Manchester Royal Infirmary. 1989
2 Gibbon JH Jr. Application of a mechanical heart lung apparatus to cardiac surgery. Minn Med 1954; 37: 171–177
3 Tuffier T. Etude experimentale sur la chirurgie des valves de coeur. Bull Acad Med Paris. 1914; 71: 293
4 Bailey CP, Ramirez HP, Larselere HB. Surgical treatment of aortic stenosis. JAMA 1952; 150: 1647
5 Hufnagel CA, Harvey WP. The surgical correction of aortic regurgitation: preliminary report. Bull Georgetown University Med Center 1953; 6: 60
6 Cutler EC, Levine SA. Cardiotomy and valvotomy for mitral stenosis. Boston Med Surg J 1923; 188: 1023
7 Harken DE, Ellis LB, Ware PF, Norman LR. The surgical treatment of mitral stenosis. N Engl J Med 1948; 239: 801
8 Bailey CP. The surgical treatment of mitral stenosis (mitral commissurotomy). Dis Chest 1949; 15: 377
9 Logan A, Turner R. Surgical treatment of mitral stenosis with particular reference to the transventricular approach with a mechanical dilator. Lancet 1959; ii: 874
10 Starr A, Edwards ML. Mitral replacement: clinical experience with a ball-valve prosthesis. Ann Surg 1961; 154: 726–740
11 Bjork VO. A new tilting disc valve prosthesis. Scand J Thorac Cardiovasc Surg 1969; 3: 1–10
12 Emery RW, Mettler E, Nicoloff DM. A new cardiac prosthesis: the St Jude medical cardiac valve: in vivo results. Circulation (Suppl) 1979; 60: 1148–1154
13 Ross DN. Homograft replacement of aortic valve. Lancet 1962; ii: 487
14 Binet JP, Duran CG, Carpentier A, Langlois J. Heterologous aortic valve transplantation. Lancet 1965; ii(425): 1275
15 Ionescu MI, Tandon AP, Silverton NP, Chidambaram M, Smith DR. Longterm durability of the pericardial valve. In: Bodnar E, Yacoub M, eds. Biologic and bioprosthetic valves. New York: Yorke Medical Books. 1986: p 165
16 Ceitlin MD. The timing of surgery in mitral and aortic valve disease. Curr Probl Cardiol 1987; 12: 69–149
17 Hugenholtz PG, Ryan TJ, Stein SW. The spectrum of pure mitral stenosis: haemodynamic studies in relation to clinical disability. Am J Cardiol 1962; 10: 773–784
18 Ross J Jr. Afterload mismatch in aortic and mitral valve disease: implication for surgical therapy. J Am Coll Cardiol 1985; 5: 811–826
19 Rapaport E. Natural history of aortic and mitral valve disease. Am J Cardiol 1975; 35: 221–227
20 Frank S, Johnson A, Ross J Jr. Natural history of valvular aortic stenosis. Br Heart J 1973; 35: 41–46
21 Abedelnoor M, Hall KV, Nitter-Hange S, Levorstad K, Lindberg H, Ovrum E. Prognostic factors for survival in surgically treated aortic regurgitation. Scand J Thorac Cardiovasc Surg 1986; 20: 221–226
22 Boskovic D, Elezovic I, Boskovic D, Simin N, Rolovic Z, Josipovic V. Late thrombosis of the Bjork-Shiley tilting disc valve in the tricuspid position: thrombolytic treatment with streptokinase. J Thorac Cardiovasc Surg 1986; 91: 1–8
23 Thoburn CW, Morgan JJ, Shanaham MX, Chang VP. Long-term results of tricuspid valve replacement and the problem of prosthetic valve thrombosis. Am J Cardiol 1983; 51: 1128–1132
24 Eng J, Ravichandran PS, Kay PH, Murday AJ. Long-term results of Ionescu-Shiley valve in the tricuspid position. Ann Thorac Surg 1991; 51: 200–203
25 Kaster RL, Lillehei CW. A new cageless free-floating pivoting disc prosthetic heart valve: design, development and evaluation. In: Jacobson B, ed. Dig 7th Int Conf Med, Biol Eng. Stockholm: Almquist and Wiksell. 1967: p 387
26 Nitter-Hange S, Enge I, Semb BKH et al. Primary clinical experience with the Hall–Kaster valve in the aortic position: results of 3 months including haemodynamic studies. Circulation 1979; 60(Suppl 2): 193

27 Nitter-Hange S, Semb BKH, Levorstad K et al. Primary results with the new
    Hall–Kaster disc valve prosthesis in the mitral position. J Thorac Cardiovasc Surg 1979;
    27: 85–91
28 Young WP, Gott LV, Rowe GG. Open heart surgery for mitral valve disease with special
    reference to a new prosthetic valve. J Thorac Cardiovasc Surg 1965; 50: 827–833
29 Senning A. Fascia lata replacement of aortic valve. J Thorac Cardiovasc Surg 1967; 54:
    465–470
30 Gerbode F. Proceedings of the first international workshop on tissue valves. Ann Surg
    1970; 172(Suppl 1) 1–24
31 Rothlin ME, Senning A. 15 years experience with fascia lata aortic valves and the outlook
    of modern bioprosthesis. In: Sebberning F, ed. Bioprosthetic cardiac valves. Munich:
    Deutsches Herzzentrum Munchen. 1979: p 172
32 Ionescu MI, Tandon AP, Many DAS et al. Heart valve replacement with the
    Ionescu–Shiley pericardial xenograft. J Thorac Cardiovasc Surg 1977; 73: 31–42
33 Arom KV, Nicoloff DM, Kersten TE, Lindsay WG, Northrup WF. 3rd St Jude medical
    prosthesis: valve related deaths and complications. Ann Thorac Surg 1987; 43(6):
    591–598
34 Baudet RL, Poirier NL, Doyle D, Dakkle G, Gauvin C. The Medtronic Hall cardiac
    valve: 7½ years clinical experience. Ann Thorac Surg 1986; 42(6): 644–650
35 Borkon AM, Soule L, Baughman KL et al. Ten-year analysis of the Bjork–Shiley
    standard aortic valve. Ann Thorac Surg 1987 43(1): 39–51
36 Martinell J, Fraile J, Artiz V, Moreno J, Rabago G. Long-term comparative analysis of
    the Bjork–Shiley and Hancock valves implanted in 1975. J Thorac Cardiovasc Surg 1985;
    90(5): 741–749
37 Karp RB, Cyrus RJ, Blackstone EH, Kirklin JW, Kouchoukos NT, Pacifico AD. The
    Bjork–Shiley valve: intermediate-term follow up. J Thorac Cardiovasc Surg 1981; 81:
    602–614
38 Nashef SAM, Stewart M, Bain WH. Heart valve replacement: thromboembolism or
    thrombosis and embolism? In: Bodnar E, ed. Surgery for heart valve disease 1990; pp
    159–165
39 Edmunds LH Jr. Thromboembolic complications of current cardiac valvular prostheses.
    Ann Thorac Surg 1982; 34: 96–106
40 Gouzales-Lavin L, Tandon AP, Chi S et al. The risk of thromboembolism and
    haemorrhage following mitral valve replacement. J Thorac Cardiovasc Surg 1984; 87:
    340–351
41 Edmunds LH. Thrombo-embolic complications of current cardiac valvular prostheses.
    Ann Thorac Surg 1982; 34: 90–100
42 Nair CK, Mohiuddin SM, Hilleman DE et al. Ten year result with the St Jude medical
    prosthesis. Am J Cardiol 1990; 65: 217–222
43 Nitter-Hange S, Abdelnoor M. Ten-year experience with the Medtronic Hall valvular
    prosthesis. Circulation 1989; Suppl 1: I43–I48
44 Barnhorst DA, Oxman HA, Connoly DC et al. Long-term follow up of isolated
    replacement of the aortic and mitral valve with Starr Edwards prosthesis. Am J Cardiol
    1975; 35: 228–233
45 Bjork VO, Henze A. Ten year experience with the Bjork–Shiley tilting disc valve. J
    Thorac Cardiovasc Surg 1979; 78: 331–342
46 Thorburn CW, Morgan JJ, Shanaham MX, Chang VP. Long-term results of tricuspid
    valve replacement and the problem of prosthetic valve thrombosis. Am J Cardiol 1983; 51:
    1128–1132
47 Moreno-Cabral RJ, McNamara JJ, Mamiya RT, Brainard SC, Chung GKT. Acute
    thrombotic obstruction with Bjork–Shiley valves. J Thorac Cardiovasc Surg 1978; 75:
    321–330
48 Ribeiro PA, Zaibag MA, Idris M et al. Antiplatelet drugs and the incidence of
    thromboembolic complications of the St Jude medical aortic prosthesis in patients with
    rheumatic heart disease. J Thorac Cardiovasc Surg 1986; 91: 92–98
49 Bernal-Ramires JA, Philips JH. Echocardiographic study of malfunction of the
    Bjork–Shiley prosthetic heart valve in the mitral position. Am J Cardiol 1977; 40:
    449–453
50 Pavac A, Bors V, Bard F et al. Surgery of prosthetic valve thrombosis. Eur Heart J 1984;
    5(Suppl 8): 39

51 Wilkinson GAL, Williams WG. Fibrinolytic treatment of acute prosthetic valve thrombosis. 5 cases and a review. Eur J Cardiothorac Surg 1989; 3: 178–183
52 Roudaut ML, Ledain L, Roudaut R et al. Thrombolytic treatment of acute thrombotic obstruction with disc valve prostheses. Experience with 26 cases. Semin Thromb Hemost 1987; 13: 201–205
53 Geraci JE, Dale AJD, McGoon DC. Bacterial endocarditis and endarteritis following cardiac operation. Wis Med J 1963; 62: 302–315
54 Dismukes WE, Karchmer AW, Buckley MJ et al. Prosthetic valve endocarditis: analysis of 38 cases. Circulation 1973; 48: 365–377
55 Rossiter SJ, Stinson EB, Oyer PE et al. Prosthetic valve endocarditis: comparison of heterograft tissue valves and mechanical valves. J Thorac Cardiovasc Surg 1978; 76: 795–802
56 Wilson WR, Jaumin PM, Danielson GK et al. Prosthetic valve endocarditis. Ann Intern Med 1975; 82: 751–756
57 Forfar JC. A 7 year analysis of haemorrhage in patients on long-term anticoagulant treatment. Br Heart J 1979; 42: 128–132
58 Hiratzka LF, Kouchoukos NT, Grunkemeier GL et al. Outlet strut fracture of the Bjork–Shiley 60° convexo-concave valve: current information and recommendation for patient care. J Am Coll Cardiol 1988; 11: 1130–1137
59 Bortolotti V, Milano A, Mazzucco A et al. Results of reoperation for primary tissue failure of porcine bioprostheses. J Thorac Cardiovasc Surg 1985; 90: 564–569
60 Antunes MJ, Santos LP. Performances of glutaraldehyde-preserved porcine bioprosthesis as a mitral valve substitute in a young population group. Ann Thorac Surg 1984; 37: 387–392
61 Salazar E, Zajorias A, Gutierez N, Iturbe I. The problem of cardiac valve prostheses, anticoagulants and pregnancies. Circulation 1984; 70(Suppl 1): 169–177
62 Vitali E, Donatelli F, Quaini E et al. Pregnancy in patients with mechanical prosthetic valves. Our experience regarding 98 pregnancies in 57 patients. J Cardiovasc Surg 1986; 27: 221–227
63 Paget S. The surgery of the chest. London: Wright. 1896: p 212
64 Galetti PM. Artificial organs: learning to live with risk. Technology Review 1988; 35: 40

Reviews of some key papers published in 1990/1992

1. Coronary artery bypass graft surgery—guidelines and indications

ACC/AHA guidelines and indications for coronary artery bypass graft surgery. Circulation 1991; 83: 1125–1173

This paper contains a wide-ranging report on the indications for, conduct of, and expected results from coronary artery bypass graft surgery. The article, however, also considers the costs and sizing of the units performing the operation and, although formulated in the USA, these can easily be transferred to this side of the Atlantic. It suggests that the data is now available to base firm recommendations and that consensus opinion is no longer applicable.

In considering the indications for intervention, as opposed to persisting with medical therapy, the article suggests that all patients should be placed in one of three classes: (1) where the operation clearly has demonstrable advantages in terms of survival and/or symptomatic relief, (2) where no such advantage can be found, and (3) where the advantages are not clear cut.

In asymptomatic patients, a great majority will have undergone non-invasive tests suggestive of ischaemia, and, at angiography, those who have either important left main stem stenosis (> 50%) or important three-vessel coronary artery disease, with a proximal left anterior descending stenosis, clearly need surgery. This indication is stronger if the stress test suggests moderate or severe ischaemia and/or if left ventricular function is depressed. When the patient is symptomatic with angina then the indications are relaxed somewhat with a left main stem stenosis and three-vessel disease clearly needing surgery. Patients with two- or one-vessel disease may need surgery if the angina is particularly severe and if left ventricular function is depressed. The article points out the prognostic importance of a proximal left anterior descending stenosis. The indications for surgery increase when the left ventricular ejection fraction decreases, but this holds true only down to greater than 20%. Totally secure evidence to suggest improved benefit in those below this level is lacking. Debility, from whatever cause, is regarded as a contraindication to surgery. Old age is not regarded as a contraindication, although morbidity and mortality are higher.

The article considers a variety of outcome events such as death, return of angina, risk of infarction and quality of life, and presents these in a time-related fashion. It suggests that at one month, one, five and ten years, 96.5%, 95%, 88% and 75%, respectively, of patients should be alive. Poor ventricular function, more severe coronary artery disease and non-use of the internal mammary artery are factors increasing the risk of death. Angina returns as time passes so that over a similar time period 0.3%, 5%, 17% and 37% experience a recurrence. Incomplete revascularization is an important factor in early return.

Finally, in relation to cost and personnel, it suggests that, in general, the cost per case is lower in larger units with the results improving with more cases. It suggests that a surgeon should be performing at least 100–150 cases per year (mostly coronary artery work). The number of intensive care beds should be numerically half of the number of cases performed per week in the unit. Surgeons' assistants should be used to replace junior surgeons to keep costs down and all deaths should be audited.

D.J.M.K.

2. W-P-W syndrome—current treatment

Bolling SF, Morady F, Calkins H et al. Current treatment for Wolff-Parkinson-White syndrome: results and surgical implications. Ann Thorac Surg 1991; 52: 461–468

This is the first report comparing the results of surgical and catheter radiofrequency ablation of accessory atrioventricular pathways within the same institution. Of the 247 consecutive patients, 123 underwent surgical ablation with endocardial approach and 124 catheter radiofrequency ablation. Radiofrequency ablation was the predominant treatment of choice in the last 12 months. The surgical series had younger patients and more patients with multiple pathways and posteroseptal pathways. During a mean follow up of 26 ± 7 months, surgical ablation was successful in 119 patients (97%), 5 of them required a second operation hours to 24 months after the first operation. One patient with multiple congenital anomalies suffered from hypoxic brain injury during a cardiac arrest after surgery and died 2 months after surgery. Other complications included: postoperative bleeding necessitating a return to the operating room; intermittent third-degree atrioventricular block requiring placement of a permanent pace-maker, cerebral vascular accident; mild mitral regurgitation; and small lateral myocardial infarction. Radiofrequency ablation was successful in 112 patients (90%) during a mean follow up of 7 ± 5 months though 11 required a second session and one required a third session. A mean of 7 ± 5 radiofrequency pulses were applied during successful ablation sessions. Complications included: occlusion of the circumflex artery due to ablating catheter positioning; perforation of a deformed aortic valve leaflet with mild aortic insufficiency; retroperitoneal haematoma; and transient neurologic deficit. The mean duration of fluoroscopy was 48 ± 30 minutes, approximately 0.52 Gy of radiation, and was similar to that of coronary angioplasty. The amount of radiation was estimated to result in 56 to 90 fatal malignancies per one million patients. The authors discussed the costs associated with long-term pharmacologic therapy, surgical ablation, and radiofrequency ablation, and also compared the technical aspects of the two procedures. They suggested that surgical ablation was more beneficial in patients undergoing concomitant cardiac procedures and might be more efficacious in treating multiple pathways.

The two methods appeared comparable in their high success rate and low incidence of complications though the study was retrospective and non-random and the follow up of the radiofrequency ablation series was not as long as that of the surgical series. The trend favouring radiofrequency ablation is obviously due to the lower cost and the less traumatic nature of radiofrequency ablation. The two methods may be equally efficacious in ablating multiple pathways as experience is gained to shorten the duration of radiofrequency ablation. Long-term follow up is necessary to determine the outcome of radiation exposure during radiofrequency ablation.

D.P.Z.

3. Intensive lipid-lowering therapy leads to regression of coronary artery disease

Brown G, Albers JJ, Fisher LD et al. Regression of coronary artery disease as a result of intensive lipid-lowering therapy in men with high levels of apolipoprotein B. N Engl J Med 1990; 323: 1289–1298

The participants in this investigation were 146 men who were selected from patients undergoing coronary angiography because they had at least one coronary stenosis of more than 50% or three of more than 30%, together with a serum level of apolipoprotein B (apo B) (the main protein component of LDL) exceeding 125 mg/dl and a family history of atherosclerosis early in life. None had yet had coronary artery surgery. All patients were given lipid-lowering dietary advice. They were randomized to three groups. One group received colestipol 10 g t.d.s. and niacin up to 1.5 g q.d.s. Another group was treated with a similar dose of colestipol combined with lovastatin 20 mg b.d. The third group (conventional therapy group) either received no treatment for hyperlipidaemia or, if their serum LDL cholesterol exceeded the 90th percentile, were given colestipol and a placebo. Coronary angiography was repeated after 2.5 years in 120 men who completed the study.

The serum cholesterol decreased by 7% in the conventional therapy group and averaged 6.55 mmol/l. On colestipol/lovastatin it decreased to 4.71 mmol/l (28% less than conventional therapy) and on colestipol/niacin to 5.41 (17% less than conventional therapy). The group receiving niacin had the greatest decrease in triglycerides and lipoprotein (a) and the greatest increases in HDL cholesterol and apo AI, although the decrease in LDL cholesterol and apo B was greatest in those men having lovastatin. The two sets of coronary angiograms were compared visually and by digitalization of hand-tracings. The average percentage stenosis of the worst lesion in each of 9 proximal segments was 34% initially. At the end of the study stenosis had progressed at the rate of 2.1% in the conventional therapy group, whereas on colestipol/lovastatin it had regressed at 0.7% and by 0.9% on colestipol/niacin, which was statistically significant by analysis of variance. In the rigorously treated men this represented half the rate of progression and three times the rate of regression of the men on conventional therapy. A combination of regression and progression occurred in only 4% of men. The men were a high-risk group, 44% having had a previous myocardial infarction and 67% angina. The rate of death, definite myocardial infarction or need for arterial bypass surgery or angioplasty was 19/100 on conventional therapy, 7/100 on colestipol/lovastatin and 4/100 on colestipol/niacin. Niacin was associated with development of diabetes, acanthosis nigricans, gout and pruritus, and presumably also flushing, and colestipol frequently caused constipation.

P.N.D.

4. Partial ileal bypass surgery—mortality and morbidity from coronary heart disease in hypercholesterolaemic patients

Buchwald H, Varco RL, Matts JP et al. Effect of partial ileal bypass surgery on mortality and morbidity from coronary heart disease in patients with hypercholesterolemia. Report of the Program on the Surgical Control of the Hyperlipidaemias (POSCH). N Engl J Med 1990; 323: 946–955

This trial involved 838 middle-aged patients (more than 90% men) who had previously sustained a myocardial infarction, and whose serum cholesterol after a lipid-lowering diet for 6 weeks either exceeded 5.7 mmol/l (220 mg/dl) or 5.2 mmol/l (200 mg/dl), if the LDL component was greater than 3.6 mmol/l (140 mg/dl). Patients in whom coronary angiography had no significant coronary disease, or at the other end of the scale had 75% or more stenosis of the left mainstem, were not eligible for the trial. Patients were randomized to two groups, one of whom had partial ileal bypass (PIB) surgery (the terminal 200 cm or the terminal third of the small intestine, whichever was greatest) and another who did not. The average serum cholesterol at randomization was 6.5 mmol/l (250 mg/dl). On average, the patients were followed for 9.7 years during which time the serum cholesterol of the PIB group was 23% lower (4.7 v 6.1 mmol/l (180 v 235 mg/dl)) and HDL cholesterol was 4% higher. There was, however, an increase of serum triglycerides and VLDL cholesterol of 20–30%. Cardiac treatment including coronary artery surgery was not withheld and the overall death rate was low (13%) so that the difference in mortality between the PIB group and the others (49 versus 62) was not statistically significant, illustrating the difficulty of using total deaths as a primary end point even in MI survivors with modern techniques for managing coronary heart disease (CHD) and when patients with left mainstem disease are excluded. The primary end point used in the Lipid Research Clinics study with combined CHD mortality and morbidity, was significantly reduced by PIB (82 versus 125). CHD deaths were 32 in the PIB group and 44 in the controls and did not achieve significance, except in those patients whose left ventricular function was not compromised (ejection fraction $> 50\%$), when there was a 39% decrease in CHD deaths. Serial coronary angiograms using a scoring system showed significantly less progression of disease in the PIB patients and significantly fewer coronary artery bypass operations were performed in them (52 versus 137).

PIB produced a lot of side-effects: diarrhoea in most, kidney stones (4% per annum), gallstones and bowel obstruction (symptomatic in 13.5%, requiring surgery in 3.6%). Cancer deaths and violent deaths were not affected by cholesterol reduction. Overall, the cardiovascular results of the trial are consistent with benefit from cholesterol reduction, but there would appear to be considerable advantages to achieving this by drug therapy (particularly as this need not adversely affect triglycerides) rather than PIB surgery, except perhaps in the exceptional patient.

P.N.D.

5. Captopril for angina pectoris and heart failure

Cleland JGF, Henderson E, McLenachan J, Findlay IN, Dargie HJ. Effect of captopril, an angiotensin-converting enzyme inhibitor, in patients with angina pectoris and heart failure. J Am Coll Cardiol 1991; 17: 733–739

The effects of captopril and placebo were compared in a double blind crossover study in 18 patients (4 female) with chronic heart failure (CHF) and angina pectoris. All patients were receiving frusemide (mean dose 120 mg/d), 10 were taking digoxin, 4 were taking nitrates, 2 were taking nifedipine and 2 were taking both nitrates and nifedipine. Mean left ventricular ejection fraction was $24 \pm 8\%$. Exercise capacity was measured using a 'slow' and a 'fast' protocol and symptoms assessed by patient treatment preference, visual analogue scores and glyceryl trinitrate (GTN) consumption. Patients preferred placebo to captopril, apparently because of increased symptoms of angina with captopril (9 preferences v 3 preferences; $P < 0.05$). GTN consumption was significantly greater on captopril than on placebo. Treadmill exercise time on the 'fast' protocol was reduced with captopril compared to placebo ($P < 0.01$). Angina became the limiting symptom significantly more frequently on captopril than on placebo (13 v 6 patients; $P < 0.05$) during the 'slow' protocol. Patients who deteriorated with captopril tended to be treated with nifedipine rather than nitrates, to have the greatest falls in diastolic blood pressure and to have stenosed coronary arteries supplying areas of myocardium with normal contraction rather than regions with diminished contraction.

This is a very important paper because it is the first to assess the effects of an ACE inhibitor on myocardial ischaemia in patients with CHF. This is a large and important subgroup of patients—over one-third of patients in the 'treatment' arm of SOLVD had current angina, approximately one-third were receiving calcium channel blockers and nearly 40% were taking nitrates. The present study appears to show that captopril aggravated angina in ambulatory patients with CHF due to cocoronary artery disease. The likely mechanism seems to have been reduced coronary perfusion due to reduced diastolic blood pressure, an effect most pronounced in patients co-prescribed nifedipine. The implications of these findings are, however, unclear as both the 'prevention' and 'treatment' arms of SOLVD reported reductions in the incidence of unstable angina and myocardial infarction (MI) with enalapril. Whether this discrepancy reflects differences in the ACE inhibitor used (captopril v enalapril), magnitude of reduction in blood pressure (possibly substantially more in the present study) or a difference in the pathophysiology of unstable angina/MI and stable symptomatic reversible ischaemia remains to be determined. There is no doubt, however, that the coexistence of angina pectoris and CHF, and the potential for drug interactions in these patients, merits urgent further study.

J.McM.

6. Aortic insufficiency—a conservative approach

Cosgrove DM, Rosenkranz ER, Hendren WJ, Bartlett JC, Stewart WJ. Valvuloplasty for aortic insufficiency. J Thorac Cardiovasc Surg 1991; 102: 571–577

This article proposes a conservative operation for the treatment of aortic insufficiency. Spurred on by the successful results of atrio-ventricular valve repair, attention has been directed towards the aortic valve. In this series presented from the Cleveland Clinic, 28 patients underwent a conservative procedure for aortic regurgitation, which represents 21% of all patients being treated for isolated aortic insufficiency at this institution. Seven (25%) had a tricuspid valve and the remainder were bicuspid; the majority related to failure of division of the right and left coronary cusps.

The repair consisted of two parts. The elongated free edge of the prolapsing leaflet was shortened by a triangular resection, and an annulo-plasty performed by taking a tuck in at each commissure, using a buttressed suture. Assessments were made before and after the repair using colour flow Doppler imaging and the degree of regurgitation was noted to be radically reduced. No significant obstruction to left ventricular outflow was imposed by the technique. There was one unrelated operative death and, during a mean follow-up period of six months, there was one patient with recurrent regurgitation who required re-operation. This patient had dehiscence of the leaflet repair which was re-repaired and the patient remained well. The other patients showed no progression of regurgitation. Long-term anticoagulation was not used.

The authors comment on the changing aetiology of aortic regurgitation with rheumatic disease being much less important and aortic root dilatation causing the majority of cases coming forward for surgery at this institution. Calcification renders repair impossible, except for the limited calcification seen in the rudimentary commissure, or raphe, present with bicuspid valves. When this alone was calcified, the authors excised this calcium as part of the prolapsing leaflet resection, and thus performed a repair.

Obviously the long term results of this repair remain to be seen and also whether or not the repaired bicuspid valves proceed to calcification.

D.J.M.K.

7. Atrial fibrillation—a definitive surgical procedure

Cox JL, Schuessler RB, D'Agostino HJ et al. The surgical treatment of atrial fibrillation. III. Development of a definitive surgical procedure. J Thorac Cardiovasc Surg 1991; 101: 569–583

This is one of a series of papers presented in the *Journal of Thoracic and Cardiovascular Surgery* in 1991 concerning the development of a new surgical procedure designed to treat atrial fibrillation. The procedure has three aims: (1) to interrupt all the potential re-entrant circuits that might lead to the development and maintenance of atrial fibrillation; (2) to restore the control of the heart beat to the atrial pacemaker; and (3) to allow the atrial generated impulse to activate the entire atrial myocardium in order to preserve atrial transport function. The principle is the creation of a maze. Atrial fibrillation is characterized by the presence of multiple transient macro re-entrant circuits occurring anywhere in the atrium. Both appendages are excised and the pulmonary veins isolated. Multiple incisions interrupt the most common re-entrant circuits and direct the sinus impulses from the sinoatrial node to the atrioventricular node along a specified route.

The operation involves an extensive dissection of the heart with mobilization of the superior vena cava, right pulmonary veins and the atrioventricular grooves. In essence, the portion of the left atrium holding the pulmonary veins is divided completely and then re-sewn. During this process the posterior atrioventricular fat is explored inferior to the mitral valve annulus and any atrial fibres are divided in addition to cryoablation of any fibres on the coronary sinus or posterior rim of the mitral annulus. The right atrial appendage is excised and incisions made laterally and medially. Similarly, the left atrial appendage is excised and the incisions joined through the atrial septum. These incisions are then closed. Two further incisions are made in the lateral wall of the right atrium, directed at creating at minimum a 1.5 cm strip of atrium extending from the superior vena cava in order for impulses to exit from the sinoatrial node. One of these right atrial incisions is taken to the tricuspid annulus, and cryotherapy applied here to ablate any additional fibres in this area.

The results are presented in 7 patients, all successfully treated, with an addendum reporting on a further 7 who have now had a successful operation. One patient required a shock to the atrial septum to abolish atrial flutter, thought to be related to fibres remaining around the coronary sinus, and this patient then remained in sinus rhythm. None had inducible atrial fibrillation. All had a tendency to early fluid retention, perhaps due to depletion of the atrial natriuretic peptide.

This paper, together with the others, presents a new operation to treat those difficult cases of atrial fibrillation. It remains to be seen what the results will be like in other hands and what the long term results will be.

D.J.M.K.

8. Aortic valve disease—a retrospective review

Davies SW, Gershlick AH, Balcon R. Progression of valvar aortic stenosis: a long term retrospective study. Eur Heart J 1991; 12: 10–14

This is a retrospective review of some patients with aortic valve disease investigated by cardiac catheterization. The patients included were those who had at least two cardiac catheterizations carried out over a period of years. There were 65 patients of mean age 54 years, of whom 40 had degenerative aetiology and 25 rheumatic; many of the latter with mitral valve disease in addition. The clinical indications for the second catheter study were, in most cases, angina or dyspnoea. In 15 cases there were other reasons such as clinical detection of a slow rising pulse and/or left ventricular hypertrophy, ECG evidence of left ventricular hypertrophy and lateral ST segment depression or, finally, increasing heart size on chest X-ray. The mean time interval between the catheter studies was 7 years (range 1–18 years). The median gradient increased from 10 mmHg (range 0–40) to 50 mmHg (range 15–120). In the vast majority of patients ejection fraction could be calculated for both catheter studies and the data needed to calculate cardiac output was available. From this data it could be shown that there was no significant change in ejection fraction or cardiac output between the first and second catheter studies. There was no correlation between change in these variables in an individual from the first to the second catheter study, and the change in the aortic valve gradient in the same patient. The mean rate of progression of the gradient was 6.5 mmHg per year. This rate was faster (7.1) if there was a gradient at the original catheter than if there was no gradient (3.9). The rate of progression was not influenced by age or sex but was influenced by the presence of aortic valve calcification and aortic regurgitation. Thus the calcified valves progressed at a rate of 9.7 mmHg while those without progressed at a rate of 4.4 mmHg. When aortic regurgitation was present the rate of progression was 8.8 mmHg as opposed to 4.6 mmHg without.

The authors rightly discuss the problem of a patient with less than severe aortic stenosis who is committed to other cardiac surgery, usually coronary artery bypass grafting, but also occasional mitral valve surgery, and give valuable rates of progression which can be used to calculate the subsequent gradients. Clearly, the presence of calcification and regurgitation indicates the likelihood of rapid progression. The study of the progression of aortic valve gradients has been made exceedingly easy with the using of Doppler echocardiography. However, one is frequently faced with a patient where another lesion necessitates semi-urgent surgery so that time cannot be spent in studying the rate of progression, and in these cases aortic valve replacement should be considered for even moderate gradients.

D.J.M.K.

9. Chest wall pain from sternal wire sutures

Eastridge CE, Mahfood SS, Walker WA, Cole FH Jr. Delayed chest wall pain due to sternal wire sutures. Ann Thorac Surg 1991; 51: 56–59

Anterior chest wall pain that continues or arises weeks after a medium sternotomy is usually attributed to incisional trauma, anxiety or non-specific musculoskeletal problems. Recently, reports have described a group of patients thought to have had scar-entrapped neuromas causing a neuralgic-type pain. Others have suggested the pain is due to a hypersensitivity reaction to nickel contained in stainless steel. This article describes 18 patients seen over an 18-year period after medium sternotomy who had delayed chest pain due to corrosion of one or more sternal wires. Recognition of this cause of pain is important, especially after coronary artery bypass operations, as the pain may be confused with recurrent myocardial ischaemia. In each of the 18 patients removal of the wires and the adjacent scar tissue gave complete relief from pain and tenderness. The sternal wires and areas that were tender to palpation exhibited a thick fibrous tissue reaction that surrounded the twisted portion of the wires. Wires from non-tender areas exhibited very little fibrous reaction. Histological sections of the fibrous tissue surrounding the wires causing pain revealed one or more sensory nerve fibres entrapped in scar tissue. The resistance of stainless steel to corrosion depends on the presence of a thin, invisible but continuous film of chromium oxide which insulates the metal from corrosive electrolytes contained in body fluids. If the protective chromic oxide coat is damaged, this area becomes anodic to the rest of the wire. In body fluids an electric current will flow from the anodic (damaged) portion to the cathodic (undamaged) portion of the wire. If oxygen is present on a cathode, it will combine with the discharged hydrogen ions to form water. In tissue ions will accumulate in the area adjacent to the anode, stimulating an inflammatory response.

G.G.

10. Treatment of recurrent ischaemia after thrombolysis

Ellis SG, Debowey D, Bates ER, Topol EJ. Treatment of recurrent ischemia after thrombolysis and successful reperfusion for acute myocardial infarction: effect on in-hospital mortality and left ventricular function. J Am Coll Cardiol 1991; 17: 752–757

This paper deals with the problem of recurrent ischaemia after thrombolysis. In a retrospective survey of 405 patients who had early (< 6 hours) thrombolytic therapy and early (< 120 minute) angiographic confirmation of their reperfusion status, 303 had adequate reperfusion with or without 'rescue angioplasty', 74 had initially successful reperfusion followed by recurrent ischaemia, and 28 patients had failed reperfusion. It is interesting to note, although not commented on in the paper, that 58.4% of the successful reperfusion group actually had immediate coronary angioplasty: a much higher proportion than would be practicable in hospitals without immediate access to catheter laboratory facilities! In-hospital mortality was 2.0% for the successful reperfusion/no recurrent ischaemia group, 14.9% for successful reperfusion/recurrent ischaemia, and 32.1% for the failed reperfusion groups. This bears out previous experience from the early days of thrombolytic therapy that in-hospital reocclusion carries a substantial mortality, and that patients who receive thrombolytic therapy but do not reperfuse are selected into a high mortality subgroup. Multivariate comparison of factors predicting death or survival in the patients with recurrent ischaemia identified absence of cardiogenic shock and early initiation of efforts at restoring coronary patency as the only independent predictors of survival. There was no mortality in patients treated within 90 minutes of the onset of reocclusion symptoms. Most patients with recurrent ischaemia were treated with 'retrieval angioplasty' (52 patients), with 3 patients receiving a repeated dose of thrombolytic drug, 11 having coronary bypass surgery, and 13 treated conservatively. Retrieval angioplasty was successful in 75% of patients.

   This paper emphasizes the need for early, aggressive treatment if the substantial mortality of recurrent occlusion is to be reduced. Clearly, early retrieval angioplasty is not going to be practicable in hospitals without angiographic facilities. On the other hand, the reocclusion rates reported are much higher than reinfarction rates from studies such as ISIS-2, ISIS-3 or GISSI-2, which were largely conducted in district hospitals.

The price to be paid for an aggressive policy of 'rescue angioplasty' is constant alertness to maintain coronary patency.

D.deB.

11. Molecular genetic studies reveal a missense mutation or 'spelling mistake' in the DNA encoding β myosin heavy chain in a family with familial hypertrophic cardiomyopathy

Geisterfer-Lowrance AAT, Kass S, Tanigawa G, Vosberg H-P, McKenna W, Seidman CE, Seidmann JG. A molecular basis for familial hypertrophic cardiomyopathy: a β cardiac myosin heavy chain missense mutation. Cell 1990; 62: 999–1006

Refined genetic mapping revealed a point mutation in exon 13 of the β cardiac myosin heavy chain in all individuals affected with familial hypertrophic cardiomyopathy from a large kindred. This missense mutation converts a highly conserved arginine residue (arginine 403) to a glutamine residue. Arginine residue 403 is one of five amino acids that is invariant in all sequences of exon 13, and is contained in a region of six amino acids which has been conserved through 600 million years of evolution. Affected individuals from an unrelated family lack this missense mutation, but instead have an α/β cardiac myosin heavy chain hybrid gene which was probably the result of unequal crossover during meiosis. Identification of two unique mutations within cardiac myosin heavy chain genes in all individuals with familial hypertrophic cardiomyopathy from two unrelated families demonstrates that defects in the cardiac myosin heavy chain genes can cause this disease. The pathology resulting from a missense mutation at residue 403 further suggests that a critical function of myosin is disrupted by this mutation. Ongoing studies should lead to the development of a molecular diagnosis and classification of familial hypertrophic cardiomyopathy.

J.T.S.

12. Alteplase v. streptokinase and heparin v. no heparin for acute myocardial infarction

Gruppo Italiano per lo Studio della Sopravvivenza nell'Infarto Miocardico. GISSI-2: a factorial randomised trial of alteplase versus streptokinase and heparin versus no heparin among 12 490 patients with acute myocardial infarction. Lancet 1990; 336: 65–71

GISSI-1 was the study which definitively established the role of thrombolysis in the treatment of myocardial infarction; GISSI-2 (the group has changed its name, but the acronym remains) was the long-awaited comparison of streptokinase and alteplase, with an additional factorial randomization to heparin (12 500 u s.c. twice daily, starting 12 hours after initiation of thrombolytic therapy) or no heparin. The heparin regimen was that used in the earlier SCATI trial.[1] Streptokinase was given in the GISSI-1 dose of 1 500 000 u i.v. over one hour, alteplase in the dose of 100 mg over 3 hours. All patients received aspirin 300–325 mg daily, and those without specific contraindications received atenolol 5–10 mg i.v. The end point was a combined one of death plus severe left ventricular damage (assessed by echocardiography). There was no significant difference in combined end point between patients receiving streptokinase or alteplase (streptokinase 22.5%, alteplase 23.1%), or between heparin and no heparin (heparin 22.7%, no heparin 22.9%). The combined end point was actually lower in the streptokinase no heparin group (22.8) than the alteplase heparin group (23.3). There was no significant difference in the rates of stroke or reinfarction between alteplase and streptokinase. Heparin increased the risk of haemorrhagic, and decreased that of embolic, stroke. Alteplase had a lower risk of hypotension or allergic reaction.

The puzzling feature of this study was why, in a large and potentially expensive trial, alteplase was used with a novel heparin regimen which had not previously been validated in terms of its contribution to the maintenance of coronary patency. The SCATI study did not use alteplase, and the differential effects of alteplase and streptokinase on systemic fibrinogen had been emphasized in a series of preceding studies. The discussion section deals with this issue in a polemical, rather than a scientific, manner. The point about the simplicity of the heparin regimen chosen is well taken, but there is little point in giving any medication unless it works! Sadly, GISSI-2 seems to have muddied the waters rather than resolved the issue as regards alteplase/streptokinase comparisons; however, it does suggest that prolonged heparin in combination with streptokinase has little effect on ultimate outcome.

REFERENCE

1. The SCATI (Studio sulla calciparina nell'Angina e nella Trombosi Ventricolare nell'Infarto) Group. Randomised controlled trial of subcutaneous calcium heparin in acute myocardial infarction. Lancet 1990; 335: 289–292

D.deB.

13. W-P-W syndrome—catheter radiofrequency ablation

Jackman WM, Wang X, Friday KJ et al. Catheter ablation of accessory atrioventricular pathways (Wolff-Parkinson-White syndrome) by radiofrequency current. N Engl J Med 1991; 324: 1605–1611

Jackman et al reported their experience in catheter radiofrequency ablation of accessory atrioventricular pathways in 166 patients who were symptomatic from atrioventricular reciprocating tachycardia and/or atrial fibrillation associated with accessory pathways. A total of 177 accessory pathways were identified and 174 (98%) were successfully ablated in the first ablation session, including all but three posteroseptal pathways. The procedure was successful in 164 patients (99%). The ablation procedure required a median of three radiofrequency pulses and a duration of 8.3 ± 3.5 h, including the time for ablating a second pathway or eliminating atrioventricular nodal re-entrant tachycardia or ectopic atrial tachycardia. In 35% of the patients, the procedure also included the initial diagnostic electrophysiologic study. There was 9% recurrence one day to 4.7 months after ablation during a follow up of one week to 27 months. All underwent a successful second ablation procedure and none had evidence of recurrence in 0.9 to 16.1 months. Follow up electrophysiologic study after a mean of 3.1 ± 1.9 months showed no evidence of accessory pathway conduction in all of the 75 patients studied. Serum creatine kinase and the MB fraction were elevated in 19 patients but there was no evidence of myocardial infarction by electrocardiograms. Echocardiographically, no thrombus was identified at the ablation site. Other complications occurred in 5 patients: complete atrioventricular block following ablation of a posteroseptal pathway at a site remote from the normal location of the atrioventricular node in a patient with corrected transposition of the great vessels and no evidence of normal atrioventricular nodal conduction before ablation; haemopericardium and cardiac tamponade after radiofrequency application in a small venous branch of the proximal coronary sinus; pericarditis without effusion; small pseudoaneurysm of the right femoral artery; and a large femoral haematoma requiring blood transfusion.

This was the first report of a large series of catheter radiofrequency ablation of accessory pathways. The authors demonstrated that catheter radiofrequency ablation of accessory pathways was safe and highly effective in experienced hands. For the posteroseptal pathways not ablatable from either the mitral or tricuspid annulus, ablation via small branches of the coronary sinus may cause pericarditis or cardiac tamponade and should be carried out with caution. However, the authors did not address the issues of adequate procedure duration and the potential risk of malignancy associated with radiation exposure from radiography and prolonged fluoroscopy.

D.P.Z.

14. Gene mapping in familial hypertrophic cardiomyopathy

Jarcho JA, McKenna W, Pare JAP, Solomon SD, Holcombe RF, Dickie S, Levi T, Donis-Keller H, Seidman JG, Seidman CE. Mapping a gene for familial hypertrophic cardiomyopathy to chromosome 14q1. N Engl J Med 1989; 321: 1372–1378

Clinical and molecular genetic techniques were used to identify the chromosomal location of a gene responsible for familial hypertrophic cardiomyopathy in members of a single family. In a large kindred of 102 individuals, hypertrophic cardiomyopathy was present in 44. Of these, 20 were surviving at the time of the study and 24 were deceased; 58 surviving family members were unaffected. Genetic-linkage analyses were performed with polymorphic DNA loci dispersed throughout the entire genome, to identify a locus that was inherited with hypertrophic cardiomyopathy in family members. The significance of the linkage detected between the disease locus and polymorphic loci was assessed by calculating a lod score (the logarithm of the probability of observing coinheritance of two loci, assuming that they are genetically linked, divided by the probability of detecting coinheritance if they are unlinked). A DNA locus (D14S26), previously mapped to chromosome 14 and of unknown function, was found to be coinherited with the disease in this family. No instances of recombination were observed between the locus for familial hypertrophic cardiomyopathy and D14S26, yielding a lod score of +9.37. These data indicate that in this kindred, the odds are greater than 2 000 000 000:1 that the gene responsible for familial hypertrophic cardiomyopathy is located on chromosome 14 (band q1).

J.T.S.

15. Quicker recovery after cardiac operations

Krohn BG, Kay GH, Mandez MA, Zubiate P, Gregory LK. Rapid sustained recovery after cardiac operations. J Thorac Cardiovasc Surg 1990; 100: 194–197

Improved surgical technique in perioperative management helps patients recover more quickly now than in the past after cardiac operation. This study sought to determine if more rapid recovery after cardiac operations and the resulting earlier discharge from hospital caused any change in subsequent re-hospitalization or death rate. Did early success mean ultimate success? The study also aimed to see if a simple exercise test could help select patients who were well enough and strong enough to go home and not require hospitalization in the following 6 months. Exercise testing was performed on the third postoperative day or sooner. Criteria for patients to be eligible for discharge home were:

1. Stable cardiac rhythm
2. Apyrexial
3. Stable haematocrits of 25% or higher.
4. Oral intake of at least 1000 calories per day
5. Successful completion of exercise test
6. Absence of significant wound problems
7. Absence of active complications
8. Confident desire to go home
9. Ability to report progress from home adequately to physician by telephone.

In 240 consecutive patients the medium length of hospital stay after operation was 4 days. Six patients (2.5%) were re-hospitalized within 6 months of discharge and 5 patients (2.1%) were re-hospitalized 6–12 months after discharge. Long initial hospitalization would not have prevented re-hospitalization. Forty of the 240 patients were discharged on the third postoperative day or earlier (1 patient). None died or were re-hospitalized in the following 2 years.

Patients discharged on the third postoperative day had a low subsequent morbidity and mortality rate. This fits with the general proposition that prognosis is best for well persons, and it is better to get well sooner rather than later. Sixteen patients aged 65 or older who were discharged on the third or fourth day after operation demonstrated that rapid sustained recovery was not reserved for the young. In the present study the rapid recovery resulted in part from preventing and quickly correcting disorders of non-cardiac organs.

G.G.

16. Optimal timing of cardiac transplantation

Mancini DM, Eisen H, Kussmaul W, Mull R, Edmunds LH, Wilson JR. Value of peak exercise oxygen consumption for optimal timing of cardiac transplantation in ambulatory patients with heart failure. Circulation 1991; 83: 778–786

All ambulatory patients referred to the Hospital of the University of Pennsylvania for cardiac transplantation assessment between October 1986 and December 1989 underwent maximal treadmill exercise testing to determine whether measurement of peak $\dot{V}o_2$ could safely identify patients in whom surgery could be deferred. Three groups of patients were prospectively identified: Group 1 ($n = 35$) were patients accepted for transplantation ($\dot{V}o_2 \leqslant 14$ ml/kg/min); Group 2 ($n = 52$) were patients considered too well for transplantation ($\dot{V}o_2 > 14$ ml/kg/min); Group 3 ($n = 27$) were patients with a low $\dot{V}o_2$ who could not undergo transplantation because of concomitant non-cardiac problems. Of relevant baseline variables only pulmonary artery occlusion pressure was significantly different between groups (lower in Group 2).

One- and two-year cumulative survival rates in Group 2 were 94% and 84% (i.e. equal to those after transplantation). The respective rates for Group 3 were 47% and 32%. One-year survival in Group 1 patients awaiting transplant was 70% (48% if transplanted patients counted as 'deaths') ($P < 0.005$ v Group 2 but n.s. v Group 1). All deaths in Group 2 were sudden. In this study peak $\dot{V}o_2$ was the best predictor of survival.

Demand for cardiac transplantation continues to far outstrip donor organ supply and even when they are accepted for surgery the cardiologist is faced with the difficult task of prioritizing his patients. This paper by Mancini et al will help simplify this decision. Their data seems to show that patients with a peak $\dot{V}o_2$ of $\geqslant 14/\text{ml}/\text{kg}/\text{min}$ can safely be deferred for surgery. It also appears that repeat testing every 3–6 months may be sufficient to detect those who deteriorate and need transplantation. Interestingly, the present study showed that all deaths in Group 2 were sudden. This raises the possibility that targetted anti-arrhythmic therapy (pharmacological or electrical) could further improve the prognosis in this group.

J.McM.

17. Effect of digoxin on paroxysmal atrial fibrillation

Rawles JM, Metcalfe MJ, Jennings K. Time of occurrence, duration, and ventricular rate of paroxysmal atrial fibrillation: the effect of digoxin. Br Heart J 1990; 63: 225–227

This retrospective study examined Holter recordings from 72 consecutive patients who had episodes of paroxysmal atrial fibrillation during the recording period. Time of onset, ventricular rate at onset, duration of prolonged attacks (exceeding 30 minutes) and ventricular rate prior to termination were recorded, along with clinical factors. A total of 139 episodes of atrial fibrillation were identified; 19% occurred between 2200 and 0600 hours and 81% were evenly spread between 0600 and 2200 hours. In the 41 patients who were not taking digoxin there were 79 episodes and in the 31 taking digoxin there were 60 episodes. Significantly more of the prolonged attacks (13/17) occurred in patients taking digoxin. The mean ventricular rate at the onset of attacks was similar in patients taking digoxin (140 ± 25) and in those who were not (134 ± 22). The effects of other treatments could not be assessed due to small numbers of patients involved.

In view of the intermittent, variable and unpredictable occurrence of attacks in paroxysmal atrial fibrillation the non-randomized and retrospective design of this observational study does not negate the pertinent findings. However, the authors failed to report the distribution of associated cardiovascular disease between the digoxin and non-digoxin groups so the observation on the frequency of prolonged attacks is open to doubt, even though there are good electrophysiological reasons for believing it may be so. The major conclusion is that pre-treatment with digoxin does not reduce the ventricular response at the onset of attacks of paroxysmal atrial fibrillation, contrary to popular opinion and practice. It was suggested that the failure of digoxin to slow the ventricular response was because the majority of attacks occurred during the daytime, in conditions of sympathetic predominance. However it is more likely that reflex increase in sympathetic activity occurs as a result of the onset of atrial fibrillation rather than the reverse, though the study did not address this point. It is a pity that there were not enough patients taking beta-blockers to compare with the other groups.

J.C.

Index